LAPAROSCOPIC COLORECTAL SURGERY

LAPAROSCOPIC COLORECTAL SURGERY

Edited by

John R T Monson MD FRCSI FRCS FACS
Professor of Surgery, University of Hull.
Head of Department, Academic Surgical Unit,
Castle Hill Hospital, Castle Road, Cottingham, North Humberside.

Ara Darzi MD FRCS FRCSI
Consultant Surgeon, St Mary's Hospital, London.
Senior Lecturer, St Mary's Hospital Medical School, Imperial College
of Science and Technology.
Tutor in Laparoscopic Surgery, Minimal Access Therapy Training Unit,
Royal College of Surgeons in England.
Honorary Consultant Surgeon, Central Middlesex Hospital, London.

Illustrated by Dee McLean

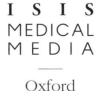

ISIS
MEDICAL
MEDIA

Oxford

© 1995 Isis Medical Media Ltd
Saxon Beck, 58 St Aldates
Oxford OX1 1ST, UK

First published 1995

British Library Cataloguing in Publication Data
A catalogue record for this title is available from the British Library

ISBN   1 899066 02 0

Monson J.R.T. (John)
Laparoscopic Colorectal Surgery/
John Monson and Ara Darzi

Always refer to the manufacturer's Prescribing Information
before prescribing drugs cited in this book

Typeset by
Creative Associates Ltd, Oxford, UK

Printed by
G.Z. Printek, S.A.L., Bilbao, Spain

Distributed by
Times Mirror International Publishers
Customer Service Centre, Unit 1, 3 Sheldon Way
Larkfield, Aylesford, Kent ME20 6SF, UK

Contents

List of Contributors

Juan Santiago Azagra MD FACS
Professor of Surgery, Department of Digestive and Laparoscopic Surgery, CHU André Vésale, 706 route de Gozee, 6110 Montigny-le-Tilleul, Belgium

Garth H. Ballantyne MD FACS FASCRS
Director, The Center for Advanced Laparoscopic Surgery; Chief of Laparoscopic Surgery, St Luke's–Roosevelt Hospital Center, New York, NY 10021, USA

Robert W. Beart Jr MD
Professor of Surgery, Department of Surgery, University of Southern California School of Medicine, 1510 San Pablo Street, Suite 514, Los Angeles, CA 90033-4612, USA

Dennis G. Begos MD
The Center for Advanced Laparoscopic Surgery and the Division of Laparoscopic Surgery, St Luke's–Roosevelt Hospital Center, New York, NY 10021, USA

Walter M. Bridges II MD
Riverview Regional Medical Center, Gadsden Regional Medical Center, Georgia Baptist Medical Center, Atlanta, GA, USA

P. Declan Carey MCh FRCSI
Senior Lecturer and Consultant Surgeon, University Department of Surgery, University of Wales College of Medicine, Heath Park, Cardiff CF4 4XN, UK

E. Carlier MD
Consultant, Department of Intensive Care, CHU André Vésale, 706 route de Gozee, 6110 Montigny-le-Tilleul, Belgium

Stephen M. Cohen MD
Department of Colorectal Surgery, Cleveland Clinic Florida, 3000 West Cypress Creek Road, Fort Lauderdale, Florida 33309, USA

Ara Darzi MD FRCSI
Consultant Surgeon, Academic Surgical Unit, St Mary's Hospital Medical School, Praed Street, London W2 1NY, UK

R. J. Delicata MD FRCS(Ed)
Research Fellow, Department of Surgery, University of Wales College of Medicine, Heath Park, Cardiff CF4 4XN, UK

Harry J. Espiner ChM FRCS
Consultant Surgeon, Royal Infirmary, Bristol, Avon BS2 8HW, UK

O. James Garden MD FRCS (Glas & Ed)
Senior Lecturer in Surgery and Honorary Consultant Surgeon, University of Edinburgh
Department of Surgery, The Royal Infirmary, Lauriston Place, Edinburgh EH3 9YW, UK

Eric Gilbart MD
Consultant , Department of Anaesthesia, CHU André Vésale,706 route de Gozee, 6110
Montigny-le-Tilleul, Belgium

Martine Goergen MD
Senior Registrar, Department of Digestive and Laparoscopic Surgery, CHU André Vésale,
706 route de Gozee, 6110 Montigny-le-Tilleul, Belgium

Pierre J. Guillou BSc MD FRCS
Professor of Surgery, Academic Unit of Surgery, Department of Molecular Medicine,
University of Leeds, St James' University Hospital, Leeds LS9 7TF, UK

John E. Hartley BSc FRCS
Research Fellow, The University of Hull, Academic Surgical Unit, Castle Hill Hospital,
Castle Road, Cottingham, North Humberside HU16 5JQ, UK

Daniel Jacobs MD
Consultant, Department of Anaesthesia, CHU André Vésale, 706 route de Gozee, 6110
Montigny-le-Tilleul, Belgium

Timothy G. John MB BCh FRCS(Ed)
Lecturer in Surgery, Department of Surgery, University of Edinburgh, The Royal
Infirmary NHS Trust, Lauriston Place, Edinburgh EH3 9YW, UK

Samuel P.Y. Kwok FRCS(Ed) FRACS FHKAM(Surgery)
Consultant Surgeon, Department of Surgery, Prince of Wales Hospital, Shatin, New
Territories, Hong Kong

Peter Lee MD FRCS
Consultant Colon and Rectal Surgeon, and Honorary Senior Lecturer, Academic Surgical
Unit, University of Hull, North Humberside, UK

Philippe Lejeune MD PhD
Professor of Medicine, Department of Intensive Care, CHU André Vésale, 706 route de
Gozee, 6110 Montigny-le-Tilleul, Belgium

Arthur K.C. Li MD FRCS FRACS FACS FPCS(Hon)
Chairman and Professor of Surgery, Department of Surgery, The Chinese University of
Hong Kong, Prince of Wales Hospital, Shatin, New Territories, Hong Kong

A.W. MacDonald MRCPath
Consultant Histopathologist, Royal Hull Hospitals NHS Trust, Hull HU3 2KZ, UK

John R.T. Monson MD FRCSI FRCS FACS
Professor of Surgery, University of Hull and Head of Department, Academic Surgical Unit,
Castle Hill Hospital, Castle Road, Cottingham, North Humberside HU16 5JQ, UK

Lucian Newman III MD
Riverview Regional Medical Center, Gadsden Regional Medical Center, Georgia Baptist Medical Center, Atlanta, GA, USA

Brian I. Rees MA FRCS
Consultant Surgeon and Director WIMAT, University Department of Surgery, University of Wales College of Medicine, Heath Park, Cardiff CF4 4XN, UK

Petachia Reissman MD
Department of Colorectal Surgery, Cleveland Clinic Florida, 3000 West Cypress Creek Road, Fort Lauderdale, FL 33309, USA

Ahmed H.S. Saleh DA FFARCSI
Consultant Anaesthetist, Department of Anaesthesia, Castle Hill Hospital, Cottingham, Hull HU16 5JQ, UK

Richard Stacey MB BS FRCS
Registrar in Neurosurgery, Walton Centre for Neurology and Neurosurgery, Walton Hospital, Liverpool L9 1AE, UK

Steven D. Wexner MD, FACS, FACRS
Chairman, Department of Colorectal Surgery, Cleveland Clinic Florida, 3000 West Cypress Creek Road, Fort Lauderdale, FL 33309, USA

Foreword

Albert Einstein once said that 'perfection of tools and confusion of aims are two characteristics of our time'. John Monson and Ara Darzi go a long way with this book towards answering the dual challenges posed by these words for the new technocrats of the laparoscopic revolution. This revolution has taken medical progress out of the hands of the profession and placed it instead in the public domain. Perhaps this is a change for the better since control shifts to patients to whom it matters most, but there is a real danger of media hype and revolutionary hyperbole overshadowing scientific evaluation and objective analysis. Predictions by the BBC that 80% of all abdominal surgery would be practised laparoscopically by the end of the century already seem wildly exaggerated. Indeed one begins to wonder whether the reports of early and probably avoidable disasters may now impede progress inappropriately just as medical ambition and media hype promoted a far faster revolution than was ever prudent. There can be no doubt that many casual practitioners of laparoscopic surgery, drawn in by the desire to compete with their colleagues, have surged forward largely on the euphoric realisation that 'it can be done therefore we will do it'. Some such careless adventurers are licking their wounds from the mauling received at the hands of the media, whilst this book thoughtfully and carefully addresses one of the most controversial areas of all - the role of the laparoscope in colorectal surgery.

Colorectal cancer is the most important surgical malignancy; it is common and it is often curable. It has an incidence of over 30,000 cases per year in the United Kingdom, and will kill more than a million people in Western Europe before the end of the century. Many of these deaths could be prevented by better surgery. Hermanek in Germany has recently analysed the enormous variations that occur between surgeons in terms of cancer cure. Local recurrence in rectal cancer varies from 5% to over 50%, with the worse figure being far nearer to the norm in everyday practice. Along with these variations in local failure, now so clearly the responsibility of the surgeon ,go variations in long term cure rate between 40% and 80% for R_0 tumours. Such variability is seen in no other malignancy and demands careful attention on the part of the surgical profession. The provocative critique of Wexner and Reissman in Chapter 8 addresses many of these issues and should be read by all potential recruits to the new technology.

In the final analysis the status of the laparoscope in colorectal surgery will be decided on the basis of whether parts of the operations can actually be performed better laparoscopically than by open surgery. For the usually middle aged patient with cancer the issues of cosmesis, and short term discomfort or hospital stay are utterly irrelevant when compared with expectation of cure, the presence or absence of a permanent stoma, or the loss of sexual or bladder function. If more perfect specimens can be removed, the inferior hypogastric plaxuses more perfectly visualised, and the plane between the low anterior tumour and the back of the prostate be more precisely developed – then these would be substantial reasons for the new technology to take over. Since the surgery is performed on a TV screen communication between one surgeon and another has never been more easy and all these issues can be demonstrated to large groups of surgeons so that they may become convinced that this is indeed the way forward.

'Among all forms of mistake prophecy is the most gratuitous' ... so said George Eliot in Middlemarch. Nevertheless my task in writing the Foreword to this excellent book must be at least to try to see forward to the next century. How many of the chapters which may seem today to be a triumph of skill over commonsense will be the established conventional methods of the future? What is clear is that the balance of power in surgery is shifting away from older surgeons towards new skills which are largely the province of the young. Many future advances will come technological innovation whilst the profession's contributions will often be reduced from prime mover to the practical application of the ideas of others. To a great extent the laparoscopic revolution has come from far sighted investment of technical skill and financial support of the surgical equipment companies. Progress has been driven forward by the public and the press whilst the purse strings of the health care economist and the politicians writhe ineffectually to contain the expensive aspirations of all but those who have to pay. The answers to most of the questions will in the end be provided by the economics of what society can afford and what is truly worthwhile in the balance between cost and major long term benefit.

R.J. Heald M.Chir. FRCS
Consultant Surgeon
Colorectal Research Unit
The North Hampshire Hospitals NHS Trust

Preface

In the field of minimal access surgery probably the most controversial topic is the application of laparoscopic techniques in coloproctology. Although laparoscopic surgery has represented an irresistible force of change in many areas such as cholecystectomy, hernia repair and fundoplication this is not the case in colorectal surgery. There are several reasons for this, some of which will be addressed in this text and some of which are likely to remain unanswered for some time to come. At the current time all forms of colorectal procedures can be performed laparoscopically from a technical standpoint with appropriate experience and training. Many of these operations are detailed in this text although we do not suggest that the list is comprehensive. Instead we have concentrated on more commonly performed operations as well as the more controversial areas. Undeniably the most contentious issue remains the laparoscopic approach to surgical cure of colorectal cancer.

Although laparoscopic surgery has been used in oncology for decades it has predominantly been applied as a diagnostic and staging technique in cancers with a poor natural history or very advanced disease (such as pancreatic and oesophageal tumours). In these instances the chance of long term cure is small and the aim is usually to avoid unnecessarily aggressive surgery. In colorectal cancer the situation is very different. The chance of surgical cure is high and therefore the consequences of inappropriate surgical technique leading to tumour recurrence and likely death are obviously unacceptable. In this text we have attempted to provide a balanced approach to this issue by detailing techniques used by a wide range of surgeons active in the field. Experience is reported from Europe, the Far East and the United States where variations in philosophy are evident. We accept that the final answers to this question will not be available for some time but hope the reader will be able to make a value judgement concerning different techniques and therefore decide whether or not to introduce them into clinical practice. It is hoped that the use of randomised controlled trials may answer some of these issues in the long term. However they are not without their difficulties and Pierre Guillou discusses this important concept in some detail. In the field of rectal prolapse we have not attempted to resolve the ongoing arguments regarding the use of transabdominal rectopexy. We have simply detailed a suitable technique that exactly mirrors one of the open procedures. Herein lies one of the major concepts within the book. As much as possible the laparoscopic operation should be the same as the open operation and we would counsel against any major changes in techniques – especially in the field of cancer.

Another difference applicable to laparoscopic colorectal surgery concerns training. It would seem unlikely that all colorectal surgery will be performed laparoscopically within the foreseeable future. Unresectable cancers, toxic megacolon, colonic obstruction, abdominal trauma, and extreme obesity all represent relative contraindications to the minimal access approach. It therefore follows that a substantial proportion of procedures will be performed in the traditional manner thus requiring appropriate conventional colorectal training for all surgeons contemplating a laparoscopic operation. As time passes this text will need to be updated as technology progresses and experience increases. Harry Espiner's ingenious and elegant struggles to facilitate specimen extraction represents just one of the major hurdles to be overcome in the future. However we feel sure that laparoscopic surgery will not pass the colorectal surgeon by and hope that this book will serve as a companion in these early days.

John RT Monson
Ara Darzi

Chapter 1
Right hemicolectomy

R.W. Beart Jr

Introduction

Laparoscopic surgery became popular in the late 1980s [1]. It is only natural that as this technique became acceptable for such procedures as colecystectomy, appendicectomy and hernia repair it would be extended to other abdominal organs. Virtually every organ in the abdomen and the retroperitoneum has been approached laparoscopically and successfully resected. The colon is a unique organ. It extends throughout the abdomen and therefore poses unique problems in its resection. The right colon can be particularly mobile and lends itself to laparoscopic resection [2]. It is the purpose of this chapter to review the background behind laparoscopic colon resection and, in particular, to address the techniques of laparoscopic right hemicolectomy.

Philosophy

It is important when performing colon resection that traditional standards of resection be preserved [3]. It is philosophically important to accept that one can perform the same operation laparoscopically that can be performed using an open technique. If the operation is going to be compromised in some way, then a completely different level of research would be needed to establish the safety and efficacy of this technique. Therefore, one must be able to maintain the same degrees of safety, achieve the same margins of resection and the procedure cannot be so unduly prolonged as to make it unsafe or cost ineffective. The procedure needs to be done effectively and within a reasonable cost range.

Credentialing and certification

As new technologies are introduced, individuals must be credentialed and certified to perform the new techniques. There has been a great deal of controversy about the credentialing of laparoscopic surgical procedures. The principles of laparoscopic colon resection are no different than those of an open colon resection. The colon is mobilized from the retroperitoneum, the vessels are ligated and the colon is removed. It can be removed intracorporeally or extracorporeally.

It is my preference to perform the resection and anastomosis extracorporeally. This allows for the extent of the resection to be clearly evaluated. The mesenteric dissection can then be completed outside the abdomen. The anastomosis can be completed using the standard technique, either stapled or handsewn. One can be assured that the anastomosis is not under tension as the anastomosis is created outside the abdomen and returned to the abdomen. Finally, it is necessary to open the abdomen to remove the colon to provide the pathological specimen. One might as well take advantage of this necessity to complete the resection and do the anastomosis. Therefore, it is my conviction that this same procedure can be done with very similar techniques whether using laparoscopic or open approaches.

Since surgeons are doing the same operation, it seems only appropriate that individuals are credentialed to do an open right hemicolectomy if they are to be trained to do a laparoscopic right hemicolectomy. If an individual has demonstrated competence with the instrumentation, then it is a reasonable extension that he or she be allowed to do it laparoscopically. One could suggest that familiarity with the instrumentation can be obtained in an animal model*, but there is no good model for human colon resection. Therefore, a careful and planned approach to the use of this procedure in human beings is appropriate. It should probably be performed initially not only by laparoscopically experienced individuals, but in combination with other individuals who have preferably had bowel resection experience. In the situations where there is no experienced individual available, two experienced laparoscopic surgeons should initiate this procedure together.

This procedure should not be so unduly prolonged that the patient is not served well. In our initial experience, we placed an alarm clock in the operating room and if we were not substantially finished with the procedure within 1 h we converted to an open procedure. Although we had a somewhat higher conversion rate initially, we felt that this was a good guideline that protected the best interests of the patient.

The same standards of open resection must be maintained. This means that margins of resection must be preserved. If the procedure is going to be unduly prolonged or in any way different than that which would be performed in an open procedure, then it should be converted to the latter.

I have emphasized the importance of maintaining traditional standards. This includes standards of resection, standards of time and standards of putting the patient's best interest first. However, if we are going to take advantage of laparoscopic procedures, then certain paradigms must be changed. In particular, one must recognize the early return of bowel function [4,5]. Typically, we offer clear liquids during the night after surgery if the procedure took place in the morning. If the procedure is performed in the afternoon, we offer a clear liquid diet the following morning. This diet is advanced as rapidly as the patient tolerates it. At the same time, as the patient is able to tolerate oral intake, oral pain medicines can be used. Typically the pain is less than with open procedures and narcotics are necessary for a shorter period of time.

Equipment

There is a large amount of equipment available on the market for colonic resections. My initial experience was before most of this was available, so I have been comfortable doing my resections with the same instruments used for gallbladder resections. I rarely find it necessary to use bowel clamps or special

---

* In some countries, including the UK, the use of animals for training is prohibited by law.

grasping instruments. Babcock instruments should not be used liberally. The corners on these instruments are prone to tear and injure the bowel. A Babcock clamp, however, is valuable if the mesentery is fat and it is not possible to hold the mesentery easily. Electrified scissors are useful for incising and mobilizing the bowel. More sophisticated instrumentation is helpful to aid in intracorporeal anastomosis and manipulation of the bowel and will be necessary if intracorporeal anastomosis is to be more commonly used.

Physiology

The physiology of colon resection is only now being worked out. However, a number of observations have been made [6,7]. The first is that extensive retroperitoneal dissections can be associated with extensive subcutaneous emphysema. We have had a number of cases with subcutaneous emphysema when we used higher pressures. In the last several years, we have used 10 mmHg intra-abdominal carbon dioxide (CO_2) pressure and this has been well tolerated. This does not seem to compromise our ability to see adequately [8,9]. The rate of absorption of CO_2 does not seem to be increased by doing a retroperitoneal dissection. Nevertheless, the patients must be watched for progressive acidosis as the length of the procedure may be longer than typically experienced with other procedures [10].

Even cardiac patients seem to tolerate laparoscopic resection well. It is unclear whether this affords cardiac patients a physiological advantage over open techniques [11]. Patients with respiratory disease can be compromised. This occurs both because of the progressive acidosis and the mechanical effects of the abdominal distension. These patients should be approached cautiously [12,13].

There has been some interest in the immune function of patients having laparoscopic surgery [14,15]. It has been well established that there is immune suppression following major abdominal procedures. There have been several reports that immune suppression may be less significant if the procedures are small. It has been an assumption that a laparoscopic colon resection is a smaller procedure than an open colon resection but this has not been clearly established. This area is currently being investigated.

Technique

The procedure is initiated with the patient in the supine position. A Foley catheter is placed, a nasogastric tube is put in position and the abdomen is prepared in the usual fashion. We prefer to place sequential compression devices on the legs [16]. After the abdomen is prepped and draped, the equipment is set up in a standard fashion. The nurse is at the foot of the table with the surgeon standing on the side of the abdomen opposite the pathology being resected. In the case of a right hemicolectomy, the surgeon would be on the patient's left and the first assistant would be next to the nurse. A camera would be placed in the left upper quadrant. The procedure is initiated using a Hassan technique to place a 10–12 mm port in the left upper quadrant. This is usually placed through the left rectus muscle under direct visualization. We have had experience over the years of placing ports in different places. When the camera is placed at the level of the umbilicus, it is right on top of the origin of the inferior mesenteric and the ileocolic vessels.

These are the primary vessels to be resected and the camera is often too close to see the area well. By placing the camera in the left upper quadrant, both colonic flexures can be seen clearly, as well as the primary feeding vessels.

Once the camera is in place, the patient is placed in the steep Trendelenburg position and rotated away from the pathology to be resected. In this case, the patient would be rotated to the left. Under direct vision, another 10–12 mm port is placed in the suprapubic area and two 5 mm ports are placed at the sites where colostomies might traditionally be performed. I am in favour of minimizing the use of 10 mm or larger ports as the fascia needs to be repaired in these port sites to minimize the risk of hernias. It is rarely necessary to have more than two 10 mm ports for a standard colonic resection. Once these three additional ports are in place, the mesentery of the small bowel is grasped and is carefully put into the left upper quadrant. Adequate exposure has been achieved when the duodenum can be visualized and/or the aorta and the origin of the inferior mesenteric ileocolic vessel can be seen.

After the small bowel has been mobilized out of the way, the peritoneum just lateral to the caecum is grasped and scissors are used to incise the peritoneum. A two-handed technique is desirable and the role of the assistant is minimal. By grasping the peritoneum and putting it under tension at that site, the line of incision can easily be identified and the peritoneum along the entire colon can be divided (Fig. 1.1). It is important to incise the terminal ileal attachments in order that the terminal ileum can be mobilized. The general approach is to incise the peritoneum and then use blunt force to elevate the mesentery and colon off the retroperitoneum. Remember, the colon is merely lying on the retroperitoneum and it can be lifted easily. As the colon is lifted, the ureters and gonadal vessels can be identified. The mobilization is carried up to and around the hepatic flexure (Fig. 1.2). The omentum can then be identified and dissected off the stomach as well to gain adequate mobilization. It is important to recognize, however, that most of this dissection can be done outside the abdomen. This is a very mobile part of the colon and it comes out easily.

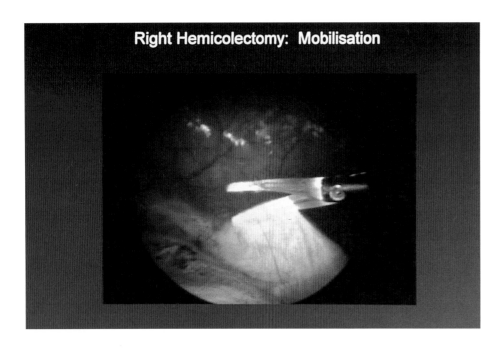

Figure 1.1
Division of the lateral peritoneal reflections of the right colon.

Figure 1.2
Mobilization of the hepatic flexure.

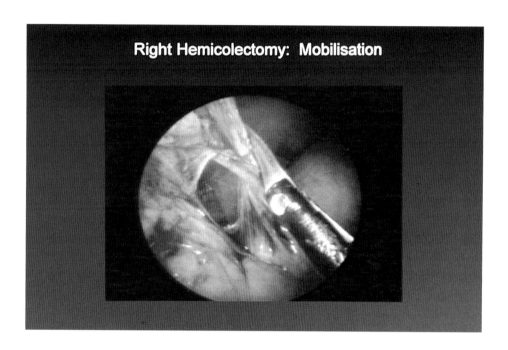

Once the terminal ileum and colon are mobilized from the retroperitoneum by pulling the colon progressively to the left, the colon is placed back in its normal position against the retroperitoneum. At this point, the mesentery is grasped at the base of the caecum and put under traction. This traction on the mesentery highlights the path of the ileocolic vessels. Unless the patient is obese, the duodenum can usually be seen through the mesentery. Where the ileocolic vessels cross near the duodenum is a good place for the former to be ligated. We therefore incise the peritoneum over the ileocolic vessels at this point and using blunt dissection expose the vessels. Once the vessels are identified, a right-angle clamp is placed through the 10 mm port and the dissection is completed with the right-angle clamp. We favour separating the artery and the vein and clipping them separately.

Initially, we both clipped and ligated the vessels. More recently, however, double clips placed proximally have been found sufficient for haemostasis [17]. Endoclips are placed proximally and distally on the artery and the artery is partially divided. It is important not to divide the artery completely until one is sure the clips are completely occluding. By cutting the vessel part way through and keeping it under tension, control is maintained. Once the surgeon is sure that the clips are adequate, the vessel is completely divided and the next vessel is clipped and divided. One should always be aware that there may be a third vessel behind these two vessels. One should not overclip or cut the area in case an unrecognized vessel is injured and bleeding is caused, which is difficult to control. One should also be aware that once the vessels have been divided they may very well retract into the fatty mesentery. This makes control of them difficult if adequate clipping has not been achieved. On both sides of the vascular pedicle there is a clear space and additional tissue can be ligated. In addition, the mesenteric window can be completed to the site of the initial dissection, achieving complete dissection through the mesentery. The dissection can be carried up along the duodenum. The next vessel to be identified is the right colic vessel and this can be similarly ligated.

Once these vessels are ligated, it is appropriate to think about bringing the bowel outside the abdominal wall. I do not routinely complete the mesenteric dissection as the mesentery closest to the bowel can be easily identified using standard techniques outside the abdomen, clamped and ligated under direct vision. Therefore, when the initial vessels have been ligated and mobility achieved, a 5 cm incision is made over the right 5 mm port side. This is carried out under direct vision. It is important to maintain careful haemostasis as the abdomen is being entered. As the abdomen is distended there is little concern about injuring the bowel and electrocautery can be freely used. A clamp is placed through the 5 mm port and the bowel is grasped so that once the abdominal cavity is entered the bowel can be identified. The abdominal cavity is entered, and the bowel is grasped with a Babcock clamp and brought into the wound. A finger can be placed into the wound, the window through the mesentery identified and the bowel lifted outside the abdomen (Fig. 1.3). The ileal attachments have then been freed completely. The small bowel comes up easily as does the right colon and hepatic flexure. The omentum can actually be drawn outside the bowel and some of the dissection can be completed under direct visualization (Fig. 1.4). The mesenteric dissection is completed, the bowel is resected (Fig. 1.5) and the anastomosis is undertaken using whichever technique the surgeon prefers.

After the anastomosis is completed, the bowel is carefully lowered into the abdomen (Fig. 1.6), the peritoneum is closed with a running monofilament absorbable suture and the abdomen is re-insufflated. The abdomen can then be carefully inspected. The anastomosis should be evaluated and care must be taken to make sure the ileum has not been rotated in the course of performing the anastomosis. The mesenteric defect can be repaired either with a hernia stapler or with sutures. I have not routinely closed the mesenteric defect in laparoscopic or in open cases.

The abdomen is then irrigated and inspected for haemostasis. If all is well, the cannulae are removed under direct vision and the left upper quadrant cannula is

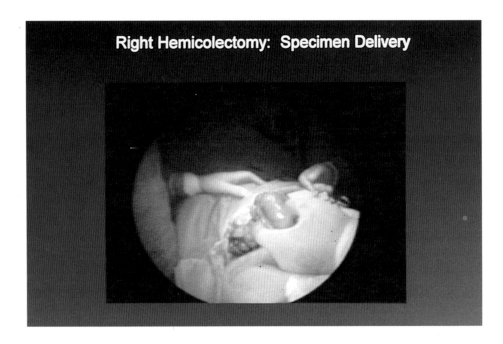

Figure 1.3
Delivery of the right colon.

Figure 1.4
Extracorporeal completion of the division of the mesentery.

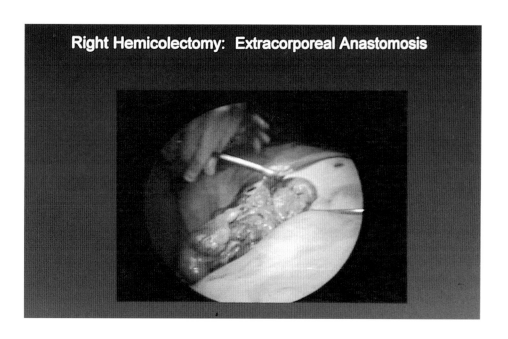

Figure 1.5
Extracorporeal resection of the specimen.

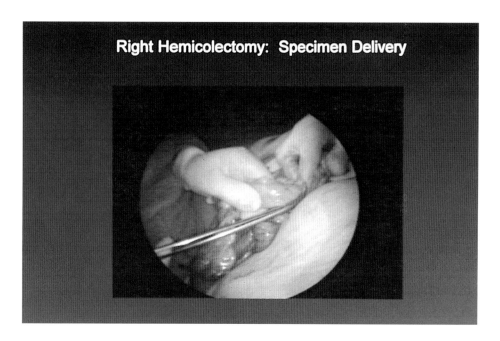

removed last. The fascia of the 10 mm defects must be closed and the skin incisions are closed with Vicryl (Fig. 1.7). Efforts should be made to remove CO_2, to minimize abdominal pain, prior to removal of the cannulae.

Postoperative recovery

Postoperatively, if the operation is completed before noon, clear liquids are offered to the patient at dinnertime. If the procedure is completed in the afternoon, clear liquids are offered the following morning. We generally give the patient a patient-controlled analgesia pump with morphine to help control pain. We advance the diet at the patient's discretion, and typically within 2–3 days the

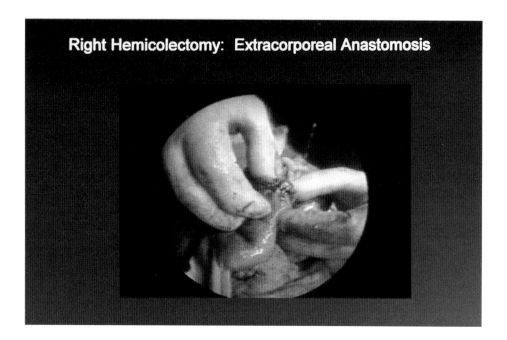

Figure 1.6
Completion of an extracorporeal anastomosis (in this case an end-to-end anastomosis).

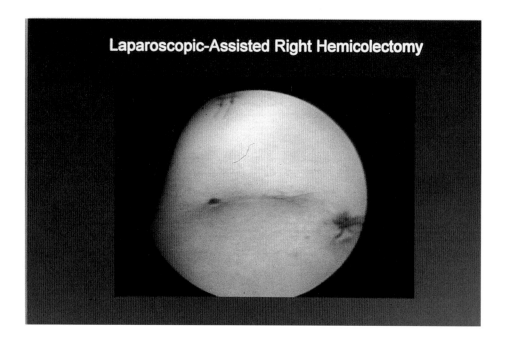

Figure 1.7
Completion of the procedure.

patient has gained confidence and can eat well. Once the patient is taking liquids well, we switch the patient to oral pain medications and encourage ambulation. Once the patient is eating a regular diet, he or she is discharged home. This may be before the patient is passing stools or flatus. Since the bowel had been sterilized and bacteria largely eliminated, it is likely that the patient will not produce much flatus in the first 4–5 days. Similarly, as the colon was clean, there will not be much stool present. For these reasons, we have been willing to discharge a patient prior to the passage of flatus and stool but do follow their progress on an outpatient basis. If there is any evidence of distension, nausea or vomiting then they will not be discharged.

Clinical results

The issue has been raised about the appropriateness of this procedure for cancer [18]. There are several theoretical concerns which have been raised based on the work of Mikulicz [19]. In the late 1800s, Mikulicz devised a procedure for advanced carcinoma. During this procedure, a small incision was made in the abdomen, the tumour was mobilized and pulled through this incision. There was a high mortality rate due to sepsis, the advanced stage of the tumours and the fact that there were no antibiotics and that most of these tumours were associated with abscesses. In those patients who did survive, there is some indirect evidence that there was an increased incidence of wound implantation. This is not clearly outlined by Mikulicz or Sistrunk. This cancer has been perpetuated through the years and it remains a legitimate concern as we draw the tumour through a small extraction site.

In addition, there have been several reports of extraction site or port site recurrences. It is difficult to understand how these implantations could occur. Nevertheless, their report is worrisome. It is appropriate to recognize that a denominator is not known. A very real incidence of wound recurrence has been reported by E.S. Hughes and is 1–2% at 1 year after surgery. Whether or not the reports in the literature can be interpreted as being greater than this incidence is unclear.

Conclusion

It is unclear at this point whether laparoscopic colon resection is in the patient's best interest. There does seem to be evidence that patients have less pain, an earlier return of bowel function, an earlier discharge from hospital and an earlier return to normal activity [20]. A benign pathology can be handled laparoscopically and in certain situations may be in the patient's best interest. The role for laparoscopic colectomy in the management of malignancy, however, remains to be defined. The advantages noted for benign disease are present but there is concern that patterns or incidence of recurrence may be changed. This will only be clearly defined with a randomized prospective study which will be initiated in 1995. In the interim, it is probably in the surgeon's best interest to use laparoscopic techniques for malignancy in only selected, favourable situations.

References

1 Bongard FS, Pianim NA, Leighton TA *et al.* Helium insufflation for laparoscopic operation. *Surg Gynecol Obstet* 1993; **177**: 140–6.

2 Chaudry IH, Ayala A. Mechanism of increased susceptibility to infection following hemorrhage. *Am J Surg* 1993; **165**: 59S–66S.

3 Coelho JCU, de Araujo RPM, Marchesini JB, Coelho ICMM, de Araujo LRR. Pulmonary function after cholecystectomy performed through Kocher's incision, a mini-incision, and laparoscopy. *World J Surg* 1993; **17**: 544–6.

4 Dalen JE. An apple a day or an aspirin a day. *Arch Intern Med* 1991; **151**: 1066–9.

5 Falk PM, Beart RW, Wexner SD *et al.* Laparoscopic colectomy: a critical appraisal. *Dis Colon Rectum* 1993; **36**: 28–34.

6 Frazee RC, Roberts JW, Symmonds RE *et al.* A prospective randomized trial comparing open versus laparoscopic appendectomy. *Ann Surg* 1994; **219**: 725–31.

7 Hoffman GC, Baker JW, Fitchett CW, Vansant JH. Laparoscopic-assisted colectomy: initial experience. *Ann Surg* 1994; **219**: 732–43.

8   Ishizaki Y, Bandai Y, Shimomura K, Abe H, Ohtomo Y, Idezuki Y. Safe intraabdominal pressure of carbon dioxide pneumoperitoneum during laparoscopic surgery. *Surgery* 1993; **114**: 549–54.

9   Kwok SPY, Lau WY, Li AKC. Prospective comparison of laparoscopic and conventional anterior resection. Reply. *Br J Surg* 1994; **81**: 625.

10 Millard JA, Hill BB, Cook PS, Fenoglio ME, Stahlgren LH. Intermittent sequential pneumatic compression in prevention of venous stasis associated with pneumoperitoneum during laparoscopic cholecystectomy. *Arch Surg* 1993; **128**: 914–18.

11 Nduka CCE. Abdominal wall metastases following laparoscopy. *Br J Surg* 1993; **81**: 648–52.

12 Nelson MT, Nakashima M, Mulvihill SJ. How secure are laparoscopically placed clips? An *in vitro* and *in vivo* study. *Arch Surg* 1992; **127**: 718–20.

13 Peters JH, Ortega A, Lehnerd SL *et al*. The physiology of laparoscopic surgery: pulmonary function after laparoscopic cholecystectomy. *Surg Laparosc Endosc* 1993; **3**: 370–4.

14 Phillips EH, Franklin M, Carroll BJ, Fallas MJ, Ramos R, Rosenthal D. Laparoscopic colectomy. *Ann Surg* 1993; **216**: 703–7.

15 Safran D, Sgambati S, Orlando R. Laparoscopy in high-risk cardiac patients. *Surg Gynecol Obstet* 1993; **176**: 548–54.

16 Safran DB, Orlando R III. Physiologic effects of pneumoperitoneum. *Am J Surg* 1994; **167**: 281–6.

17 Sandler RS, Lyles CM, McAuliffe C, Woosley JT, Kupper LL. Cigarette smoking, alcohol, and the risk of colorectal adenomas. *Gastroenterology* 1993; **104**: 1445–51.

18 Scoggin SD, Frazee RC, Snyder SK *et al*. Laparoscopic-assisted bowel surgery. *Dis Colon Rectum* 1993; **36**: 747–50.

19 Sistrunk, WE. The Mikulicz operation for resection of the colon. *unknown* 1994; **00**: 597–606.

20 Wolf JS Jr, Stoller ML. The physiology of laparoscopy: basic principles, complications and other considerations. *J Urol* 1994; **152**: 294–302.

Chapter 2

Laparoscopic left hemicolectomy and anterior resection

D.G. Begos and G.H. Ballantyne

Introduction

The widespread acceptance of laparoscopic cholecystectomy by the general surgical community, combined with advances in laparoscopic technology, has facilitated the development of techniques for performing other surgical procedures laparoscopically. Laparoscopic colon and rectal operations are a direct result of this new use for a century-old technology [1–3]. Although these procedures are technically more difficult than laparoscopic cholecystectomy, a properly trained colorectal surgeon, or general surgeon who performs frequent colon and rectal resections, should be able to become proficient in laparoscopic colon and rectal surgery. It is important to remember, however, that advanced laparoscopic surgery is still in an evolutionary stage, and that the procedures described are being continually refined as technology improves and as more experience is gained in operative strategies and patient selection.

This chapter will focus on two specific procedures: laparoscopic left hemicolectomy and anterior resection. The indications for performing these operations are the same as for open surgery. Patient selection criteria suggest in which patients these operations will more readily accomplished. Those patients who are converted from laparoscopic to open procedures have the 'worst of both worlds': the added operative time and expense of the laparoscopic procedure, with the morbidity associated with a large ventral incision.

Preoperative management

Patient selection

Laparoscopic procedures can be performed in almost any patient. The carbon dioxide pneumoperitoneum alters cardiovascular function very little. The carbon dioxide causes a respiratory-type acidosis, which mildly improves myocardial contractility, stroke volume and cardiac output. The major effects on the cardiovascular system by the operation are produced by changes in the position of the patient and are independent of the pneumoperitoneum. Lowering the patient down into the Trendelenburg position increases cardiac venous return and increases cardiac output. In contrast, raising the head of the table into a reverse Trendelenburg position diminishes venous return and decreases cardiac output. In contrast, patients with severe restrictive pulmonary disease may not tolerate the hypercapnia induced by the carbon dioxide pneumoperitoneum.

There are several factors that make the performance of a laparoscopic bowel resection more difficult. Obesity may significantly impair visibility within the abdomen. This is more of a problem in men than in women. Obese men often have thick mesenteries, thick omentums and numerous epiploic fat tags. Previous operations may have generated adhesions that interfere with exposure. Thus, laparoscopic bowel resections tend to be easier to perform in patients without significant restrictive pulmonary disease who are female, thin and have not undergone previous abdominal operations.

Laparoscopic colectomy is appropriate for the treatment of the same diseases that are treated by traditional open operations. The treatment of colorectal cancers, however, remains somewhat controversial because of the lack of long-term follow-up at this point. Nonetheless, the information that is available at the present time supports the use of minimally invasive techniques in this group of patients. Quantitative measurements of the specimens obtained in laparoscopic procedures compare favourable with those of specimens obtained by open techniques in the same institution. The length of the proximal and distal margins, the length of resected mesentery and the number of harvested lymph nodes is similar in both groups [4,5].

Some concern has arisen about wound implantation by metastatic lesions following laparoscopic resections for colorectal malignancies [6,7]. Nonetheless, among patients entered into the laparoscopy registry of the American Society of Colon and Rectal Surgeons, the rate of wound implantation to date is strikingly similar to that reported after open operations [8]. This rate is about 0.4% for both groups. Although these early results compare favourably with previous reports from open operations, minimally invasive techniques for the resection of colorectal malignancies are still within a period of evaluation. This should be stressed with patients to whom this technique is offered.

Preoperative preparation of the patient

The patient is evaluated in the same manner as prior to traditional open operations. In patient afflicted with colorectal malignancies, we obtain computed tomography (CT) scans of the abdomen in the perioperative period for the purpose of future comparison should recurrent disease be suspected. Similarly, the bowel preparation is the same as for open colorectal operations. Most patients undergo a mechanical bowel preparation with polyethylene glycol solution and receive a Nichols–Condon type of antibiotic bowel preparation with neomycin base and erythromycin.

Ureteral stents

The indications for the insertion of ureteral stents are the same as for open operations. Ureteral stents are placed in patients who have had previous pelvic surgery such as oophorectomy or hysterectomy. In addition, ureteral stents may prove helpful in patients with a history of pelvic inflammation such as diverticulitis. The older, more rigid stents are more easily palpated with laparoscopic instruments. Some surgeons find illuminated stents to be helpful. These stents, however, can only be illuminated for short periods of time because the heat generated by them can injure the ureters.

Preoperative localization of the lesion

In patients afflicted with colorectal neoplasms, preoperative localization of the lesions can reduce total operative time. If the lesion was first identified with a barium enema adequate information may already be available since a left hemicolectomy will adequately treat any lesion distal to the splenic flexure and proximal to the rectosigmoid junction. If a segmental resection if planned, however, more accurate localization will be required. This can be accomplished either preoperatively or during the operation. The colonoscopy should not be performed on the day of the operation because the distended bowel may be perforated during the insertion of the trocars and may interfere with exposure. A colonoscopist can mark the location of the lesion before the operation with indian ink. This is injected in at least three places around the circumference of the bowel lumen with a sclerotherapy needle. Injections in only one place may be obscured by the mesentery or epiploic fat tags. Methylene blue can be used but it sometimes dissipates too quickly or spreads too widely along the bowel wall.

Setup of the operating room

A large operating room facilitates the performance of a laparoscopic colorectal resection. A small room is rapidly cluttered with the many re-usable and disposable laparoscopic instruments, traditional surgical instruments and various electronic devices required for these operations. The video camera, insufflator and light source are stacked vertically within a mobile cart. Two high-resolution monitors are required. One is placed between the legs of the patient and the second by the left shoulder of the patient (Fig. 2.1). The Mayo stand is positioned laterally to the right leg of the patient. A colonoscope is often necessary for intraoperative identification of the colorectal lesion. The light source, video camera and monitor for the colonoscope is place laterally to the patient's left leg. For rectal lesions, a rigid sigmoidoscope may be sufficient.

Figure 2.1
Distribution of personnel and equipment in the operating room.

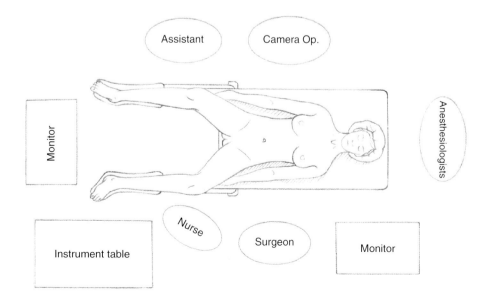

Instruments and equipment

Very few laparoscopic instruments are required. These include:

1 one pair of laparoscopic electrocautery scissors;
2 one laparoscopic atraumatic grasping instrument;
3 two laparoscopic Babcocks;
4 one laparoscopic surgical clip applier;
5 one laparoscopic linear stapling device with multiple cartridges;
6 one laparoscopic suction and irrigation device;
7 one laparoscopic fan retractor (optional);
8 one laparoscopic atraumatic bowel clamp (optional).

Nevertheless, a full array of laparoscopic instruments should be readily available in the operating room should unexpected findings be encountered.

A 10 mm 0° telescope is generally sufficient for performing the procedure. A 10 mm 30° telescope may improve visualization deep in the pelvis in some cases and facilitate mobilization of the splenic flexure.

A recent generation of video equipment improves visualization during the operation. Generally, a three-chip video system is preferable to a one-chip system. A three-dimensional system greatly improves orientation within the abdomen (Fig. 2.2). Moreover, the improved depth perception allows more

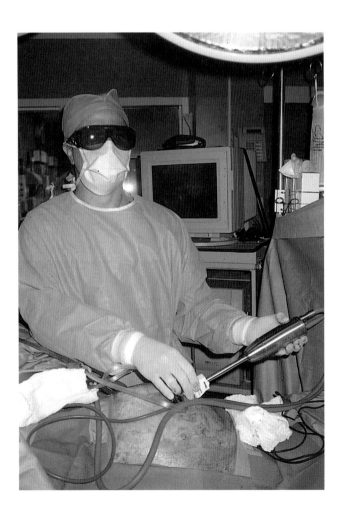

Figure 2.2
The use of three-dimensional video systems helps the surgeon maintain his or her orientation in a complex three-dimensional anatomical field of dissection. This 3-D Scope™ system requires the surgeon to wear polarizing lenses which allow only the right image to reach the right eye and the left image to reach the left eye.

deliberate dissection and diminishes the risk of pointing injuries. The cavernous space of the abdomen is best illuminated with a 300 W xenon bulb light source. A high-flow insufflator that achieve rates of 15–20 l/min maintains an adequate pneumoperitoneum even if leaks develop around the cannulae. A device for heating the carbon dioxide may diminish fogging of the telescope's lens.

A full set of traditional surgical instruments for abdominal operations should also be available within the operating room. These are supplied in case the operation cannot be completed laparoscopically or uncontrollable haemorrhage is inadvertently precipitated.

Placement of the operative team

Certain aspects of laparoscopic procedures determine the principles that lead to the best strategies for placement of the operative team around the table. These features are quite different from those that have established the standard placement of personel during open operations. The first characteristic of laparoscopic operations that must be taken into account is that the cannula is fixed in position in the abdominal wall. These cannulae can only move within a cone-shaped space. The second factor is that most laparoscopic instruments are straight and have no ability to articulate. These two factors severely limit the degrees of freedom of movement of laparoscopic surgical instruments. As a result, the ability of a specific instrument to perform a task may be severely handicapped if it is placed through one cannula, while placement through another one may facilitate the task. This problem stands in sharp contrast to the situation in an open operation, where the surgeon can use almost any instrument from one position because of the great flexibility of stance and various joint movements. Thus, in a laparoscopic procedure it is often much easier for the surgeon to change position around the table rather than to struggle with a manoeuvre that is thwarted by the fixed angle of attack dictated by the position of a particular cannula.

Strategy for a two-member team
The placement of the surgical team will vary somewhat depending on the number of individuals available for the operation. If only two people are available, the surgeon will usually stand on the side of the patient opposite to the area of dissection. A four-puncture technique provides access for the instruments and camera for each of the hands of the surgeon and assistant surgeon. The surgeon uses a Babcock in his non-dominant hand to pull the bowel towards himself thus putting tension on the tissues. Electrocautery scissors are used in the surgeon's dominant hand. The camera person stands on the opposite side. One hand works the camera while the other uses a Babcock or grasping instrument to provide countertraction.

Strategy for a three-member team
When three people are available for the surgical team, more hands are available and a different strategy may prove advantageous. A five- or six-puncture technique allows use of the extra set of hands. Initially, the surgeon stands on the patient's left side, using endoscopic electrocautery-equipped shears and a grasping device (see Fig. 2.1). The grasping instrument pulls the tissues anteriorly and laterally toward the left side of the patient. This sets up a favourable angle of attack for these straight instruments to identify the ureter as it

crosses the left iliac vessels. The assistant surgeon stands on the patient's right. The assistant uses two Babcocks to elevate the bowel and to retract it medially toward the right side of the patient. The tension and countertraction produced by the opposite actions of the surgeon and assistant open the planes of dissection. The camera person stands by the head of the patient on whichever side has more room.

Positions of the team change during the operation. Access to the presacral space and right pelvic wall is easier from the right side of the patient. Insertion of the straight electrocautery scissors through cannulae on the right side of the patient establish an advantageous angle of approach. The surgeon uses his other hand to push the mesorectum anteriorly or medially. The assistant surgeon stands on the left side of the patient, and uses two Babcocks in tandem to elevate the rectosigmoid and proximal rectum anteriorly and toward the left side of the patient. The camera person stands by the head of the patient on either the left or right side.

During mobilization of the splenic flexure, the axis of orientation of the operative team changes (Fig. 2.3). The surgeon stands between the legs of the patient and views the dissection on the video monitor near the left shoulder of the patient. Insertion of the electrocautery scissors through trocars on the left side of the patient provides an excellent angle of approach. The assistant surgeon stands on the right side of the patient and uses two Babcocks in tandem to retract the splenic flexure medially and caudally. The camera person may find it easier to stand by the right leg of the patient.

Patient position

The patient is placed in a modified Lloyd-Davies position with one or both arms tucked in (Fig. 2.4). The thighs remain straight while the knees are gently flexed. Even small amounts of flexion of the thighs block the excursion arcs of the video laparoscope and laparoscopic surgical instruments and may interfere with access

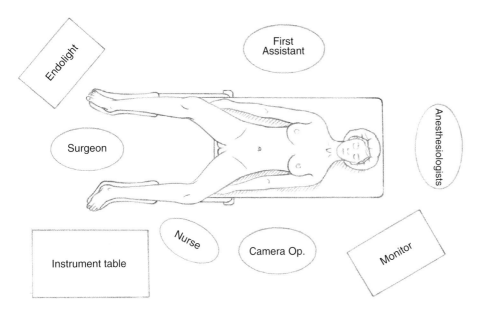

Figure 2.3
Placement of personnel during mobilization of the splenic flexure.

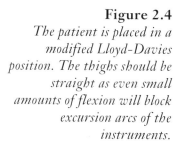

Figure 2.4
The patient is placed in a modified Lloyd-Davies position. The thighs should be straight as even small amounts of flexion will block excursion arcs of the instruments.

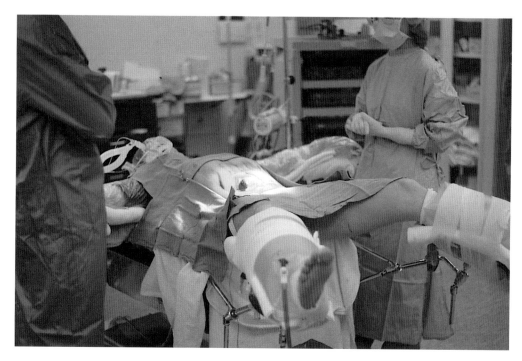

to the left and right upper quadrants. This position allows access to the anus for the introduction of a colonoscope to identify and to localize the lesion and for the insertion of a circular stapling device in the rectum. It also allows the surgeon or assistant surgeon to stand between the legs of the patient while taking down the splenic flexure.

All patients receive a nasogastric tube and urinary catheter. Ureteral stents can be placed once the patient is asleep, if they are to be used. All patients have pneumatic compression boots placed and receive one dose of subcutaneous heparin preoperatively for prophylaxis of deep venous thrombosis.

Port site placement

A five-puncture technique will be described (for a description of four-puncture techniques see references [9]). Four 10 mm cannulae and one 12 or 15 mm cannula are used. Pneumoperitoneum is established in the usual fashion with a Veress needle. A 10 mm cannula is inserted through a supra-umbilical incision. The video laparoscope is inserted through the 10 mm cannula. The abdomen is inspected for evidence of visceral injury during initial cannula placement. Four more cannulae are placed, two in each lower quadrant lateral to the rectus sheath (Fig. 2.5). The caudad right lower quadrant port is usually the best site for the insertion of the stapling devices.

Under some circumstances, an additional cannula is placed in a suprapubic position. If dissection proceeds below the anterior peritoneal resection, the standard length laparoscopic instruments may not reach from the craniad cannulae. Insertion of the instruments through this port will permit deeper dissection within the pelvis. Also, introduction of the laparoscopic linear stapling device through the suprapubic cannula will allow a much lower transection of the rectum.

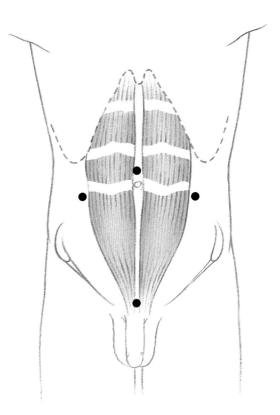

Figure 2.5
Port site placement: five-puncture technique. The umbilical port is used by the telescope. This leaves two ports available for the surgeon and two for the assistant surgeon.

Staging laparoscopy

After cannula insertion, the abdomen is explored. The pelvis is examined first since the patient is already in the Trendelenburg position. Then, using atraumatic bowel clamps (e.g. Endo-Babcock™, United States Surgical Corporation, Norwalk, CT, USA), the entire small bowel is examined. The terminal ileum is identified as it enters into the caecum. Using the laparoscopic Babcocks in tandem, the small bowel is followed back to the ligament of Treitz.

The liver can be examined best with the patient in the reverse Trendelenburg position. In this position the liver drops away from the diaphragms revealing the anterior surface of the left and right lobes. Babcocks can be used to lift the edges of the liver lobes to expose the inferior surface of the lobes. Small metastatic lesions are easily observed on the surface of the liver (Fig. 2.6). Unfortunately, large lesions within the liver parenchyma can easily remain undetected since the surgeon cannot palpate the liver. Use of laparoscopic ultrasonography overcomes this problem.

Laparoscopic ultrasound

Laparoscopic ultrasound probes are available which can effectively image the liver parenchyma. The surgeon places the ultrasound probe directly onto the liver surface (Fig. 2.6). The sensitivity of these systems for the identification of metastatic lesions exceeds that of any currently available computed tomography scanner [10–13]. In addition, the ultrasound system can identify gallstones within the gallbladder or common duct. Early studies suggest that laparoscopic ultrasonography will also prove useful for intraoperative staging of the depth of penetration of colorectal neoplasms.

Figure 2.6
Intraoperative laparoscopic ultrasonography visualizes the lesions within the parenchyma of the liver. This compensates for the surgeon's inability to palpate the liver.

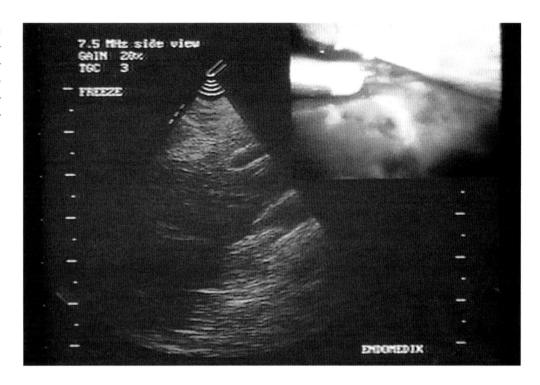

Radioimmuno-guided surgery (RIGS)

Another technology has recently emerged that may permit accurate intraoperative assessment of liver and lymph node involvement with metastatic disease. Monoclonal antibodies against colorectal cancers such as CC49 are radiolabelled with ^{125}iodine. Patients are injected with the antibodies 2 weeks prior to the operation. The monoclonal antibody binds the primary lesion as well as any metastatic lesions. During the 2-week waiting period the radiolabelled antibody clears from the bloodstream, liver and other tissues. This time interval significantly reduces background noise from non-specific binding and circulating radiolabelled antibodies. A prototype device now allows detection of gamma emissions from the ^{125}iodine during the staging laparoscopy (Fig. 2.7). The surgeon may be able to detect the primary lesion as well as metastatic lesions in lymph nodes, the abdominal cavity and within the liver with the laparoscopic gamma detector. Preliminary clinical trials with this device are currently in progress.

Intraoperative localization of the lesion

If the location of the lesion was demonstrated before the operation by a barium enema or not discovered during the staging laparoscopy, the location of the lesion should be identified. Blind resections should not be undertaken based on preoperative colonoscopy reports.

The table is dropped into a deep Trendelenburg position. The left side of the table is rolled up. The endoscopist stands between the legs of the patient. The surgeon stands on the right side of the patient for a lesion in the left colon. The surgeon obstructs the colon proximal to the presumed location of the lesion with an atraumatic bowel clamp. This prevents troublesome distension of the proximal bowel. The intensity of the laparoscopic light is turned down.

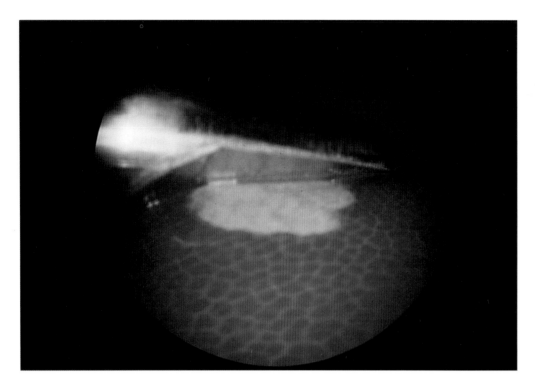

Figure 2.7
Prototypes are now available of laparoscopic (RIGS) gamma detectors that locate ^{125}iodine-labelled monoclonal antibodies bound to colorectal cancers. This system can be used to find the primary lesion, lymph node metastases and also liver metastases.

The endoscopist performs a digital examination and then inserts the colonoscope. In most patients the light of the colonoscope is visible through the wall of the colon once the colonoscope is advanced proximal to the anterior peritoneal reflection. The laparoscopist monitors the advancement of the colonoscope. Once the lesion is reached, the laparoscopic surgeon marks its proximal and distal extent. A laparoscopic clipping device is inserted. The colonoscopist can observe the silhouette of the instrument through the bowel wall and then the indentation produced by the open jaws of the instrument as it is pushed into the colonic wall. The endoscopist directs the surgeon to move the clipping device to the desired location. Surgical clips are used as they remain easily visible throughout the remainder of the operation. After the lesion is marked, the colonoscopist aspirates as much air as possible from the lumen of the bowel. In addition, if the bowel preparation was inadequate, the colonoscopist can supplement it at this time through the irrigation port of the colonoscope.

Operative technique

Irrigation with heparinized saline

Before dissection commences, the operative field is flushed with heparinized saline. If haemorrhage occurs during dissection, the heparin will prevent clot formation. This will allow the laparoscopic suctioning device to aspirate the blood. It is important to maintain perfect haemostasis and to keep the operative field free of blood. Even small amounts of blood stain the tissues and obscure the planes of dissection. Moreover, the haemoglobin absorbs the light and rapidly dims the video laparoscopic image.

Lysis of adhesions

Adhesions between the viscera and the abdominal wall found anywhere within the abdomen should be sharply divided with electrocautery scissors (Fig. 2.8). These adhesions may prevent the movement of the viscera within the abdomen and limit exposure of the planes of dissection. Similarly, adhesions between the small bowel and the pelvic structures, such as encountered after hysterectomies, should be divided. These adhesions will prevent the small bowel from sliding out of the pelvis when the patient is lowered into a deep Trendelenburg position.

Exposure through changes in the patient's position

Exposure of vital anatomic structures is often accomplished by changes in the position of the patient.

Pelvis

Exposure of the pelvis requires lowering the patient into a deep Trendelenburg position. Once a critical angle is reached, the small bowel slides out of the pelvis past the sacral promontory and out of view. There is a critical angle, however, at which this occurs. If this steep angle is not reached, the small bowel remains within the pelvis and tortures the surgeon throughout the procedure.

The pelvis in women

The uterus may hinder visualization of the distal rectum. In these cases, it can be retracted anteriorly with a heavy suture passed on a Keith needle through the abdominal wall, uterus and back through the abdominal wall. Alternatively, a transvaginal uterine elevator can be used.

Figure 2.8

Adhesions between the omentum and previous abdominal incisions should be divided early in the operation. This allows the viscera to slide more freely within the abdomen and helps to improve exposure.

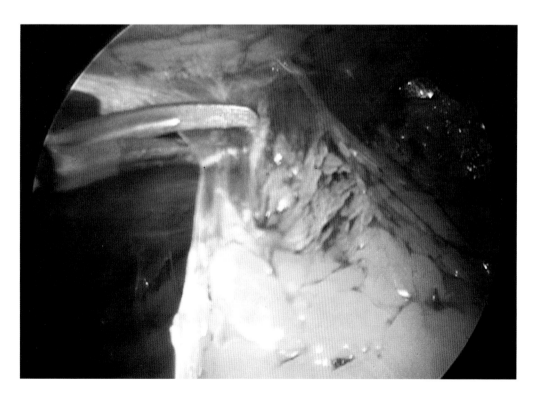

Upper abdomen

The upper abdomen is exposed by raising the head of the bed into a reverse Trendelenburg position. This angle is more gentle than for exposure of the pelvis. The liver, spleen and stomach drop away from the diaphragms. The lesser sac widens as the transverse colon separates from the stomach. This action also has the advantage of pushing these organs closer to the lower abdominal ports and, thereby, bringing them within reach of standard length laparoscopic instruments.

Left gutter

The table is elevated into a slight reverse Trendelenburg position. This causes the viscera to slide back down towards the lower abdominal ports and gains functional length for the laparoscopic instruments. The left side of the table is rolled up. This opens the space between the descending colon and left lateral abdominal wall.

The root of the mesentery

The patient is lowered into a deep Trendelenburg position. This causes the small bowel to slide back up towards the diaphragms. The left side of the table is rolled up. This helps keep the small bowel away from the mesocolon. A fan retractor may be needed to assist in keeping the small bowel off the root of the mesentery. The origin of the inferior mesenteric artery is almost directly under the umbilicus. In some patients, visualization may be improved by insertion of the camera through a left lateral trocar. The surgeon stands either between the legs or on the right side of the patient. The dissection is observed on the secondary monitor at the patient's left shoulder. Although the dissection can be accomplished from other positions, this orientation obviates the need for reversal of instrument movement on the video monitor.

Initial steps of the procedure

Exposure of the left ureter

The limited field of view obtained through laparoscopic telescopes often causes the surgeon to become disoriented within the abdominal cavity. Identification of the ureter early during the operation provides a useful landmark for orientation throughout the remainder of the operation. Following the ureter back to the hilum of the kidney ensures that the surgeon follows the proper planes of dissection during mobilization of the left colon and splenic flexure. It is very easy during laparoscopic procedures to veer laterally and posteriorly and to go behind Gerota's fascia during this dissection. Moreover, its identification early in the procedure permits its protection during mobilization of the left colon and division of the mesentery.

The head of the bed is dropped into a deep Trendelenburg position. The assistant surgeon grasps the rectosigmoid and proximal rectum with two Babcocks inserted into the abdomen through the two right lower quadrant trocars (Fig. 2.9). The assistant drops the handles of the Babcocks down using the abdominal wall as a fulcrum to elevate the rectosigmoid anteriorly. Swinging the handles of the Babcocks along an arc medially causes the grasped bowel to be retracted laterally towards the right. This places traction on the posterior peritoneum overlying the iliac vessels.

The surgeon stands on the left side of the patient using electrocautery scissors and a grasping instrument. The peritoneum over the iliac vessels is elevated

Figure 2.9
*The left ureter is identified
early in the operation.*

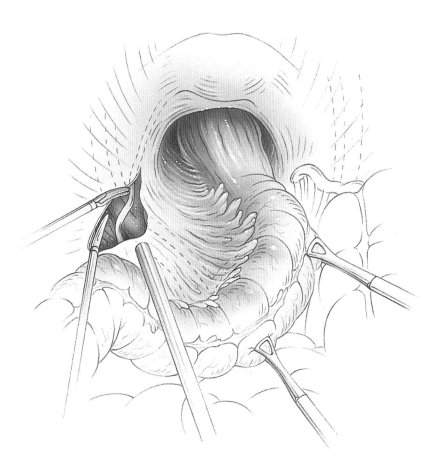

anteriorly and retracted laterally towards the patient's left. The surgeon incises
the peritoneum allowing air to dissect under the peritoneum. The spatula-shaped
tips of the scissors are slid under the peritoneum, advanced down the pelvic side
wall toward the anterior peritoneum reflection, and used to elevate the
peritoneum. This tissue is only divided after it has been elevated in this manner.
The incision in the peritoneum is extended up the left gutter over the psoas. The
flat side of the scissors are used to push the mesorectum and mesosigmoid
medially off the other retroperitoneal structures. It should be noted that it is very
easy to follow the plane between the posterior visceral peritoneum of the
mesosigmoid and the posterior parietal peritoneum because of the extreme
magnification produced by the video laparoscope. The ureter can only be
identified, however, if the parietal peritoneum is incised and the retroperitoneum
exposed. The ureter is found as it crosses the iliac vessels just as in open
operations (Fig. 2.10). Once it is found, it is traced proximally as far as possible.
Exposure of the proximal portion is only accomplished, however, during the
mobilization of the descending colon.

Left pelvic dissection
With the patient in the Trendelenburg position, exposure of the pelvis is
excellent. Consequently, after identification of the left ureter, it makes sense to
continue the dissection down into the left side of the pelvis. Using two Babcocks,
the assistant grasps the rectum as low as possible by alternatively grasping,
pulling and then repositioning the clamps. The rectum is retracted cephaladally
and anteriorly. From the left side of the patient, the surgeon has a excellent angle

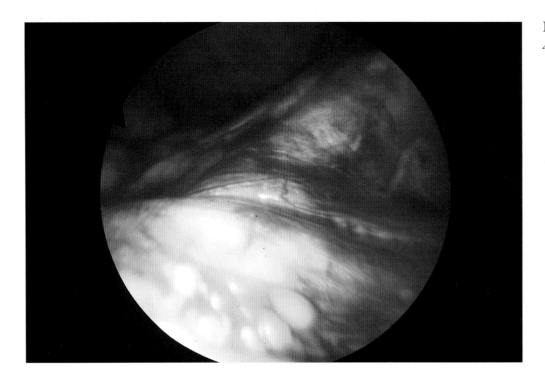

Figure 2.10
A left ureter after exposure.

of attack for this dissection. The curved scissor blades are slid under the peritoneum and used to elevate it. The mobilized peritoneum is divided with cautery. This continues until the midline is reached of the anterior peritoneal resection. The course of the left ureter is traced around the pelvic side wall to its insertion into the trigone of the bladder.

Meticulous haemostasis is critical in the pelvis, as even small amounts of blood can impair exposure and become quite frustrating. Consequently, all tissues are divided with cautery. Any accumulated blood is irrigated with heparinized saline and aspirated.

The presacral space is entered over the sacral promontory. This bony prominence is easily palpated with the tip of an instrument. The magnification provided by the video laparoscope facilitates identification of the sympathetic nerves as they arise from the pre-aortic ganglion and course down into the pelvis. A plane of dissection is selected anterior to these nerves as nothing is gained by division of these nerves in the treatment of a colonic neoplasm.

The areolar plane between the fascia propria, which envails the mesorectum and Waldeyer's fascia, is easily followed down into the pelvis along the sacrum. The surgeon pushes the mesorectum anteriorly with a grasping instrument or a fan retractor (Fig. 2.11). Electrocautery scissors divide the tissues. The assistant continues to elevate the proximal rectum with two Babcocks working in tandem.

Mobilization of the sigmoid and descending colon
The surgeon moves to the right side of the patient and the assistant to the left. The camera remains within the umbilical port. The assistant grasps the sigmoid with two Babcocks displacing it medially and anteriorly to the patient's right side of the camera. The surgeon incises the while line of Toldt (Fig. 2.12). This is best done with the scissors inserted through the caudad right lower quadrant trocar. From this position, the scissors can be slid under the peritoneal reflection along

Figure 2.11
Exposure of the presacral space from the left side. A fan retractor is elevating the mesorectum. The left ureter is visible on the left as it courses around the pelvic brim.

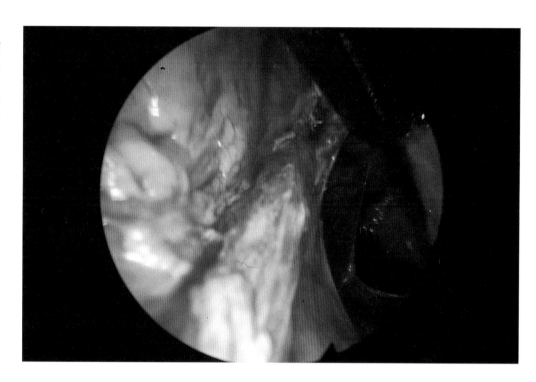

Figure 2.12
Mobilization of the descending colon.

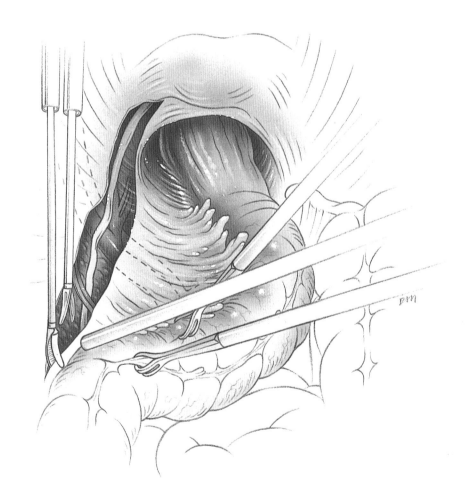

the left gutter. The peritoneum is elevated and divided with electrocautery. The gonadal vessels are identified and bluntly pushed laterally.

The assistant continues to exert median traction on the sigmoid and descending colon. With sweeping motions of the lateral surface of the shaft of the scissors, the surgeon bluntly pushes the mesocolon medially and off the retroperitoneum. The sigmoid is mobilized to the midline over the aorta. As the mesosigmoid is swept medially, the proximal portion of the left ureter is exposed. This ensures that the proper plane of dissection is followed.

Division of the white line of Toldt is continued towards the splenic flexure while exposure remains satisfactory and while the instruments continue to reach the point of dissection. Once dissection becomes tedious, the position of the patient is altered and mobilization of the splenic flexure commences.

Mobilization of the splenic flexure
The patient is placed into a reverse Trendelenburg position, which drops the transverse colon away from the spleen and stomach. In addition, this change of position causes the viscera to slide down towards the lower abdominal trocars. This permits the laparoscopic instruments to better reach the splenic flexure. On occasion in tall individuals, it proves necessary to insert additional trocars so that the standard size instruments can reach the planned area of dissection. Some long instruments are now available and prove beneficial under these circumstances.

The surgeon stands between the patient's legs and inserts the instruments through the left lateral trocars. The assistant moves to the right side of the patient and retracts the splenic flexure towards the umbilicus with the two Babcocks. The surgeon incises the lateral attachments of the descending colon up to the splenic flexure.

The splenic flexure is now approached along the transverse colon. The assistant flips the edge of the omentum up towards the stomach. If necessary the angle of the operating table is modified to one that causes the omentum to remain in place cephalad to the transverse colon. The assistant lifts the omentum anteriorly with one Babcock while displacing the transverse colon posteriorly with the other Babcock (Fig. 2.13). This exposes the avascular plane between the omentum and transverse colon. Electrocautery is used to penetrate this plane and to enter the lesser sac. This is accomplished most easily just to the left of the midline. This plane is followed until the splenic flexure is reached.

The assistant retracts the splenic flexure towards the umbilicus. One Babcock grasps the distal transverse colon and one the proximal splenic flexure. The lienocolic, gastrocolic and splenocolic ligaments are then divided with the cautery scissors. These structures appear as distinct structures due to the magnification of the video laparoscope. The mesocolon is elevated off Gerota's fascia with sweeping motions of the blunt shaft of the surgeon's scissors. This process is continued until the aorta is reached medially. At this point the entire sigmoid, descending and transverse colon are fully mobilized to the midline.

Posterior and right pelvic dissection
The surgeon stands on the patient's right side. The assistant stands on the opposite side. The patient is placed in a deep Trendelenburg position with the right shoulder rolled up. The assistant grasps the rectum and sigmoid over the sacral promontory and provides anterior, left lateral and cephalad traction. The

Figure 2.13
Entering the lesser sac.

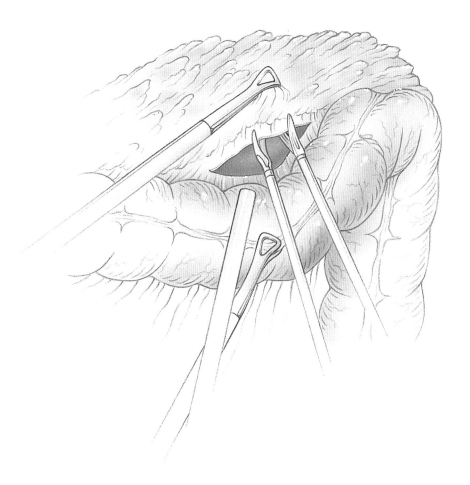

surgeon inserts the scissors and grasping instrument through the right lower quadrant trocars. The sacral promontory is easily palpated. The presacral space is entered at this point. Dissection follows the same plane as selected on the left side: behind Waldeyer's fascia or in the avascular plane between it and the fascia propria. The mesorectum can be bluntly elevated off the sacrum with a fan retractor or with sharp dissection. With either technique haemostasis is important in the pelvis. Frequent irrigation and aspiration helps maintain accurate visualization of tissue planes. The peritoneum is incised down the anterior peritoneal reflection. The right ureter is identified as it crosses the iliac vessels. Ureteral stents aid its identification but are not required in most patients.

Dissection in the pelvis is completed by connecting the left and right planes of dissection behind the mesorectum in the presacral space. A second telescope can be inserted through a left lateral port to provide transillumination of the mesorectum and mesosigmoid. This may help to identify the inferior mesenteric vessels. Also, the second telescope allows the surgeon to visualize the left ureter during this dissection. Depending on the depth of the planned level of rectal transection, the right suspensory ligaments are divided. Cautery is generally sufficient for this, but clips are occasionally required. Dissection continues until an adequate clearance of the lesion is achieved.

Anterior pelvic dissection
When transection of the rectum is planned near the anterior peritoneal resection, mobilization of the distal rectum may be required. The patient remains in a deep

Trendelenburg position. The surgeon and assistant can stand on either side of the patient. The dissection is viewed on the monitor between the legs of the patient. Anterior dissection may prove difficult because of the problems with anteriorly retracting the uterus and vagina or bladder and prostate. In a woman, the uterus can be sutured to the anterior abdominal wall or retracted anteriorly with a weighted uterine sound. A second assistant can place a finger in the vagina to provide anterior traction so as to open up the plane between the rectum and vagina. A rigid proctoscope can provide posterior countertraction. Both of these techniques, however, demand an additional assistant. In a man, once the anterior pelvic reflection is incised, a fan retractor can be placed in this plane to elevate the bladder and prostate. A 10 mm 30° telescope may improve visualization of the pelvis.

The surgeon incises the parital peritoneum just anteriorly to the peritoneal reflection. The planes of dissection on the left and right are connected across the midline. The areolar plane between the bladder/prostate or vagina and rectum is easily identified and followed in a caudad direction. In men, the seminal vesicles appear as surprisingly large structures because of the magnification of the video laparoscope. After each advance of about 1–2 cm along this plane, the fan retractor is repositioned. Mobilization can proceed as needed down to the level of the prostate or midway down the vagina.

Ligation of the inferior mesenteric vessels

Inferior mesenteric artery

The inferior mesenteric vessels can be divided early in the operation or after mobilization of the left colon and proximal rectum. Some surgeons prefer to accomplish this as the initial step of the operation so as to prevent dissemination of the tumour through the portal system during mobilization of the lesion [14]. Any alleged benefit of this strategy, however, has never been demonstrated [15]. Indeed, most atlases of surgical techniques show division of the vessels after mobilization of the colon [16–20]. Similarly, differences in patient outcome based on the level of division of the vessels have not been confirmed. Mobilization of the left colon and identification of the course of the left ureter first, however, certainly protects the left ureter from injury during division of the vessels. Nonetheless, surgeons should proceed with the operative sequence to which they are accustomed.

With the left colon fully mobilized, the inferior mesenteric vessels are easily divided. The surgeon remains on the right side of the patient. The assistant surgeon moves to between the patient's legs. The dissection is observed on the video monitor near the patient's left shoulder. The patient remains in a deep Trendelenburg position. The left side of the table is rolled up. The assistant elevates and retracts to the left side the distal sigmoid and rectosigmoid with two Babcocks (Fig. 2.14). The avascular plane between the inferior mesenteric artery and the aorta is followed from the aortic bifurcation back to the origin of the inferior mesenteric artery. The avascular window cephalad to the origin of the inferior mesenteric vessels is found. The assistant may need to adjust the Babcocks to a point more proximal along the sigmoid to expose the area. In addition, a fan retractor may help keep the small bowel out of the operative field. The window is opened with electrocautery scissors.

Figure 2.14
*Ligation of the inferior
mesenteric artery.*

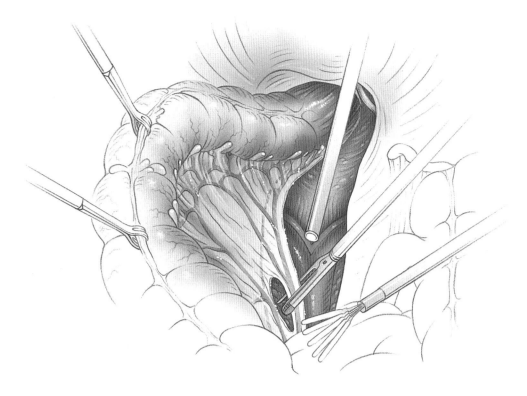

The caudal right lower quadrant trocar is replaced with a 12 or 15 mm trocar to accommodate the laparoscopic linear stapling device. The inferior mesenteric artery is seized with an Endo-Gauge™ (United States Surgical Corporation). Usually, division of these vessels requires vascular staples. The linear stapling device is inserted and positioned at the level of the planned transection of the artery. As it is atraumatic, its jaws are closed. The full length and tips of the stapling device are inspected to ensure that no contiguous tissues were inadvertently enclosed within it. In particular, the left ureter is inspected. The artery is transected. The stapling device is opened after a grasping device has been positioned nearby. Occasionally, a small pumper succeeds in overcoming the triple staple line closure. This is grasped with the instrument and reinforced with a surgical clip.

Inferior mesenteric vein

The inferior mesenteric vein is also divided near its insertion into the splenic vein. The operating table is flattened or placed in a slight reverse Trendelenburg position. This allows some of the small bowel to slide back down into the pelvis, thereby decompressing the upper abdomen. The left side of the table remains rolled up. This helps to keep the small bowel of the mesocolon. The assistant surgeon remains between the legs of the patient, and uses a Babcock to elevate the splenic flexure anteriorly and then retract it laterally to the left side. The assistant's left hand uses a fan retractor to keep the proximal jejunum out of the operative field. The surgeon stands on the right side of the patient. Dissection is observed on the video monitor by the left shoulder of the patient. The surgeon provides countertraction with a Babcock or atraumatic grasping instrument. Dissection is accomplished with electrocautery scissors.

The incision in the parietal peritoneum over the right side of the aorta is extended to the lower border of the third portion of the duodenum. Exposure may be improved by taking down the duodenojejunal flexure. With the inferior mesenteric artery already divided, tension on the colonic mesentery usually reveals the course of the inferior mesenteric vein. If an anatomical left hemicolectomy is planned, the inferior mesenteric vein is isolated cephalad to the insertion point of the large vein that drains the area of the splenic flexure. The avascular windows on either side of the inferior mesenteric vein are opened. The linear stapling device with a vascular cartridge is closed around the vein near the caudal or inferior edge of the pancreas. The tips of the stapling device are checked. The vein is divided and the stump is inspected for haemostasis.

Division of the bowel

Distal margin of resection

When anterior resection is performed for proximal rectal lesions or left colectomy for rectosigmoid lesions, the distal margin of resection should be checked prior to transection of the bowel. If the lesion is advanced and penetrating the bowel wall, video laparoscopic selection of the distal margin of resection is easily accomplished. In patients afflicted with early lesions, however, the laparoscopist may not be able to gather any visual or tactile clues as to the distal extent of disease. Intraoperative colonoscopy permits accurate identification of the distal extent of disease and determination of an adequate margin of resection.

The patient is lowered into a deep Trendelenburg position. The small bowel is swept out of the pelvis. With the rectum fully mobilized, a colonoscope or rigid proctoscope is inserted through the anus. By dimming the laparoscopic light source, the light from the colonoscope becomes visible through the bowel wall. The distal extent of the lesion is marked with surgical clips or rechecked if accomplished earlier in the procedure. Clips should not be placed at the planned level of transection as the heavy surgical clips cannot be cut by the stapling device and will cause the stapling device to misfire.

The thickness of the rectum at the distal margin of resection is gauged. In thin patients, the linear stapling device will be easily applied. In obese patients, however, application of the stapling device will be difficult because of the thickness of the mesorectum. It may be necessary to open a window in the mesorectum so that the mesorectum can be divided separately.

The linear stapling device is inserted through the caudal right lower quadrant trocar when the distal margin of resection is above the peritoneal reflection. If a low anterior resection is required, the stapling device should be inserted through a suprapubic port. This will permit a lower application of the stapling device. If the right lower quadrant trocar is selected, the 10 mm trocar is removed and replaced with a 12 or 15 mm trocar depending on the calibre of the stapling device that will be used. The rectum is transected with two or three applications of the 30 mm stapling device or one application of the 60 mm stapling device. A 3.5 mm (blue) cartridge is usually used but the bowel thickness should be gauged. The remaining mesorectum is divided either with the stapling device or with cautery and clips.

Retrieval of the specimen

Mobilization of the rectum and left colon are checked. The mesentery is elevated to ensure that no posterior points of fixation have been missed. The level of planned proximal resection is grasped with a Babcock and pulled down to the intended site of the abdominal incision as well as to the rectal stump. This should reach without tension. Any additional mobilization that may be required is accomplished at this time.

The incision can be made conveniently at two sites. If the rectum was transected proximally leaving a long rectal stump, a muscle-splitting incision is made in the left lower quadrant beyond the caudal trocar. If the rectal stump is short because of a lower level of resection, a suprapubic incision is preferred. Exteriorization of the specimen through the suprapubic incision will ensure that adequate mobilization of the proximal colon has been achieved to allow construction of a tension-free anastomosis. A wound protector can be inserted at this time (Fig. 2.15). Retrieval of the specimen into an impermeable bag may obviate problems of wound seeding.

The patient remains in a deep Trendelenburg position. The surgeon inserts a Babcock through the caudal left lower quadrant trocar. The staple line on the specimen side of the rectum is grasped. The surgeon makes an oblique or transverse incision through the trocar site. The muscle fibres are bluntly split. The abdominal cavity is entered. The pneumoperitoneum is decompressed. The

Figure 2.15
Withdrawal of the specimen into a wound protector and sleeve may prevent wound implantations from colorectal malignancies.

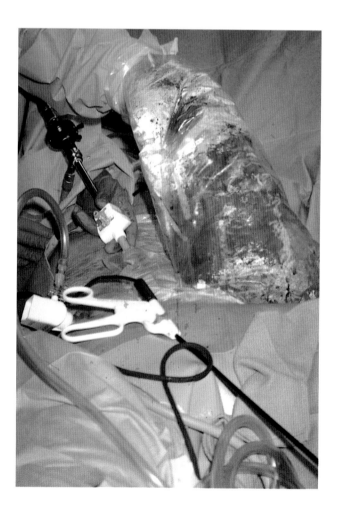

incision is widened to a length that will easily accommodate the specimen. The incision must be at least 3.5 cm long so that the anvil of the circular stapling device can be dropped with the colon into the abdomen. A wound protector may be positioned at this time. The specimen is withdrawn.

The proximal margin of transection is selected. The remaining mesentery is divided at this point and ligated with silk ties. A 2.5 cm segment of the bowel wall is cleared of mesenteric fat. A purse-string device is applied at the distal extent of the cleared zone. A monofilament purse-string suture is applied. A crushing bowel clamp is placed across the colon distal to the purse-string device. The bowel is transected and handed off the field to a pathologist and the specimen is opened within the operating room. The margins of resection are examined.

Construction of the anastomosis

The edges of the transected colon are opened. Three Allis clamps grasp the edge of the bowel holding it open by triangulation. If required, the bowel lumen is dilated. The surgeon's thumb is a delicate instrument to accomplish this task. Alternatively, a 30 ml balloon-tipped urinary catheter can be used. The lumen of the bowel is sized and the diameter of the circular stapling device is selected. A 31 mm cartridge is preferred. The anvil and shaft assembly of the Premium CEEA™ (United States Surgical Corporation) stapler is inserted into the colon, and the purse-string suture tied.

The abdomen is liberally irrigated and suctioned dry through the incision. The colon is replaced into the abdomen. It is important to maintain the proper orientation as the colon is replaced. Rotation of the colon should be avoided. The tip of the anvil–shaft assembly is placed deep in the pelvis and the incision is closed.

The pneumoperitoneum is re-insufflated. The antimesenteric taenia of the colon is traced back from the distal margin to the proximal point of mobilization. This will reveal any unsuspected twists of the colon. The shaft of the anvil is grasped with a Babcock placed through the caudal right lower quadrant trocar.

The assistant dilates the anus of the patient so that it admits four fingers. A 00 suture is placed through the small hole in the tip of the stapling device's white trocar and tied to form a loop. The Premium CEEA™ stapler is inserted through the anus and advanced to the staple line of the rectal stump. The stapler is aligned in the middle of the staple line with video laparoscopic guidance. The white trocar is screwed out through the centre of the staple line (Fig. 2.16). The suture loop in the tip of the trocar is grasped by the surgeon with a grasping instrument, withdrawn from the stapling device and retrieved through a 10 mm or larger trocar. This exposes the orange collar on the stapling device (Fig. 2.17). The anvil–shaft assembly is docked into the stapling device. The mesocolon is checked for rotation and the stapling device is screwed closed. The stapler is fired, unscrewed and removed. The tissue rings are examined and should be intact. The anastomosis is checked by visual inspection and air insufflation after filling the pelvis with irrigation.

Closure

The irrigation fluid is aspirated and the trocars are removed one at a time. The fascial defects are closed with figure-of-eight sutures of a 00 absorbable suture.

Figure 2.16
The white trocar of the circular stapling devices penetrates the wall of the rectal stump.

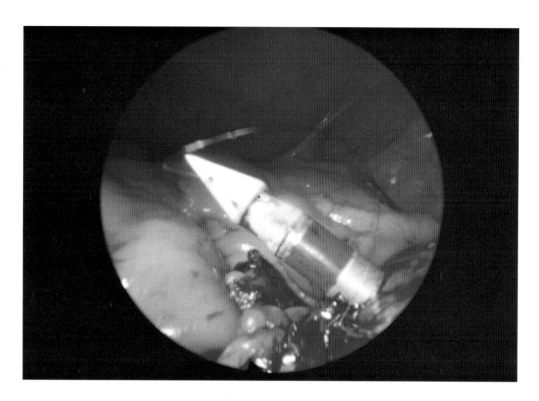

Figure 2.17
The anvil–shaft assembly is docked into the head of the circular stapling device.

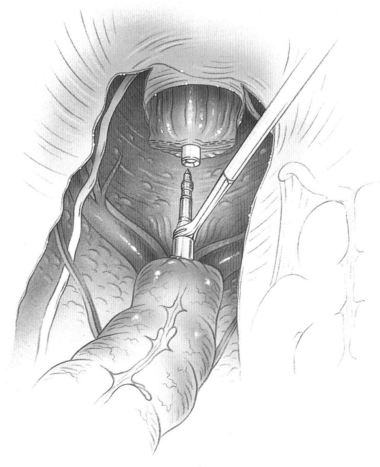

All but the final incision is done under direct video laparoscopic observation with maintenance of the pneumoperitoneum. This minimizes the risk of a Richter's hernia. The skin incisions are closed with skin staples and adhesive tape, and the wounds are covered with sterile dressings.

Postoperative management

The nasogastric tube is removed on the first postoperative morning or in the recovery room. The urinary catheter is kept in place for 3–5 days if an extensive pelvic dissection was performed. The patient is allowed to take clear liquids on the first postoperative day if desired, and is then advanced to a regular diet as tolerated. Most patients tolerate a regular diet by the second or third postoperative day. Pain is generally minimal compared with open procedures and is easily controlled with small doses of narcotics. Patient-controlled analgesia (PCA) is not required and usually slows the progress of the patient.

The pneumatic compression boots are removed when the patient is moving around. Administration of subcutaneous heparin is continued until discharge; the patient is discharged when bowel movements resume and the diet is regular, usually by the fifth postoperative day.

Learning curve

The learning curve for laparoscopic colorectal operations is more prolonged than that for laparoscopic cholecystectomy. This stems from the more complex anatomy involved with colorectal operations and the additional skill required to perform these operations. Whereas cholecystectomy is accomplished in a very limited anatomical zone that is nearly two-dimensional, colorectal operations are performed throughout much of the abdominal cavity within a complex three-dimensional environment. This jump from a two-dimensional area of dissection to a three-dimensional one challenges the surgeon's sense of orientation on the two-dimensional video monitor. Also, the movement of instruments during a cholecystectomy is very limited and the operation can be performed with a one-hand technique. During a laparoscopic colorectal operation the surgeon must move instruments throughout the abdomen. Moreover, the surgeon must operate with two instruments, one in each hand. The added challenge of a laparoscopic colorectal operation should not surprise anyone. Cholecystectomy is an operation surgeons learn early in their training, whereas colectomy is saved until the resident or registrar has accumulated years of experience with easier operations.

We initiated our experience with laparoscopic colorectal operations in 1991. At that time, techniques of dissection and mobilization were not well established. We have maintained a policy of attempting minimally invasive techniques on virtually all patients under elective conditions. Figure 2.18 shows our rates of conversion in groups of 10 patients for our first 100 consecutively attempted laparoscopic colorectal operations. Early in our experience we converted a majority of procedures to a traditional open technique. This resulted from strict time limitations that we implemented: if the operation was not nearing completion within a 2-h time period we converted to an open operation. After the first 20 operations, we have been able to accomplish about 90% of operations with the planned laparoscopic technique. The most common reason for

Figure 2.18

The learning curve for laparoscopic colorectal operations is longer than that observed for laparoscopic cholecystectomy. In an unselected series of 100 patients treated on an 'all comers' basis, one of the authors (GHB) experienced a high rate of conversions to open operations during his initial 20 procedures. During the next 80 operations, a high rate of success was maintained.

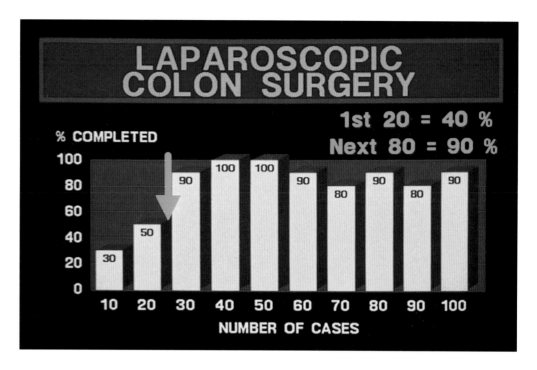

conversion was poor exposure due to the obesity of the patient or adhesions from previous operations. Other reasons included difficulty in transection of the rectum during low anterior resection, adhesion of the bowel to the left ureter, inability to identify the ureter and undue length of operative time. Careful selection of patients during one's early experience might significantly decrease the rates of conversion.

Complications

Minimally invasive techniques for colorectal operations are used to accomplish exactly the same operations as performed with open techniques. Consequently, patients sustain exactly the same spectrum of complications after laparoscopic colorectal·operations as after open operations. Table 2.1 lists the complications suffered by 100 patients who underwent laparoscopic colorectal operations in a veterans' administration (VA) medical centre (*n*=55) and in private hospitals (*n*=45). The patients in the VA hospital were consecutive and unselected. The patients in the private hospital were treated as part of a preceptor programme and were heavily preselected. The details of most of these patients have been published previously [21,22]. The average age of these patients was 65 years with a standard deviation of 16 years. Seventy percent of the patients were male and 30% female. This male preponderance reflects the sex bias of the VA hospital. These operations included six polypectomies, four colostomy constructions, nine closures of colostomies and 81 colorectal resections. Seventeen of the 55 operations performed at the VA hospital and five of the operations performed at private hospitals were converted to open operations. The high conversion rate at the VA hospital stems from the high rate of conversion during our early attempts (see above). There were no deaths in this series of patients. Of particular note in Table 2.1 is the absence of wound infections among the patients who underwent

Complications	No. of patients
Laparoscopy group (*n*=77)	
Death	0
Wound infection	0
Anastomotic dehiscence	0
Enterotomies	2
Ethanol withdrawal	1
Tachyarrhythmia	1
Postoperative prolonged ileus	2
Postoperative fever	1
Cardiac ischaemia requiring coronary artery bypass grafting	1
Urinary retention	1
Urinary tract infection	1
Allergic reaction	1
Sloughed colostomy mucosa	1
Venous laceration requiring transfusion (2 units)	1
Pelvic abscess requiring percutaneous drainage	1
Retained perineal drain	1
Total number	15
Laparoscopies converted to open operations (*n*=23)	
Death	0
Anastomotic dehiscence	0
Wound infection	1
Wound dehiscence	1
Postoperative bleeding	1
Postoperative prolonged ileus	1
Total number	4

Table 2.1
Complications sustained by 100 patients who underwent attempted laparoscopic colorectal operations. The patients are listed in two groups: 77 patients who underwent successful laparoscopic procedures and 23 who required conversion to open operations.

successful laparoscopic procedures. The total rate of complications of 19% (15/77) compares favourably with rates seen after open operations.

The data presented in Table 2.1 do not result from a randomized prospective trial. Consequently, comparisons of complication rates with those of open operations cannot be vigorously offered. Nonetheless, this information suggests that patients do well after laparoscopic colorectal operations, that the range of complications is similar to that seen after open operations and that wound complications are infrequently encountered.

References

1   Filipi CJ, Fitzgibbons RJ Jr, Salerno GM. Historical review: diagnostic laparoscopy to laparoscopic cholecystectomy and beyond. In: Zucker KA (ed.) *Surgical Laparoscopy*. Quality Medical Publishing, St Louis, 1991: 3–22.
2   Reddick EJ, Olsen DE. Laparoscopic laser cholecystectomy. *Surg Endosc* 1989; **3**: 131–3.

3 Falk PM, Beart RW Jr, Wexner SD *et al*. Laparoscopic colectomy: a critical appraisal. *Dis Colon Rectum* 1993; **36**: 28–34.
4 Senagore AJ, Luchtefeld MA, MacKeigan JM, Mazier WP. Open colectomy versus laparoscopic colectomy: are there differences? *Am Surg* 1993; **59**: 549.
5 Monson JRT, Darzi A, Carey PD, Guillou PJ. Prospective evaluation of laparoscopic-assisted colectomy in an unselected group of patients. *Lancet* 1992; **340**: 831.
6 Alexander RJT, Jaques BC, Mitchell KG. Laparoscopically assisted colectomy and wound recurrence. *Lancet* 1993; **341**: 249.
7 Walsh DCA, Wattchow DA, Wilson TG. Subcutaneous metastases after laparoscopic resection of malignancy. *Aust N Z J Surg* 1993; **63**: 563.
8 Hughes ES, McDermott FT, Polglase AI, Johnson WR. Tumor recurrence in the abdominal wall scar tissue after large-bowel cancer surgery. *Dis Colon Rectum* 1983; **26**: 571.
9 Leahy PF. Low anterior resection. In: Ballantyne GH, Leahy PF, Modlin IM (eds) *Laparoscopic Surgery*. WB Saunders, Philadelphia, 1994: 575–89.
10 Castaing D, Emond J, Bismuth H *et al*. Utility of operative ultrasound in the surgical management of liver tumors. *Ann Surg* 1986; **204**: 600–5.
11 Machi J, Isomoto H, Hurohiji T *et al*. Detection of unrecognized liver metastases from colorectal cancers by routine use of operative ultrasonography. *Dis Colon Rectum* 1986; **29**: 405–9.
12 Rifkin MD, Rosato RE, Branch HM *et al*. Intraoperative ultrasound of the liver. *Surg* 1987; **205**: 466–72.
13 Parker GA, Lawrence W, Horsley JS *et al*. Intraoperative ultrasound of the liver affects operative decision making. *Ann Surg* 1989; **209**: 569–77.
14 Jagelman DG. Colectomy for malignant disease of the colon: the 'no-touch' isolation technique. In: Fielding LP, Goldberg SM (eds) *Rob and Smith's Operative Surgery: Surgery of the Colon, Rectum and Anus*, 5th edn. Butterworth-Heinemann, London, 1993: 359–68.
15 Davis MD, Ballantyne GH. Colorectal surgery. In: Ballantyne GH, Leahy PF, Modlin IM (eds) *Laparoscopic Surgery*. WB Saunders, Philadelphia, 1994: 233–65.
16 Grant JP. Left colectomy. In: Sabiston DC Jr (ed.) *Atlas of General Surgery*. WB Saunders, Philadelphia, 1994: 420–5.
17 Enker WE. Operative treatment for carcinoma of the abdominal colon. In: Block GE, Moosa AR (eds) *Operative Colorectal Surgery*. WB Saunders, Philadelphia, 1994: 193–219.
18 Keighley MRB, Williams NS. *Surgical Management of Carcinoma of the Colon and Rectum (with Particular Reference to Colon Cancer)*. WB Saunders, Philadelphia, 1993.
19 Gordon PH. Malignant neoplasms of the colon. In: Gordon PH, Nivatvongs S (eds) *Principles and Practice of Surgery for the Colon, Rectum and Anus*. Quality Medical Publishing, St Louis, 1992: 501–65.
20 Rothenberger DA. Conventional colectomy. In: Fielding LP, Goldberg SM (eds) *Rob and Smith's Operative Surgery: Surgery of the Colon, Rectum and Anus*, 5th edn. Butterworth-Heinemann, London, 1993: 347–58.
21 Begos DG, Ballantyne GH. Laparoscopic colectomy at a VA hospital: the first 50 cases. *J Surg Res* 1994 (in press).
22 Sgambati S, Ballantyne GH. Preceptoring laparoscopic colectomy: is it effective? *Surg Endosc* 1994 (in press).

Chapter 3

Anterior resection: the total laparoscopic approach

J.S. Azagra, M. Goergen, E. Gilbart, D. Jacobs, P. Lejeune
and E. Carlier

Introduction

The triple-stapled technique (TST) is a new, entirely mechanical, end-to-end colorectal anastomosis that eliminates the problem of specimen extraction or placing a purse-string suture in one or both ends of the anastomosis. It was first described by F.M. Steichen in 1988 at the First European Congress on Stapling in surgery. We have satisfactorily adapted this technique in colorectal surgery since September 1988.

The steps of TST anastomosis by classic laparotomy are presented in Table 3.1. This chapter presents a technique of standardized anterior resection with end-to-end colorectal anastomosis using TST by the total laparoscopic approach (TLA).

Materials and methods

From October 1991, the authors performed 39 anterior resections using TST by TLA on 19 men and 20 women with an average age of 53 years (range: 23–83 years). Sixteen patients had cancer, 15 had rectal prolapse, four had diverticulitis and four had associated volvulus with idiopathic refractory constipation. Twelve patients had undergone previous abdominal surgery: six hysterectomies, one splenectomy, seven appendicectomies and two cholecystectomies. All of these procedures were successful.

1 Distal end of the rectum closed with a linear stapler
2 Anvil stem introduced into the proximal colon
3 Proximal colon closed with a linear stapler
4 Stem of the anvil pushed through the centre of the proximal staple line
5 Curved circular stapler with trocar advanced transanally to pierce the distal staple line
6 Anvil stem connected to the stapler stem
7 Circular stapler closed and fired
8 Totally stapled colorectal end-to-end anastomosis created

Table 3.1

Steps of the TST technique in anterior resection of the rectum by laparotomy.

Technique

A standard mechanical bowel preparation using 3 l of polyethylene glycol was administered 1 day prior to surgery and a prophylactic dose of parenteral antibiotic was administered 30 min before surgery.

The patients were placed in a supine position with the legs placed in low stirrups to facilitate transanal extirpation of the operative specimen and stapling of the anastomosis. The operating room setup is shown in Fig. 3.1. The surgeon stood on the right and the assistant on the left side of the patient. The instrumentation is shown in Table 3.2 and the positions of the cannulae in Fig. 3.2.

The pneumoperitoneum was created after insertion of a Veress needle at the umbilicus using approximately 14 mmHg of intra-abdominal pressure. A disposable cannula was placed in an infra-umbilical position.

After removal of the trocar, the endocamera was introduced. Two other cannulae were placed under videoscopic control in the right and left flanks at the level of Spieghel's line. All introduction sites were 12 mm in diameter thus permitting total manoeuvrability of the laparoscopic instruments.

The use of bowel graspers permitted the identification of the lesion to be resected (Fig. 3.3) and the localization of the origin of the inferior mesenteric

Figure 3.1
The operating room setup and patient monitor.

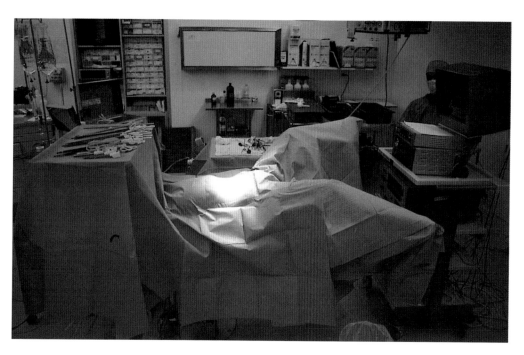

Table 3.2
Total instrumentation employed in anterior resection using the TST technique by TLA.

Optique: 10 mm 0°
4 cannulae: 12 mm
2 atraumatic bowel graspers
1 endoshears with monopolar coagulation
1 endostapler
1 circular stapler

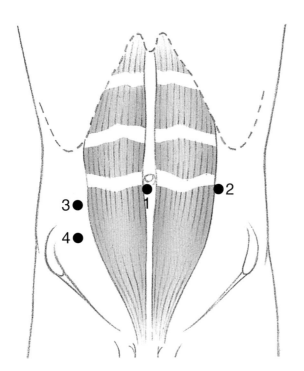

Figure 3.2
Sites for placement of the cannulae: (1) laparoscope 0° 10 mm in the infra-umbilical position; (2) bowel grasper in the left subcostal position; (3) bowel grasper or endostapler in the right subcostal position; (4) shears, clips, endostapler and endo slip knots in the right lower quadrant position.

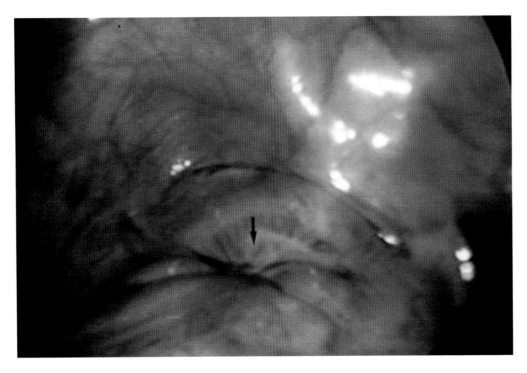

Figure 3.3
Identification of the lesion (arrow).

artery (Fig. 3.4), as well as the examination of both surfaces of the liver and the rest of the abdominal cavity.

If there was any doubt as to the localization of the lesion intraoperatively, a peroperative colonoscopy was performed to determine the site of the lesion. Because of the inability to palpate, especially the liver, laparoscopic ultrasonography with a laparoscopically guided liver biopsy, if appropriate, was employed for staging cancer.

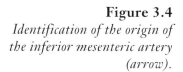

Figure 3.4
Identification of the origin of the inferior mesenteric artery (arrow).

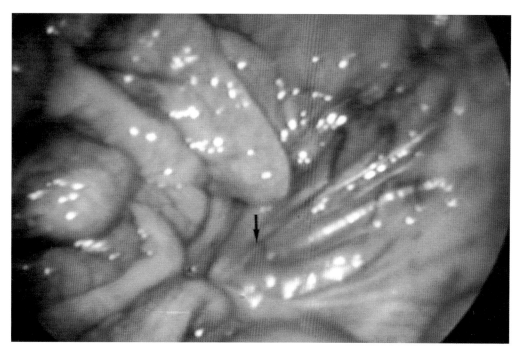

After the preliminary inspection and estimation of the feasibility of the procedure, a fourth cannula was introduced in the right lower quadrant in order to allow the passage of the endoshears, endoclips, endostapler and slip knot.

Colorectal dissection and mobilization was carried out using the classic technique and was accomplished exclusively by using the endoshears with monopolar thermocoagulation. First the left peritoneal reflection of the rectosigmoid was mobilized (Fig. 3.5) and the left ureter visualized. The retrorectal space was then mobilized down to the presacral fascia (Fig. 3.6). This

Figure 3.5
The left peritoneal reflection is dissected and the left ureter (arrow) identified.

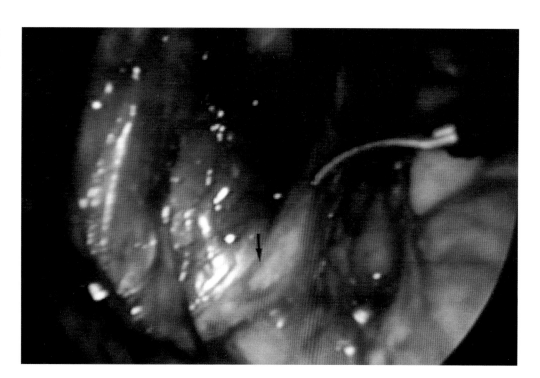

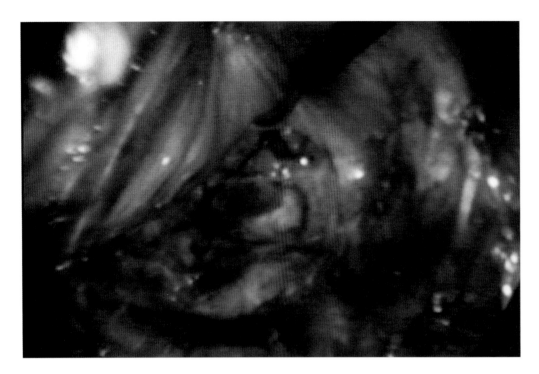

Figure 3.6
Dissection of the retrorectal space.

dissection is particularly facilitated by the laparoscopic approach. The sacral nerves were usually identified and preserved. Laterally, the dissection allows the visualization of the middle rectal vessels, which were coagulated. The dissection of the anterior wall of the rectum was performed by sagittal traction on the uterus in women or the bladder in men (Fig. 3.7).

A complete *en bloc* mobilization of the rectum was attempted 2–3 cm from the anal verge by monopolar electrocoagulation. The completely mobilized rectosigmoid was elevated to the abdominal wall by a bowel grasper and held in

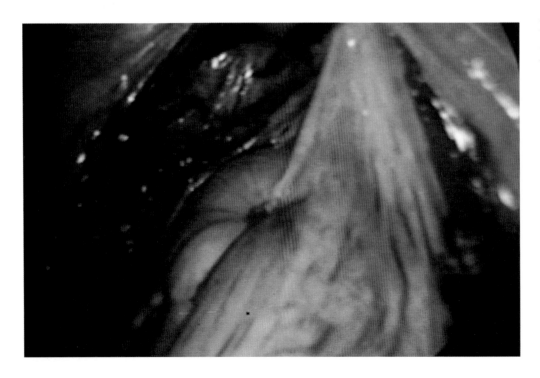

Figure 3.7
Dissection of the anterior wall of the rectum.

this position by the assistant. This allowed an easy dissection of the pre-aortic area, which was continued to the origin of the inferior mesenteric artery. Vessel ligation was by an endostapler or endoclips or with slip knots (Fig. 3.8). Figures 3.9–3.22 show the sequence of systematic and standardized steps of the procedure.

The size of the anastomosis was 31 mm in 32 patients and 28 mm in the remaining seven cases. None of the anastomoses were protected by colostomy. The last 24 patients had no in-dwelling drains. The integrity of the anastomosis was checked by methylene blue and air tests.

Figure 3.8
High pedicular section of the inferior mesenteric artery; the lymph node (arrow) can be seen.

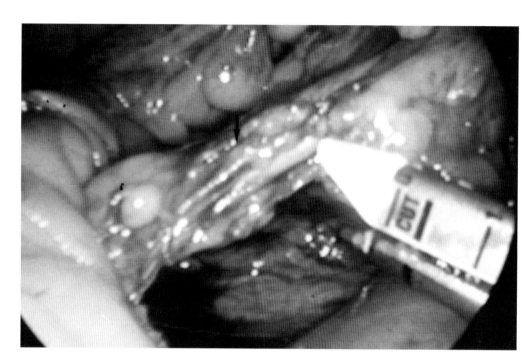

Figure 3.9
Section of the proximal colon by endostapler.

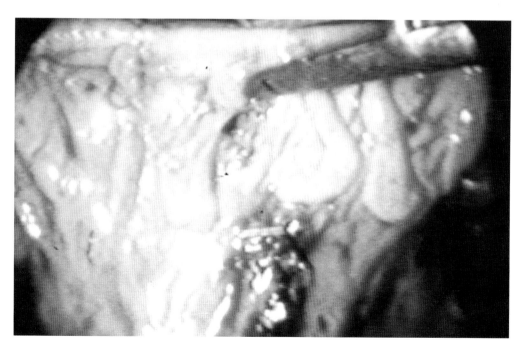

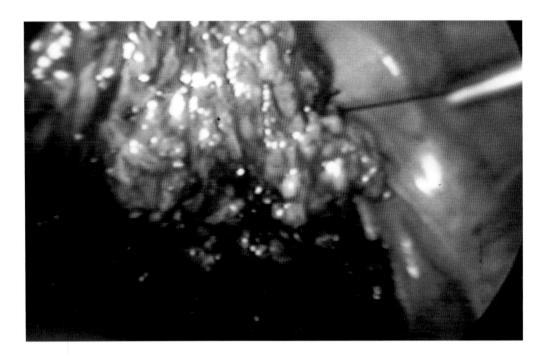

Figure 3.10
Closure of the distal colon by endo slip knots.

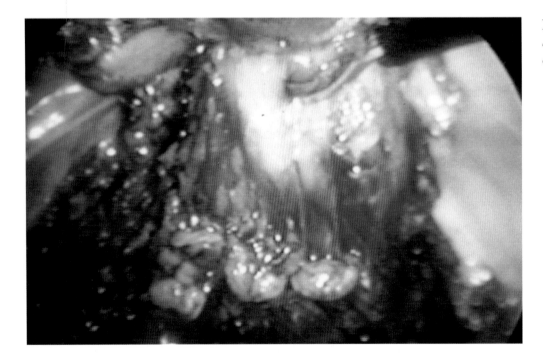

Figure 3.11
Section of the posterior wall of the rectum by endoshears.

Figure 3.12
Transanal introduction of the circular stapler and intra-abdominal withdrawal of the anvil.

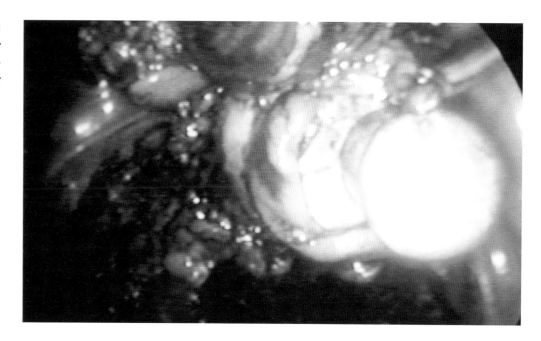

Figure 3.13
Transanal evacuation of the specimen is performed using plastic bags introduced transanally (arrow) in (a)).

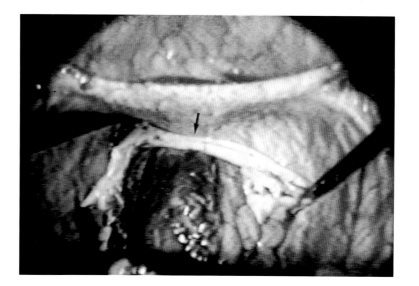

(a)

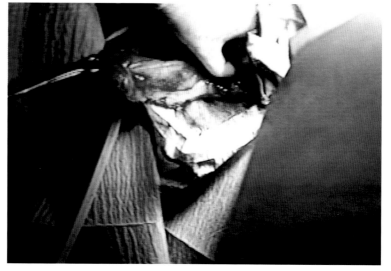

(b)

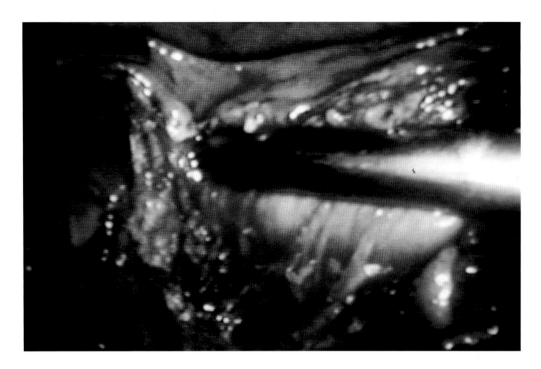

Figure 3.14
Closure of the rectal stump by endostapler.

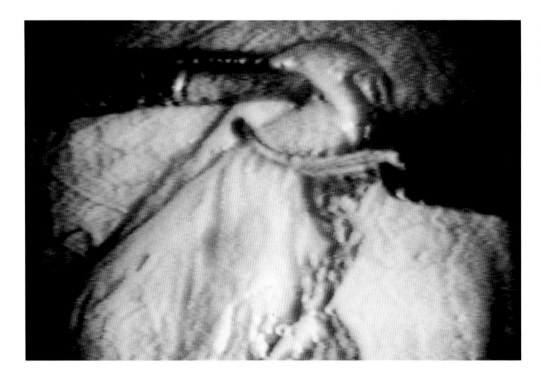

Figure 3.15
Partial antimesenteric incision of the proximal colon by endoshears.

Figure 3.16
Introduction of the anvil into the proximal colon anchored by a suture to the anterior wall, proximal to its closure.

(a)

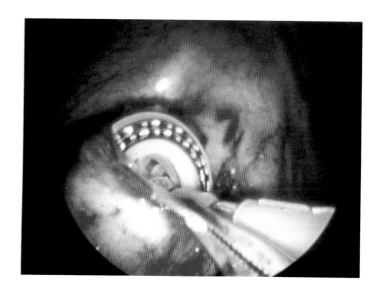

(b)

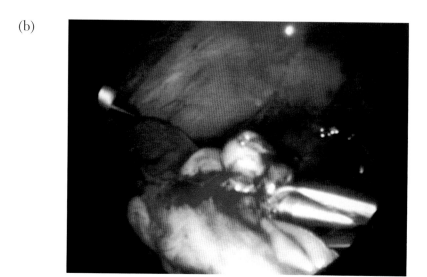

(c)

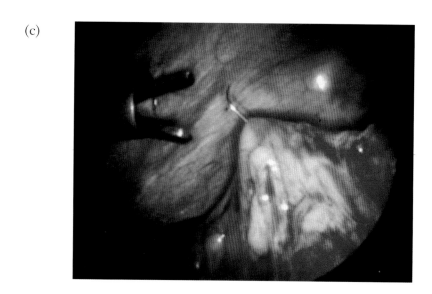

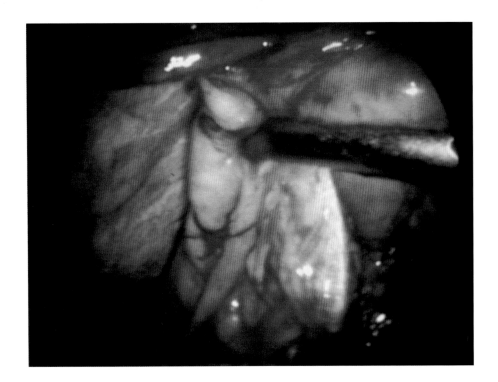

Figure 3.17
Closure of the proximal colon by endostapler.

(a)

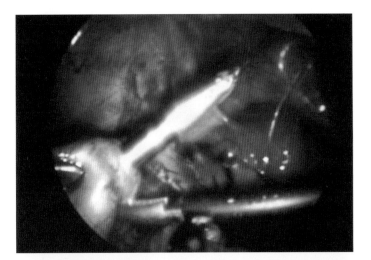

Figure 3.18
Traction on the anchoring suture advances the pointed anvil stem through the endostapler line into the abdominal cavity using the laso to exteriorize the stem of the anvil.

(b)

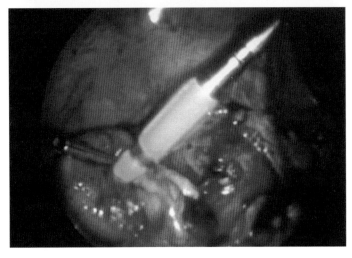

Figure 3.19
Transanal introduction of the circular stapler and trocar perforation of the distal staple line.

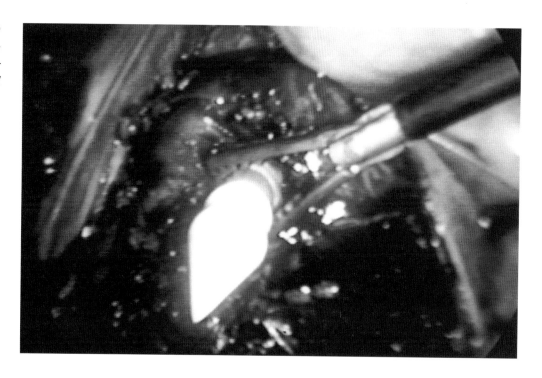

Figure 3.20
Connection of the anvil stem into the hollow stapler rod.

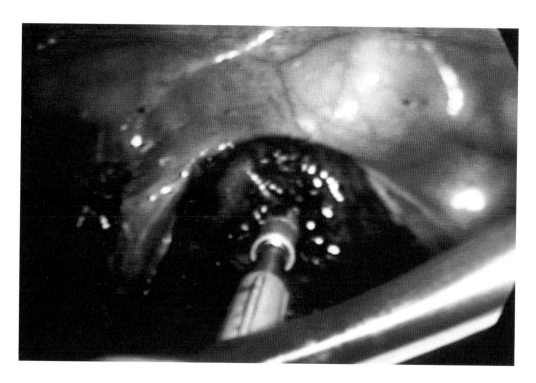

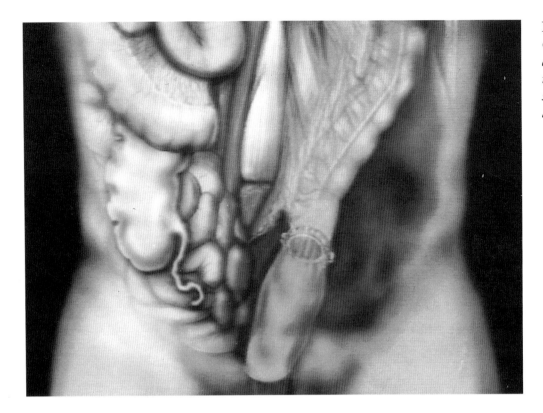

Figure 3.21
Closing and firing of the circular stapler, creating the totally laparoscopically stapled colorectal end-to-end anastomosis.

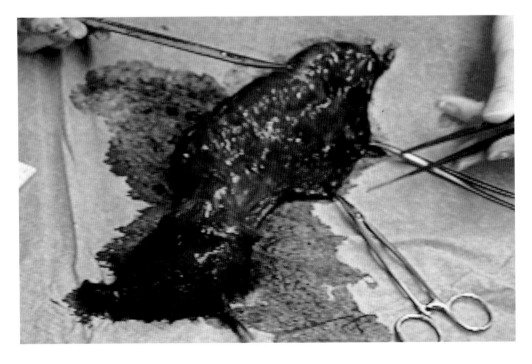

Figure 3.22
The specimen.

Results

An entirely laparoscopic approach was abandoned in three of the 39 patients. In two patients, accidental division of the suture on the stem of the anvil (Fig. 3.18) obliged us to perform a short laparotomy to extract it and then to perform an intraperitoneal anastomosis using endovision. In the third patient, the tissue rings were not complete and, in spite of a negative methylene blue test, we opted for a new anastomosis using the Pfannenstiel incision.

Consequently, of the 39 patients operated on using the described technique, the procedure was successful in 36, which is an overall success rate of 92%. The average operating time was 220 min (range: 150–330 min). The peroperative blood loss averaged 350 cm³ (range: 200–1000 cm³). Twenty anastomoses were radiologically checked at approximately the eighth postoperative day using water-soluable contrast medium. Mortality rate, and perioperative and postoperative complications up to the 30th day are shown in Table 3.3 and late complications are given in Table 3.4.

In patients undergoing colectomy for malignant disease, the mean tumour diameter was 4 cm. Of 16 cases, one was Dukes' stage A, eight Dukes' stage B, five Dukes' stage C and two Dukes' stage D. The average number of nodes identified in the resected specimen was nine (range: 4–17). The mean distance of the tumour from the proximal margins of resection was 15 cm and from the distal margins 6 cm.

One patient developed a postoperative haemorrhage revealed by the Penrose drain and successfully treated by simple transfusion. No patients developed

Table 3.3
Perioperative and postoperative complications of the TST technique by TLA in anterior resection (30th day after operation).

Complications	No. of patients
Clinical fistulae	1 (using the laparoscopic Hartmann procedure, death from MOF)
Radiological fistula	0
Perioperative faecal spill	0
Perioperative haemorrhage	0
Postoperative haemorrhage	1 (medical treatment)
Deep abscess	0
Wound infection	0
Prolonged ileus	0
Lung infection	0
Urinary infection	0
Methylene blue test	0
Air test	0
Intact tissue rings	38
Accidental section of laso	2
Great omentum evisceration	2
Duration of operation	220 min (range: 150–330 min)

MOF, multiple organ failure.

Late complications	No. of patients
Stricture	1
Wound dehiscence	1
Impotence	0
Retrograde ejaculation	0
Faecal incontinence	0
Briddle occlusion	1 (laparoscopic treatment)
Local recurrence	0

Table 3.4
Late complications of the TST technique by TLA in anterior resection.

wounds, or urinary or pulmonary infection. Two patients developed a wound dehiscence on the fourth day after operation which was repaired under local anaesthesia. One patient developed a postoperative anastomotic stricture treated successfully by endoscopic dilatation. One patient developed intestinal obstruction from adhesions on the seventh postoperative month which was treated laparoscopically. The one death in our series was an 83-year-old female with generalized sigmoid carcinoma staged as ASA (American Society of Anaesthesiology) 3. She developed a fistula which caused multiple organ failure resistant to treatment.

Discussion

Anaesthetic implications of laparoscopic anterior resection

Preoperative evaluation of the patient
The evaluation of a patient scheduled for a laparoscopic procedure is not fundamentally different from the preoperative assessment of a patient undergoing a traditional laparotomy for colectomy.

Contraindications
In view of the pathophysiological changes associated with the laparoscopic approach, some contraindications can be stated: shock (whatever its origin might be), bullous emphysema, severe restrictive or obstructive pulmonary diseases, unstable angina, intracranial hypertension and ventriculoperitoneal shunts.

Intraoperative monitoring
Routine intraoperative monitoring is mandatory for the management of the patient — an electrocardiogram monitor, a non-invasive blood pressure monitor and a pulse oximeter are all needed. The patient is placed in the supine position, with his or her arms along the body. A capnograph is also necessary, not only as a routine anaesthetic alarm, but also to follow the progression of hypercarbia during the insufflation manoeuvre and during maintenance of the pneumoperitoneum [1]. A urinary catheter is inserted for decompression of the bladder and to reduce the risk of perforation when the trocar is introduced. A gastric tube is required for decompression of the stomach.

An oesophageal rather than a rectal temperature probe is inserted to monitor any hypothermia, which is always possible in long surgical procedures. A warming blanket is routinely used to minimize heat loss, as well as a special irrigation–suction device, which injects heated saline solution to rinse out the peritoneal cavity.

A routine radial arterial cannulation is recommended for monitoring arterial blood gases and ventilation. Its usefulness is reinforced by the fact that changes in end-tidal carbon dioxide (CO_2) tension ($PeCO_2$) are not parallel to those of arterial CO_2 tension ($PaCO_2$), and adjustment of ventilation cannot be made on capnograph criteria alone [2]. In cases of recognized cardiopulmonary disease, an arterial line and, eventually, a pulmonary catheter are necessary. A precordial or oesophageal stethoscope is recommended to detect any gas embolization.

Surgical implications of laparoscopic anterior resection

Described by Steichen [3] in 1988, at the First Congress on Stapling in Luxembourg, the end-to-end colorectal anastomosis using TST is simple, rapid and entirely mechanical. It allows a systematic approach to the placement of 'high-risk' staples, such as those used in the anterior resection of the rectum, by completely avoiding the manual or mechanical introduction of a purse-string suture. This type of anastomosis is reproducible from one case to another with no problems arising from colorectal differences in size and wall thickness. This would seem to increase the security of the anastomosis.

As of 1989, Julian *et al.* [4] reported a series of experimental data that validate the TST technique and suggest a high success rate in anterior resection of the rectum. We reported our experience with 95 patients in 1992 at the Congress of Minimally Invasive Surgery and New Technology in Luxembourg [5].

Since 1988, general surgeons have adopted laparoscopy for intra-abdominal procedures: cholecystectomy, appendicectomy and herniorrhaphy. Laparoscopic colorectal surgery has appeared since 1990. The possibility of performing different types of colectomy using different techniques has been demonstrated in diverse papers and video tapes [6–11]. It seems that the TST technique is particularly well adapted to coelioscopic surgery because it allows the performance of rectosigmoid colectomies avoiding laparotomy.

In our series, anterior resection using TST by TLA was possible in most (36 of 39) of the attempted cases. In three cases, it was necessary to convert to a short laparotomy. Failure was due in two cases to the accidental division of the anchoring suture of the anvil. In the third case, we found incomplete tissue rings of the circular stapled suture, which are an indication of a new anastomosis performed by a short Pfannenstiel laparotomy.

Transanal evacuation of the specimen is difficult for low subperitoneal rectal tumours in which a small pelvis and a large tumour hinder the closing of the rectal stump by an endostaper. For these cases, we suggest Welter's [12] anterior perineal approach with an anterior perineal colorectal anastomosis as a suitable alternative to anterior resection by TLA.

The transanal evacuation of the specimen is performed using plastic bags introduced transanally (see Fig. 3.13). This prevents all contact between the tumour and the rectal stump and, thus, eliminates the risk of tumour seeding.

The absence of an intra-abdominal infection in our series confirms the low degree of contamination in this technique. However, there are two points of potential contamination in the TST technique. The first is the moment of opening of the posterior wall of the rectum in order to introduce the anvil transanally in the abdominal cavity. This manoeuvre is carried out on a closed rectal stump using a slip knot or endostapler on the side of the specimen, which permits vigorous rectal lavage. The other is the opening of the proximal colon in order to introduce the anvil. This step is brief and has never yet led to faecal spillage.

We have encountered the most difficulty in dissection in patients with diverticulitis or in colons having abundant and fatty epiploic appendices. Obesity makes colon mobilization difficult and vascular dissection tedious. The use of an endostapler or an ultrasonic dissector is especially helpful in these cases.

In the excision of malignant tumours, a laparoscopic approach seems to be acceptable given the operative specimen obtained. These have been evaluated by their free margins of resection and the nodal harvest. To date, none of our patients (16 TST by TLA and 28 laparoscopically assisted) have had local recurrences. However long-term evaluation is necessary to analyse this objectively.

Postoperative discomfort seems to be less than that in patients treated using traditional procedures. Analgesia can be provided with traditional agents. However, as a rule, patients who have undergone laparoscopic colectomy require less analgesic drugs than patients who have undergone a laparotomy [13]. Nonetheless, shoulder tip pain, secondary to irritation of the diaphragmatic peritoneum, is commonly encountered.

The laparoscopic approach for cholecystectomy has been shown to produce less reduction in pulmonary function than cholecystectomy by subcostal incision [14]. We undertook a prospective study to compare postoperative pulmonary function tests between patients undergoing laparotomy, laparoscopically assisted minilaparotomy and TST by TLA for colectomy (seven patients in each group). Peak expiratory flow, vital capacity and forced expiratory volume (FEV_1) were measured using bedside spirometry preoperatively and 1, 4, 8, 12, 24, 36 and 48 h after surgery and 2, 3, 4, 5, 6 and 7 days postoperatively and before leaving hospital (time = 8 days). The results showed no difference between the groups (Fig 3.23), suggesting that the laparoscopic approach cannot reduce postoperative pulmonary complications in patients undergoing colectomy. Our results are in accordance with the results of a recent study by Erice and co-workers [15] who demonstrated an impairment of diaphragmatic function after laparoscopic cholecystectomy or laparoscopic hernia repair.

Most patients are ambulatory within 48 h after the procedure with intestinal transit restored in 3 days. The patients are discharged, on average, at the eighth postoperative day (range: 6–14 days).

The two cases with herniation through the port site have led us to close these wounds by suturing the fascia [16].

Conclusion

Anterior resection with end-to-end anastomosis using triple stapling and a systematic, entirely laparoscopic, approach is a reliable procedure. It does not seem to increase the risk of developing anastomotic complications such as fistulae or stenosis. TST has a real place in laparoscopic colorectal surgery, allowing us to achieve secure anastomosis while avoiding laparotomy.

Figure 3.23
Peak expiratory flow (PEF) data (mean ± SE) for group 1 (▲) (anterior resection by laparotomy, n = 7), group 2 (■) (anterior resection using TST by TLS, n = 7) and group 3 (●) (laparoscopically assisted anterior resection, n = 7).

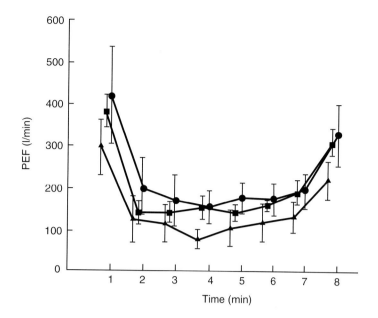

References

1   Hall O, Goldstein A, Tynan E, Braunstein L. Profound hypercarbia late in the course of laparoscopic cholecystectomy: detection by continuous capnometry. *Anesthesiology* 1993; **79**: 173–4.

2   Yamanaka MK, Sue DY. Comparison of arterial-end-tidal pCO_2 difference and dead space/tidal volume ratio in respiratory failure. *Chest* 1987; **92**: 832–5.

3   Steichen FM. Changing concepts in surgical techniques. In: Ravitch MM, Steichen FM, Welter R (eds) *Current Practice of Surgical Stapling*. Proceedings of the Second International Symposium and First European Congress on Stapling in Surgery, Luxembourg, 1988. Lea & Febiger, Philadelphia, 1990: 23–7.

4   Julian TB, Kolachalam RB, Wolmark N. The triple stapled colonic anastomosis. *Dis Colon Rectum* 1989; **32**: 989–95.

5   Azagra JS, Goergen M, Ceuterick M. The triple-stapled technique: further progress in colorectal surgery. In: Steichen FM, Welter R (eds) *Minimally Invasive Surgery and New Technology*. Second European Congress, Luxembourg, 1992. Quality Medical Publishing, St Louis, 1994: 456–63.

6   Azagra JS, Alle JL, Goergen M. Colorectal surgery by laparoscopy. Preliminary results of 64 cases. *Hepatogastroenterology* 1993; **1**: 219.

7   Brune IB, Schouleben K. Laparoskopische Sigma Resektion. *Chirurgie* 1992; 63: 342–4.

8   Jacobs M, Verdeja GD, Goldstein DS. Minimally invasive colon resection (laparoscopic colectomy). *Surg Laparosc Endosc* 1992; **1**: 144–50.

9   Monson JRT, Darzi A, Dedean PC, Guillou PY. Prospective evaluation of laparoscopic-assisted colectomy in an unselected group of patients. *Lancet* 1992; **340**: 831–3.

10 Schlinkert RT. Laparoscopic-assisted right hemicolectomy. *Dis Colon Rectum* 1991; **34**: 1030–1.

11 Werner SD, Johansen OB, Vogueras JP, Jagelman DG. Laparoscopic total abdominal colectomy. A prospective trial. *Dis Colon Rectum* 1992; **35**: 651–5.

12 Welter R. Exérèse du rectum par voie combinée abdomino-périnéale antérieure. In: Welter RT, Patel JCh (eds) *Chirurgie Mécanique Digestive*. Masson, Paris, 1985: 283–94.

13 Lin J, Durf Y, White PF, Feinstein R, Shear JM. Effects of Ketorolac on postoperative analgesia and ventilatory function after laparoscopic cholecystectomy. *Anesth Analg* 1993; **76**: 1061–6.

14 Frazee RC, Roberts JW, Okeson GC. Open versus laparoscopic cholecystectomy. A comparison of postoperative pulmonary function. *Ann Surg* 1991; **213**: 651–4.

15 Erice F, Fox GS, Salib YM, Romano E, Meakins JL, Magder SA. Diaphragmatic function before and after laparoscopic cholecystectomy. *Anesthesiology* 1993; **79**: 966–75.

16 Goergen M, Azagra JS. Herniation at the site of cannula insertion after laparoscopic cholecystectomy. Letter 2. *Br J Surg* 1993; **80**(11): 1488.

Chapter 4

Conventional colon and rectal resection

P. Lee and A.W. MacDonald

Introduction

The planning and execution of any colon and rectal resection should be based on a comprehensive understanding of three groups of principles:

1 the applied surgical pathology of the disease;
2 the correct surgical technique;
3 the patient's requirements.

Because the majority of colon and rectal resections are for malignant disease, in this chapter these principles are applied to resections for colon and rectal cancer. However, they can and should be equally applied to non-malignant conditions such as inflammatory bowel disease or diverticular disease.

Applied surgical pathology

Pathological diagnosis of the tumour

Before embarking on a colon and rectal cancer resection the surgeon requires confirmation of the diagnosis by a pathologist. Tumour type and degree of differentiation are not always essential as it may well be non-representative of the tumour as a whole. Exceptions to this may be when local excision is being considered or in estimating the acceptable clearance margins with a low anterior resection [1].

Tumour spread and biology

There are four routes of tumour spread which need to be considered:

1 direct spread;
2 extramural lymphatic spread;
3 haematogenous spread;
4 transcoelomic spread and implantation.

Direct spread

By definition all invasive tumours spread by direct extension, thus access is gained to lymphatics, blood vessels, serous cavities and contiguous structures. The surgical resection must clearly provide margins clear of the macroscopic tumour which are likely to be free from direct tumour extension. Previously a safety margin, both distal and proximal, of 5 cm was advocated by Grinnell [2] particularly if the tumour was poorly differentiated, but with the advent of low restorative anterior resection of the rectum it has been shown that a distal margin of much less than this, perhaps 2 cm or even less, is sufficient [3]. It would appear from the work of Quirke *et al.* [4] and Heald and Ryall [5] that the circumferential margin is equally important and that in the rectum at least, from the practical point of view, this should be made as wide as possible.

Where the direct extension is into other organs there is clear evidence that *en bloc* dissection without disruption of the tumour plane can provide an excellent prognosis [6]. The tumour biology of colon and rectal cancer would indicate that the size of the tumour and the degree of extraluminal extension are not necessarily a guide to poor prognosis and hence, wherever possible, radical excision is considered to be worthwhile.

Lymphatic spread

The basis of a radical curative resection for colon and rectal cancer continues to be the removal of the tumour itself and the entire related lymphatic field. This considers lymphatic involvement in simple anatomical terms with tumour emboli passing via afferent lymphatics to regional nodes and by their efferent lymphatics to distal nodes and beyond. Although this does in fact occur, such an approach belies a much more complex active tumour–host interaction. The lymphatic channels of the colon and rectum closely follow the blood vessels supplying that particular segment. Thus the resection is based on the wide removal of all extramural lymphatics which accompany the main colic blood vessels supplying the segment of colon or rectum involved. In tumours of the caecum, ascending colon, hepatic flexure and right half of the transverse colon, which are all supplied via the superior mesenteric artery, the ileocolic, right colic and middle colic arteries are all divided close to their origin and the right colon and half the transverse colon, removed as an extended right hemicolectomy (Figs 4.1–4.3). When the growth involves the transverse colon, splenic flexure, and descending and sigmoid colon, which all derive their blood supply from the inferior mesenteric artery, the resection involves ligation of the appropriate feeding main colic arteries close to their origin from the inferior mesenteric artery with removal of the associated segment of colon (Figs 4.4 and 4.5).

Haematogenous spread

Colon and rectal tumours spread by the bloodstream particularly to the liver and more rarely to the lungs, adrenals, kidneys, bone and brain. It is facile to imagine this spread as passive embolism because of the selectivity of the tumour for certain organs. From the practical point of view, however, this surgical pathology should be applied to assessment of the likely areas of distal spread in order that whenever possible preoperatively this knowledge can be included in the planning of the surgery.

Transcoelomic spread and implantation

If a tumour perforates the bowel there will be viable tumour cells within the peritoneal cavity and, irrespective of lymph node status, prognosis will be poor.

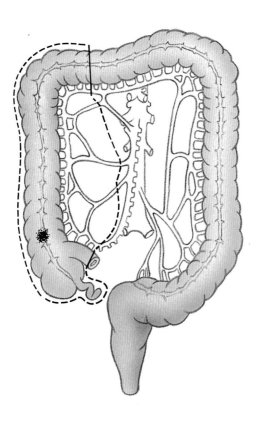

Figure 4.1
Resection lines for carcinoma in the caecum and ascending colon.

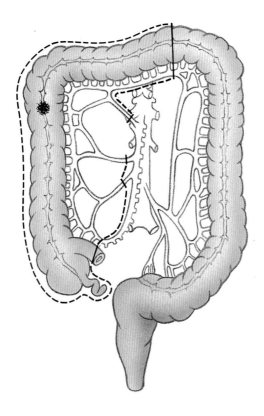

Figure 4.2
Resection lines for carcinoma in the hepatic flexure.

Figure 4.3
*Resection lines for carcinoma
in the transverse colon.*

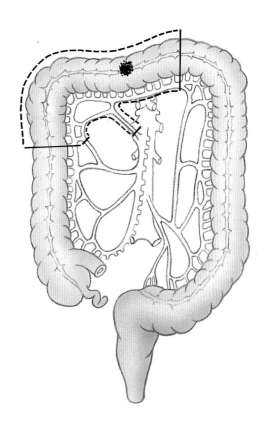

Figure 4.4
*Resection lines for carcinoma
in the splenic flexure.*

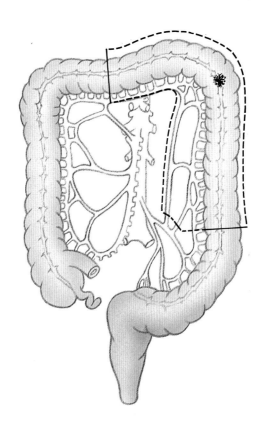

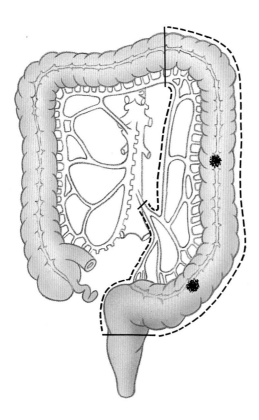

Figure 4.5
Resection lines for carcinoma in the descending and sigmoid colon.

Tumour cells may be released into the peritoneal cavity in the absence of obvious perforation by serosal extension but another important means is by the surgery itself. Cutting through the tumour or spillage of the poorly cohesive malignant cells from the margins of the specimen can result in subsequent peritoneal seedings.

On the above applied pathology is based the rationale for gentle tissue handling, non-disruption of tumour planes and care to avoid tumour spillage. It should be admitted, however, that there is little in the literature to advocate the use of peritoneal cytotoxic washouts, local washing of wound edges to prevent implantation, or covering of wound edges for a similar reason.

Preoperative extent of tumour spread

The preoperative extent of spread of the tumour must be defined as accurately as possible in order to plan the proposed surgery. Clearly if the postoperative pathological data obtained from the specimen histology were to be available preoperatively it would be easier to choose the correct surgical resection and, perhaps even more importantly, the necessary adjuvant therapy in terms of radiotherapy or chemotherapy or both. Already modern day imaging, aimed at the likely site of spread, is beginning to provide more acute data — thus a combination of endoanal ultrasound and magnetic resonance imaging (MRI) of the pelvis may soon provide accurate preoperative lymph node staging, and a combination of computed tomography (CT), MRI and intraoperative ultrasound an accurate assessment of the presence or absence of liver metastases.

Postoperative assessment of the tumour

Postoperative assessment of the tumour type, degree of differentiation, nodal involvement and macroscopic tissue plane invasion will all help to provide pointers to the probable success of the operation [7] and help in the decision regarding the necessity for and type of adjuvant therapy required.

Correct surgical technique

Requirements

The surgeon's guiding aim should be to provide the maximum chance of cure with minimal morbidity and mortality. This may be achieved with the help of the guidelines given in Table 4.1.

Clearly the patient should arrive at the operating theatre in the optimal condition for success of the surgery. Thus preoperative blood parameters should be corrected where necessary; cardiac and respiratory problems appropriately dealt with; adequate bowel preparation should be provided together with appropriate prophylactic measures such as perioperative antibiotics and anti-deep venous thrombosis prophylaxis. The patient should have been fully informed about the procedure and have signed a consent form, and have been counselled regarding the possibility of a stoma with appropriate site marking where necessary.

Optimal anaesthetic relaxation together with peroperative monitoring of central venous pressure and urine output should be provided. The patient should be placed on the operating table in the position most likely to provide maximal exposure of the operative site; thus for an anterior resection or abdominoperineal excision the patient will be in the Lloyd-Davies position with a head-down tilt as required (Fig. 4.6). The incision should be suitably placed to provide adequate

Table 4.1
Requirements for the correct surgical technique.

1 Optimal preparation of the patient
2 Optimal anaesthesia
3 Accurate perioperative monitoring with appropriate moderation
4 Optimal exposure of the operative site
5 Initial comprehensive assessment of the intraoperative findings — tumour extent, spread and associated pathology
6 Careful initial planning of the requisite surgical procedure
7 Adequate extent of resection to cover the assessed and possible tumour extension
8 Isolation and gentle handling of the tumour to avoid spillage or spread
9 Avoidance of disruption of tissue planes
10 Dissection along anatomical planes to minimize tissue trauma and blood loss
11 Optimal anastomotic technique (if indicated)
12 Optimal stoma placement (if indicated)
13 Appropriate additional protective mechanisms if required, e.g. covering stoma, drainage, washout, antibiotics
14 Optimal postoperative monitoring and corrections
15 Appropriate adjuvant therapy

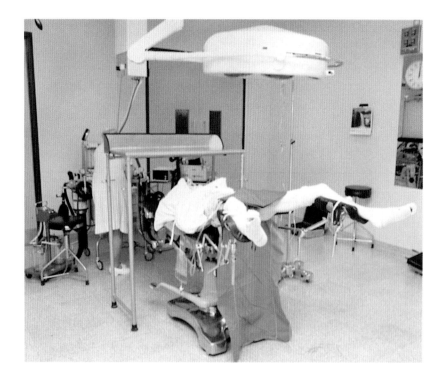

Figure 4.6
Lloyd-Davies position for anterior resection/abdominoperineal exision of the rectum.

access to the operation site and will, therefore, often involve a full-length midline incision. Exposure can, if necessary, be helped by packing the small intestine into a plastic intestinal bag (Fig. 4.7), the provision of a second assistant between the patient's legs and appropriate retraction with, for example, Goligher lipped retractors.

An initial comprehensive assessment of the intraoperative findings should then be carried out; thus the site of the tumour is confirmed and the extent of spread, both locally and distally, assessed. Intraoperative ultrasound scanning of the liver should be included. Synchronous tumours or polyps of the large bowel should be excluded as far as possible by careful palpation, and the presence of non-associated intra-abdominal pathology noted. Careful initial planning of the requisite surgical procedure is then made. It is possible that at this stage the tumour may be deemed inoperable or non-curative, for example if peritoneal metastases are present, and that a lesser procedure aimed simply at palliation or relief of symptoms will be carried out.

If the operation is deemed curative or potentially curative, then the proposed extent of resection should be decided. This is especially important if other organs are involved, e.g. the uterus, ovaries, bladder or anterior abdominal wall, as it is essential that *en bloc* resection should be carried out without disruption of tumour planes.

The extent of the resection will be decided initially by the site of the tumour. As discussed in the previous section the dissection must include adequate margins to cover local extension, both within and without the bowel lumen, together with excision of the lymph node-bearing areas associated with the tumour. Some surgeons have placed particular emphasis on early ligation of the feeding blood vessels to avoid possible tumour spillage via the bloodstream. Hence the vogue for Turnbull's no-touch technique of colonic resection [8], which involves

Figure 4.7
Plastic bowel bag used to aid exposure.

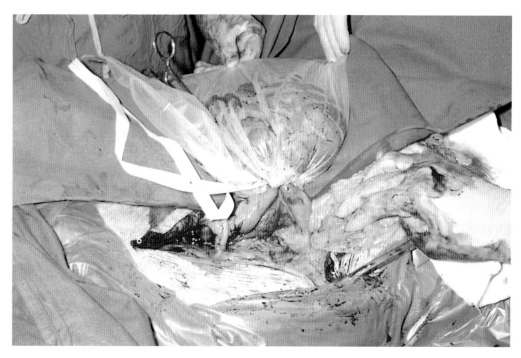

minimal handling and mobilization of the bowel before the feeding blood vessels have been ligated as high as possible in the route of the relevant mesentery. It should be pointed out, however, that there has been no confirmation of increased survival figures for the no-touch technique and that it is commonly held that the increased survival figures quoted by Turnbull are equally matched by a correct radical tumour and lymphatic excision as recommended in this chapter (as opposed to the limited wedge-type resection often favoured by non-cancer surgeons). A similar situation exists for the taping of the lumen of the bowel on either side of the tumour to avoid direct tumour spillage and implantation within the lumen. Although this may seem a plausible adjunct to the resection there does not seem to be any evidence in the literature to vindicate its necessity [9].

Five situations relating to the extent of resection in rectal cancers are worthy of special mention.

1 *High tie of the mesenteric vessels.* It is generally accepted that in the mobilization of the rectum and left colon for restorative anterior resection the inferior mesenteric vessels should be tied high (Fig. 4.8). The assumption for this recommendation is that a greater number of potentially tumour-bearing lymph nodes will be excised. There is no evidence, however, that a high tie of the inferior mesenteric artery provides better survival figures [10]. Nonetheless, a high tie of the vessels (the inferior mesenteric artery close to the aorta and the inferior mesenteric vein close to the lower border of the pancreas) is still recommended, but for a different reason, in that it allows the mobilized descending colon and splenic flexure of the colon to be brought down to the rectal anastomosis without tension (see below).

2 *Radical para-aortic and internal and external iliac node dissection.* Some authors, particularly the Japanese school of surgery [11], have suggested that a radical lymphadenectomy involving the para-aortic chains and those alongside the

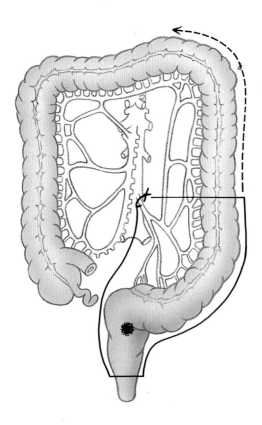

Figure 4.8
Resection lines for restorative anterior resection of the rectum. Note the high tie of the inferior mesenteric artery and the full mobilization of the splenic flexure.

internal and external iliac arteries will provide enhanced survival for rectal cancer. There does not seem to be confirmation of this in the European and North American literature — rather the contrary, in that it promotes a greatly increased morbidity particularly in relation to bladder dysfunction.

3 *The routine mobilization of the splenic flexure for carcinoma of the middle and lower third of the rectum.* It is now generally accepted that in performing a resection for a carcinoma of the middle and lower third of the rectum it is appropriate at an initial stage of the operation to fully mobilize the sigmoid colon, the left colon, the splenic flexure of the colon and part of the transverse colon. The reasons for this recommendation are threefold. Firstly, the blood supply of the descending colon is superior to that of the sigmoid colon. Secondly, the lumen of the descending colon is wider and often of better 'quality' than the narrower, often diverticular disease-affected, sigmoid colon. Thirdly, mobilization of the colon to this extent allows tension-free colon to be brought down to the anastomosis with the excess redundant colon filling up the potential dead space left in the sacral hollow.

4 *Total mesorectal dissection.* Recent impressive results from Heald's unit in Basingstoke [5], from the point of view of both increased long-term survival figures and, in particular, the very low incidence of local tumour recurrence, would indicate that a total mesorectal dissection should be carried out for all tumours of the middle and lower third of the rectum [12]. The essential features of this technique are that a meticulous and wide excision of the rectum should be carried out, remaining far out on the side walls of the pelvis until the level of the fade out of the mesorectum is reached (Fig. 4.9).

Figure 4.9
Total mesorectal excision.

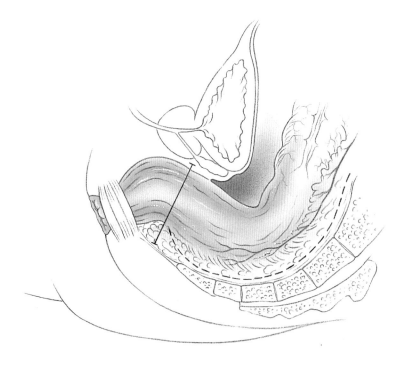

At the same time care is taken to avoid damage to the erigent nerves responsible for ejaculatory and bladder function. The Heald-type mesorectal dissection means that the tumour-bearing rectum is excised with a wide lateral margin of tissue and a non-disrupted mesorectal fat pad. Backed up by fastidious postoperative pathological dissection of the specimens as performed by the Leeds pathologist, Quirke, it would appear that this circumferential clearance of the tumour is as important as the distal clearance of the tumour, if not more so, particularly in relation to the incidence of local recurrence [13].

5 *Anterior restorative resection of the rectum vs abdominoperineal excision of the rectum.* Until the work of Williams *et al.* [3], it was generally accepted that in a rectal excision for cancer of the rectum it was preferable to have a distal clearance of the lower tumour margin of 5 cm. Clearly this meant that any tumour lying in the lower middle third or lower third of the rectum would, by definition, require an abdominoperineal excision of the rectum to provide adequate clearance. It is now, however, generally accepted that a 2 cm distal clearance of the tumour is adequate. Heald has even intimated that a distal clearance of even less than this may be adequate if accompanied by a full mesorectal dissection. Several series are available comparing anterior resection and abdominoperineal resection indicating that the supposed wider clearance of an abdominoperineal excision does not confer a reduced local recurrence rate or better prognostic figures provided the distal clearance recommended above is achieved [14,15].

Having decided on the extent of resection necessary the surgeon carries out the dissection strictly adhering to basic surgical principles in terms of isolation and gentle handling of the tumour to avoid spillage and spread, avoidance of disruption of tumour planes and dissection along the anatomical planes of the abdomen to minimize tissue trauma and blood loss.

Once the tumour has been adequately mobilized and excised the next consideration is that of optimal anastomotic technique. The requirements for a successful colon and rectal anastomosis are no different from those of an anastomosis in any other part of the body. They are:

1 that a good blood supply to the two ends of the bowel should exist;
2 that accurate apposition of the ends of the bowel should be achieved;
3 that tension-free apposition of the bowel ends should be present;
4 that faecal contamination of the anastomosis should be as little as possible.

There are several aspects of the above criteria which require special emphasis in relation to the technique of colon and rectal anastomosis. It is well recognized that the blood supply of the colon and rectum is more precarious than that of other parts of the gastrointestinal tract. It is essential, therefore, either that the cut ends of the large bowel prepared for the anastomosis should be seen to show free pulsatile arterial bleeding or that the small arteries immediately adjacent to the proposed anastomotic level on the mesenteric border of the colon should be shown to be pulsating. The lumena of the bowel prepared for the anastomosis should be as wide as possible in order to minimize the likelihood of stenosis, and the anastomosis itself, especially if handsewn, is much more satisfactory if the width of the two lumena are equal. Achievement of this may, on occasion, involve a cut-back technique such as the Cheetle split.

In both the animal and the human situation [16] there is evidence to suggest that an inverting type of anastomosis has a significantly lower leak rate in colonic anastomoses. Provided that the anastomotic technique is fastidious, accurate and carried out under the optimal conditions described above there is no evidence that a two-layer inverting, one-layer inverting, one-layer extramucosal or stapled anastomosis is advantageous provided that it is properly carried out. Having said this, it would be foolish to disregard the practical advantages of the stapling instruments, particularly the use of the circular stapling devices for low anterior resection. Whether using a double purse-string technique (Fig. 4.10) or a double stapling technique with transverse stapling of the rectal stump (Fig. 4.11), the vast majority of colon and rectal surgeons would testify to their advantages both in terms of ease of anastomotic performance and in terms of the height of anastomosis (the distance from the anal verge) safely achievable.

Once the anastomosis has been satisfactorily performed and where possible tested, for example by insufflation of air or Betadine solution into the rectum of a low anterior resection (Fig. 4.12), a decision must be made as to whether or not a covering stoma is required. This has particular application to the low anteior resection. Many surgeons would consider that any anastomosis formed in the lower third of the rectum, i.e. between 0 and 6 cm, should be covered by either a right upper quadrant loop colostomy or a right lower quadrant loop ileostomy. Although it is generally accepted that the performance of a covering stoma will not *per se* reduce the incidence of anastomotic leaks, there is every indication that faecal diversion will reduce the morbidity and mortality associated with these leaks. It is essential that not only the temporary stoma but also the permanent stoma, say accompanying an abdominoperineal excision, should be sited in the optimal position for postoperative patient management. This position should have been decided preoperatively by discussion between the patient and either the operating surgeon or the stoma nurse.

In addition to the defunctioning stoma, certain other protective mechanisms may be employed where appropriate. It is common practice to irrigate the rectal

Figure 4.10
Restorative anterior resection of the rectum: double purse-string technique.

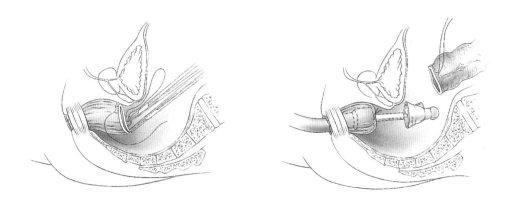

Figure 4.11
Restorative anterior resection of the rectum: double stapled technique.

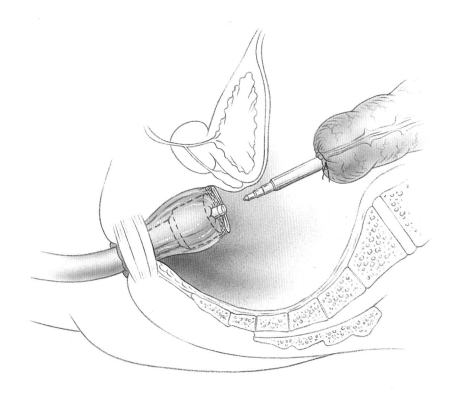

stump during a restorative resection to destroy any exfoliated cells and thereby hope to reduce the likelihood of implantation. Mustine hydrochloride was Goligher's choice of irrigant but 1% cetrimide solution is probably equally effective. Anastomotic drainage is often routinely performed for an extraperitoneal anastomosis (i.e. a rectal anastomosis) or for an intraperitoneal colocolic or small bowel to colon anastomosis where there has been contamination with either pus or faeces, or where a collection of blood is anticipated. As far as this author is concerned the place of drainage in the conventional colon and rectal anastomosis, be it either to drain or not to drain (and if to drain, the type of drain employed), remains unanswered in the literature. Similarly, the employment of cytocidal agents in the cleaning of the bowel ends to be anastomosed or in peritoneal washouts remains unanswered and is largely a question of individual surgeon preference.

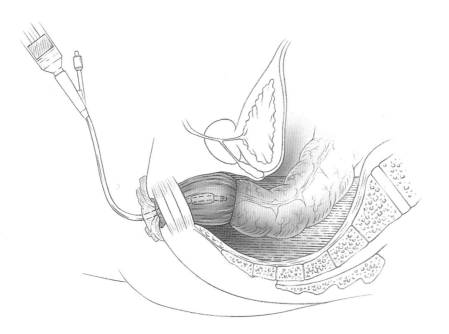

Figure 4.12
Restorative anterior resection of the rectum: testing the anastomosis.

Once the intraoperative part of the conventional colon and rectal anastomosis has been completed the patient must then be subjected to optimal postoperative monitoring and treatment. Preferably this should initially be carried out in either an intensive care unit or a high dependency unit with continuous measurement of urine output, central venous pressure and, in specific cases, arterial pressure and blood gas monitoring. In addition, care must be taken that the appropriate prophylactic antibacterial and antithrombotic measures are provided in addition to the more specific needs of the patient with respiratory, cardiac or diabetic problems.

Finally, the conventional colon and rectal resection cannot be complete without due consideration of the necessity for adjuvant therapy, be this in the form of radiotherapy or chemotherapy. Clearly the necessity for this will be defined not only by the intraoperative findings but also by accurate and comprehensive pathological examination of the tumour by an interested pathologist.

Patient requirements

The patient requirements for a successful colon and rectal resection may be summarized as 'maximal chance of cure with minimal morbidity and mortality' — exactly the same as the surgeon's requirements but perhaps expressed in a different manner and with different emphasis (Table 4.2).

It is essential, therefore, that the operating surgeon should be cognizant of each individual patient's expectations of the operation and that the operation should be tailored to fulfil as many of these expectations as possible, bearing in the mind that to the patient the quality of life is often paramount.

Finally, no chapter describing conventional colon and rectal cancer resection would be complete without mention of the word audit. Without all surgeons disciplining themselves to record details of their operations and to provide honest

Table 4.2
Patient requirements.

1 A safe operation
2 A curative operation
3 As few complications as possible
4 As little pain as feasible
5 As short a hospital stay as appropriate
6 The ability to resume normal life and work as quickly as possible with minimal disruption or permanent alteration to quality of life

and accurate follow-up data of complications, local recurrence and survival, the questions inevitably posed by this book will never be adequately answered.

References

1 Penfold JCB. A comparison of restorative resection of carcinoma of the middle third of the rectum with abdomino-perineal excision. *Aust N Z J Surg* 1974; **44**(4): 354–6.
2 Grinnell RS. Distal intramural spread of carcinoma of rectum and rectosigmoid. *Surg Gynecol Obstet* 1954; **99**: 421–30.
3 Williams NS, Dixon MF, Johnston D. Reappraisal of the 5 centimetre rule of distal excision for carcinoma of the rectum: a study of distal intramural spread and of patients' survival. *Br J Surg* 1983; **70**(3): 150–4.
4 Quirke P, Durdey P, Dixon MF, Williams NS. Local recurrence of rectal adenocarcinoma due to inadequate surgical resection. Histopathological study of lateral tumour spread and surgical excision. *Lancet* 1986; **2**: 996–9.
5 Heald RJ, Ryall RD. Recurrence and survival after total mesorectal excision for rectal cancer. *Lancet* 1986; **1**: 1479–82.
6 Gall F, Tonak J, Altendorf A. Multivisceral resections in colorectal cancer. *Dis Colon Rectum* 1987; **30**: 337–41.
7 Shepherd NA. The pathological staging of colorectal cancer. *Surgery (Oxf)* 1991; **88**: 2115a–d.
8 Turnbull RB Jr, Kyle K, Watson FR, Spratt J. Cancer of the colon: the influence of the no-touch isolation technic on survival rates. *Ann Surg* 1967; **166**(3): 420–7.
9 Cole WH, Packard D, Southwick HW. Carcinoma of colon with special reference to prevention of recurrence. *JAMA* 1954; **155**: 1549–53.
10 Pezim ME, Nicholls RJ. Survival after high or low ligation of the inferior mesenteric artery during curative surgery for rectal cancer. *Ann Surg* 1984; **200**(6): 729–33.
11 Hojo K, Sawada T, Moriya Y. An analysis of survival, voiding and sexual function after wide iliopelvic lymphadenectomy in patients with carcinoma of the rectum, compared with conventional lymphadenectomy. *Dis Colon Rectum* 1989; **32**(2): 128–33.
12 Heald RJ. Anterior resection of the rectum. *Surgery (Oxf)* 1990; **83**: 1991–2.
13 Adam IJ, Mohamdee MO, Martin IG *et al.* Role of circumferential margin involvement in the local recurrence of rectal cancer. *Lancet* 1994; **344**: 707–11.
14 Nicholls RJ, Ritchie JK, Wadsworth J, Parks AG. Total excision or restorative resection for carcinoma of the middle third of the rectum. *Br J Surg* 1979; **66**(9): 625–7.
15 Williams NS, Johnston D. Survival and recurrence after sphincter saving resection and abdomino-perineal resection for carcinoma of the middle third of the rectum. *Br J Surg* 1984; **71**(4): 278–82.
16 Goligher JC, Morris C, McAdam WA, DeDombal FT, Johnston D. A controlled trial of inverting versus everting intestinal suture in clinical large bowel surgery. *Br J Surg* 1970; **57**(11): 817–22.

Chapter 5

Laparoscopic abdominoperineal resection

J.E. Hartley, A. Darzi and J.R.T. Monson

Introduction

Continual improvements in laparoscopic instrumentation, and the increasing skill and enterprise of surgeons trained in laparoscopy, ensure that no area of the colon or rectum is exempt from the laparoscopic approach to resection. However, as evident elsewhere in this volume, most such operations are best termed 'laparoscopically assisted', since an abdominal incision, albeit reduced in size, is usually required. Laparoscopic abdominoperineal excision of the rectum, first described in 1992 [1], provides one of the few examples of a 'truly laparoscopic' procedure in current colorectal practice, since the necessity for an abdominal incision is avoided. The operation remains in the preliminary stages of evaluation and to date only 37 procedures have been reported in the world literature [2–9]. Much of what follows is therefore necessarily anecdotal but reflects the authors' personal experience with this procedure as well as the published experience of others. After some initial comments on case selection and preoperative considerations, this chapter will concentrate on the operative details, before discussing some of the results achieved to date.

Case selection and preoperative preparation

The introduction of operative techniques whose aim is to conserve the anal sphincter mechanism have led to a re-appraisal of the indications for excision of the rectum. Stapling devices have revolutionized the practice of rectal surgery and facilitate safe intrapelvic anastomoses, whilst intersphincteric colorectal anastomosis preserves the anal sphincter. In addition, early carcinomas of the rectum can be curatively treated by disc excision, using transanal microsurgical techniques, thereby preserving the rectum [10]. The latter procedure has yet to be embraced by the coloproctological community as a whole; however, these two major advances mean that the proportion of rectal cancers currently treated by abdominoperineal excision lies somewhere between 10 and 20% [11].

In principle the indications for laparoscopic abdominoperineal resection should be identical to those for conventional open procedures. The resection of low rectal cancers (a maximum of 4–5 cm from the dentate line) therefore provides the principal indication for this technique. The most important preoperative consideration is, in our view, the decision as to whether or not to submit the patient to a laparoscopic abdominoperineal resection or anterior resection. During conventional surgery the final decision may be made at operation with the additional benefit of a trial pelvic dissection, and it is commonplace to counsel the patient appropriately. There is no such facility during the laparoscopic approach where, if the above strict selection criteria are applied, the abdominal surgeon is unlikely to visualize the tumour. The surgeon must therefore be absolutely certain as to the intended resection prior to surgery. In our practice no patient is submitted to anaesthesia with a view to laparoscopic abdominoperineal excision without unequivocal histology and, in the majority of cases, a proper assessment of the tumour under general anaesthesia. Preoperative counselling by the stoma therapist is, of course, mandatory in all patients consenting to abdominoperineal resection and the patient's notes must be marked accordingly. The patient must also be aware of the possibility of conversion to an open procedure and must have given consent for this eventuality.

There are as yet no conclusive data available regarding the morbidity or mortality rates associated with the laparoscopic approach. However, knowledge of the potential hazards of laparoscopic surgery leads us to make some general recommendations regarding case selection. Firstly, a protracted pneumoperitoneum, with its attendant cardiovascular and respiratory effects, is required. We would therefore advocate avoidance of the laparoscopic approach in those with significant cardiorespiratory compromise. In such patients the decrease in venous return consequent upon the pneumoperitoneum may lead to a significant reduction in cardiac output [12]. In addition, with a prolonged pneumoperitoneum significant absorption of carbon dioxide (CO_2) occurs. This can normally be dealt with by appropriate increases in the respiratory minute volume, guided by end-tidal CO_2 measurements [13]. Where the patient's pulmonary reserve is limited such compensation may not be possible. Under these circumstances accumulation of CO_2 may lead to the development of a respiratory acidosis which may in turn provoke cardiac arrhythmias [12]. We therefore perform a baseline arterial blood gas estimation in those patients with a significant respiratory history.

Secondly, the technical problems associated with laparoscopy in the grossly obese or those with previous lower abdominal surgery justifiably influence both preoperative and intraoperative decision making. Neither of these factors, in our practice, constitutes an absolute contraindication to the laparoscopic approach. However, those inexperienced in this field would do well to avoid abdominoperineal resection in such patients since the pelvic dissection in particular is likely to prove technically demanding.

Finally, although locally advanced disease with invasion of the contiguous pelvic structures does not preclude laparoscopic surgery, it is likely to render it a difficult and perhaps hazardous venture. The oncological safety of the laparoscopic approach in such circumstances is, as discussed elsewhere in this volume, also far from clear. Attempts at preoperative staging are therefore appropriate. The choice of imaging modalities depends to a large extent on the facilities available but includes pelvic computed tomography [14], magnetic resonance imaging [15] and endoanal ultrasonography [16]. In addition, synchronous lesions, especially in the absence of serosal involvement, may be overlooked at laparoscopy. It is our practice, therefore, to undertake preoperative contrast examination of the entire colon in order to exclude the presence of additional primary tumours.

Most of the preoperative preparation of patients who are to undergo laparoscopic colorectal surgery is thereafter identical to that undertaken for patients subjected to open surgery. There is some suggestion that the laparoscopic approach may be associated with an excess of thromboembolic complications, presumably as a result of venous stasis, again due to the prolonged pneumoperitoneum. Our thromboembolic prophylaxis, comprising subcutaneous heparin and graduated compression stockings, is commenced on admission and continued postoperatively until the patient is fully mobile. We administer standard regimens of bowel preparation and antibiotic prophylaxis identical to those which we would use for conventional surgery.

Equipment and instrumentation

Full video laparoscopy facilities are required including two video monitors. For the majority of the procedure a 10 mm 0° telescope is adequate. However, in selected patients a 10 mm 30° telescope may facilitate the pelvic dissection.

There can be no absolute guidelines for the number and size of laparoscopy trocars required for success in this procedure. We have found four 10 mm ports (in the configuration shown in Fig. 5.1) to be sufficient in the majority of cases. These are then replaced by larger ports to permit the use of instruments such as the Endo-GIA linear stapling devices (United States Surgical Corporation, Norwalk, CT, USA) as required. A 12 mm port will admit an Endo-GIA 30, whilst a 15 mm port is required for the Endo-GIA 60.

The current enthusiasm for the colorectal applications of laparoscopy ensures that the range of instrumentation is wide and undergoing constant expansion and upgrading. Those essential for abdominoperineal resection are as follows:

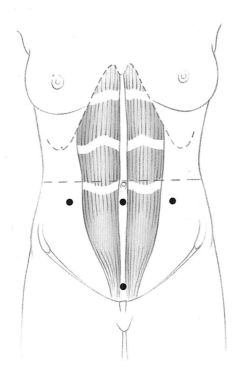

Figure 5.1
Port sites for abdominoperineal resection.

1 two Babcock-type bowel-grasping instruments;
2 curved disposable scissors and hooked endoscopic scissors, which have the advantage of holding tissues away from potentially important structures before cutting with diathermy;
3 DeBakey-type dissecting forceps;
4 one linear stapling device (Endo-GIA 30 or 60) with additional cartridges;
5 one multifire endoscopic clip applicator;
6 long laparoscopy scissors for use in pelvic dissection;
7 one suction device.

An endoscopic gauge is optional and allows the bowel wall thickness to be measured prior to selection of the appropriate-sized stapling device.

A new generation of articulating and steerable instruments are now available and seem likely to facilitate many aspects of laparoscopic surgery. In addition, flexible telescopes will probably become available in the near future and will greatly improve the visualization of all areas of the peritoneal cavity.

Positioning the patient and arranging the operating theatre

In positioning the patient adequate exposure of both the perineum and the abdomen is vital. We place the patient in a modified lithotomy position in which the legs are kept almost straight (Fig. 5.2), the rationale being that when the hips are held in flexion the patient's legs tend to intrude upon the movements of the long-handled laparoscopy instruments. A nasogastric tube and urinary catheter are inserted and these reduce the risk of a Veress needle or trocar injury to the

Figure 5.2
Patient positioning for abdominoperineal resection.

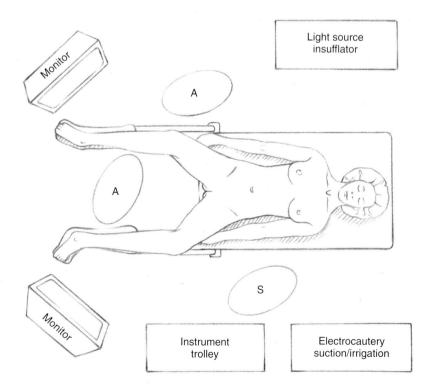

viscera. As will be seen, much of the exposure and retraction during the procedure is achieved by altering the inclination and tilt of the table thus allowing gravity to displace the small bowel from the operating field. The operating table must therefore be of the type capable of being lowered into steep Trendelenburg or reverse Trendelenburg positions, as well as being capable of being rotated to the left or right. We place the patient on a bean bag which helps prevent the patient from sliding off the table in these positions.

We use two video monitors. These are most easily viewed during the pelvic dissection if placed on either side of the patient's knees (Fig. 5.2)

Laparoscopic abdominoperineal resection

The abdominal stage

This is best considered as a sequence of logical steps. Under general anaesthesia the abdomen and perineum is prepared and draped and the anus is closed with a stout purse-string suture, our preference being number 1 silk. Carbon dioxide pneumoperitoneum to a pressure of 15 mmHg is then achieved using either a closed or open technique [17] as described elsewhere. A 10 mm trocar is then inserted whereupon the 10 mm telescope is introduced and the absence of Veress needle or trocar injury to the viscera quickly confirmed. Visceral injury can only be consistently avoided if all subsequent trocars are inserted under direct vision. The site and dimensions of these further trocars will vary slightly from case to case. The configuration which we most commonly utilize is shown above (see Fig. 5.1). The suprapubic port is ideally situated to permit elevation of the rectosigmoid as the dissection proceeds, as outlined below. At the appropriate stage of the procedure one of the ports is replaced by a 12 or 15 mm port through which the Endo-GIA will be used.

Preliminary laparoscopy is now performed paying attention first to the pelvic organs. There is a critical angle of Trendelenburg, varying from patient to patient, beyond which the small bowel will fall out of the pelvis. Any adhesions between the small bowel and pelvic structures will prevent this occurring and must therefore be divided at an early stage in the procedure. The table is then returned to a neutral position and the remainder of the peritoneal cavity examined. In particular the liver must be carefully examined for the presence of metastases. The upper surface of this organ is most readily scrutinized with the patient in a few degrees of reverse Trendelenburg. Alternatively, a 30° telescope may prove useful. A range of ultrasound transducers capable of being used through a 10 mm port are now available and can aid in the detection of parenchymal liver lesions [18–20]. We routinely perform laparoscopic ultrasound examination of the liver before commencing the procedure proper (Fig. 5.3).

Elevation and retraction of the sigmoid and mobilization of the rectum are facilitated by early ligation and division of the inferior mesenteric pedicle, a manoeuvre which also helps reduce blood loss during the subsequent pelvic dissection. Since we perform this operation, almost without exception, for malignancy it is our practice to identify and skeletonize these vessels near their origin. Laparoscopic ultrasound may assist in the identification of mesenteric vessels in the obese (Fig. 5.4). One of the lower quadrant ports is then replaced with a 12 mm port and the artery and vein are separately ligated and divided. The Endo-GIA 30 stapling device, with a vascular cartridge, is emminently suited to

Figure 5.3
Laparoscopic ultrasound examination of the liver.

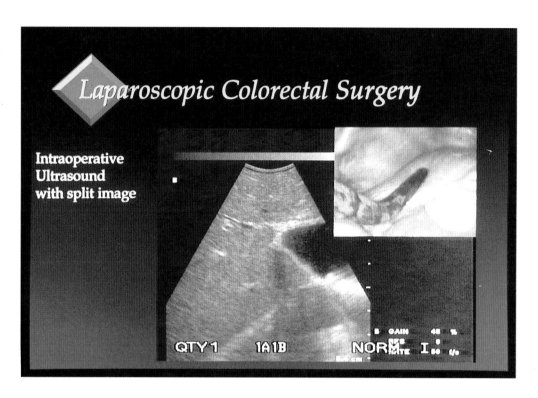

Figure 5.4
Identification of vessels using laparoscopic ultrasound.

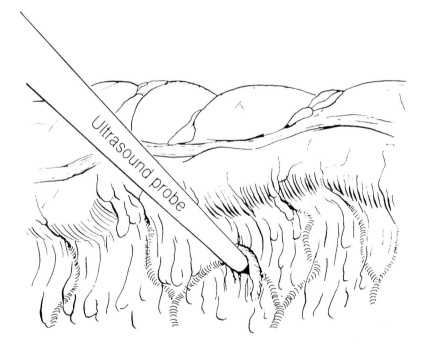

this role and places six rows of staples, three on each side of the incision (Figs 5.5 and 5.6).

The sigmoid mobilization is now commenced. This is most readily performed with the patient in the steep Trendelenburg position and rolled to the left, i.e. with the left shoulder uppermost. The surgeon stands on the right side of the table with the assistant opposite. The apex of the sigmoid loop and the

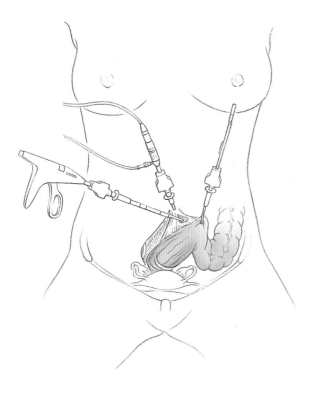

Figure 5.5
Inferior mesenteric artery flush ligation using the Endo-GIA (United States Surgical Corporation).

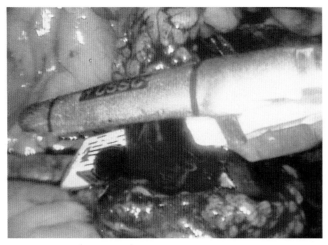
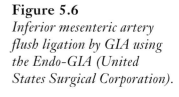
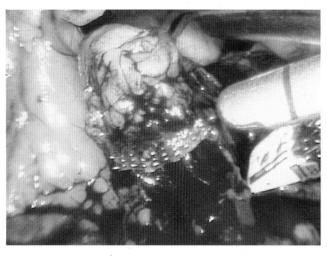

Figure 5.6
Inferior mesenteric artery flush ligation by GIA using the Endo-GIA (United States Surgical Corporation).

rectosigmoid are held with Babcocks by the assistant, and the surgeon, whilst applying countertraction with some form of grasping instrument, incises the lateral peritoneal reflection of the sigmoid along the white line of Toldt using electrocautery scissors (Fig. 5.7). As this manoeuvre progresses the mesosigmoid is pushed gently towards the midline. This lateral incision is continued over the pelvic brim and along the left pelvic side wall to the midline, in either the rectovesical or rectovaginal pouch, all the while pushing the mesorectum medially.

Identification of the left ureter at an early stage in this procedure is of paramount importance if iatrogenic injury is to be avoided. In thin patients it may be readily visible through the transparent posterior parietal peritoneum. However, most often it must be deliberately sought, either at the point where it crosses the common iliac vessels or in the retroperitoneum after the left colon has been mobilized medially. Luminous ureteric stents can be placed preoperatively and may assist in the identification of this structure [21]. In our experience these illuminate the ureter beautifully at all points except those at which it is likely to be divided! Identification of the ureter in difficult circumstances may prove to be within the remit of laparoscopic ultrasonography.

Mobilization of the rectum is continued by carrying the above dissection into the avascular areolar tissue of the presacral plane, the so-called 'holy plane' of rectal surgery [22]. Still with the patient in a steep Trendelenburg position, the patient's right shoulder is now rolled upwards and the surgeon stands on the left side of the table. The critical angle of Trendelenburg is of vital importance in keeping the small bowel out of the operating field during this phase of the

Figure 5.7
Laparoscopic mobilization of the sigmoid and left colon.

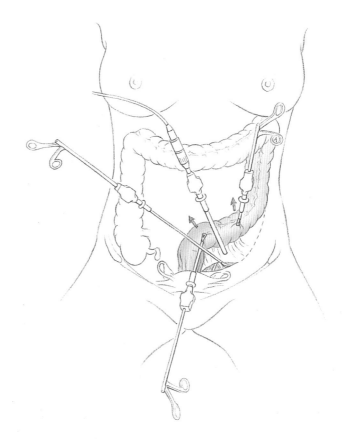

procedure. The assistant standing opposite the surgeon grasps and elevates the sigmoid and proximal rectum with Babcocks (Fig. 5.8). Alternatively the sigmoid apex can be slung or sutured from the abdominal wall, or in the female the uterus or fallopian tubes can be stapled temporarily to the anterior abdominal wall to achieve the same effect (Fig. 5.9). The surgeon applies countertraction to the retroperitoneum and incises the parietal peritoneum over the sacral promontory, thus entering the presacral areolar tissue (Fig. 5.10). The plane is developed in this way down into the pelvis, incising the peritoneum along the right pelvic side wall until the midline is reached in the rectovesical or rectovaginal pouch. The right ureter must be identified and preserved. During this phase of the procedure the laparoscope is often best used via a right-sided port since the mobilized rectum lifted out of the pelvis tends to obscure the view from the subumbilical port. The right-sided plane of dissection is finally connected to that on the left through the presacral space avoiding the left ureter.

Having connected the peritoneal incisions from the left and right sides of the pelvis, the surgeon retracts the rectum towards the sacrum by grasping the cut edge of the peritoneum with a Babcock (Fig. 5.11). If necessary a finger in the rectum or a rigid proctoscope may be used to assist in this. In males, we make use of an additional suprapubic port to retract the posterior wall of the bladder and the vasa efferentia anteriorly using an Endo-Retract. The fascia of Denonvilliers is then incised and, after this plane is opened, the dissection is completed by the perineal operator. In females, a finger in the vagina can be used to provide anterior retraction. Alternatively the uterus and adnexa can be suspended from the abdominal wall by clips, or the uterus alone may be suspended from the

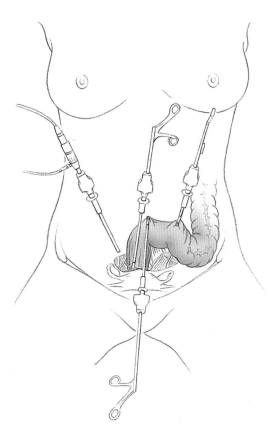

Figure 5.8
Elevation of the sigmoid and proximal rectum with Babcocks.

Figure 5.9
The sigmoid slung by a suture from the abdominal wall.

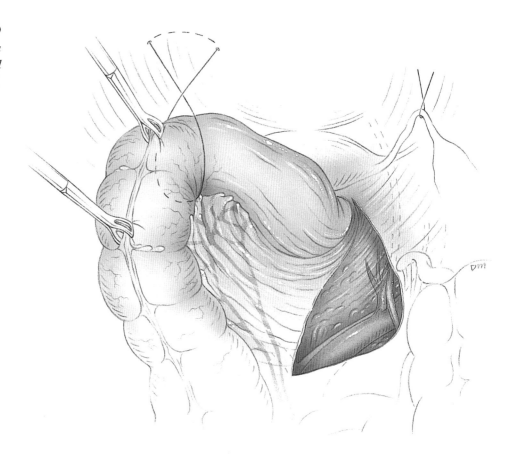

Figure 5.10
Laparoscopic dissection of the presacral plane.

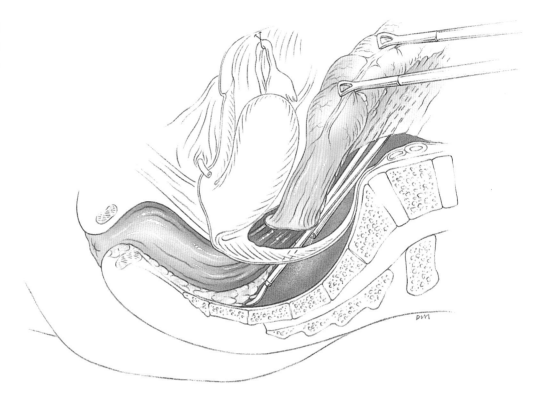

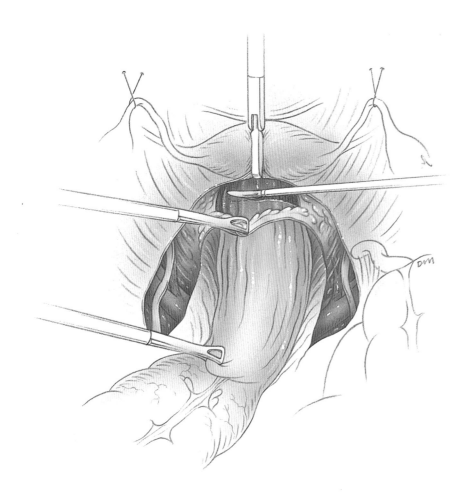

Figure 5.11
Anterior rectal dissection.

abdominal wall by a suture. Again, the perineal surgeon is best able to complete the anterior dissection in the female.

The assistant retracts the rectum out of the pelvis and laterally with two Babcocks from the opposite side of the table to the surgeon. The lateral ligaments are then divided by electrocautery under direct vision. The dissection now proceeds easily down to the level of the middle rectum and, provided meticulous attention is paid to haemostasis throughout, this rectal dissection can be carried all the way down to the level of the levators under direct vision. The perineal operator is then well positioned to complete the dissection from below.

Having completed the above mobilization the proximal colon must be transected before the perineal dissection is commenced, as it would be impossible to safely complete this without an adequate pneumoperitoneum. The colon is elevated and held with Babcocks proximal and distal to the chosen point of transection. It is not necessary to fashion a mesenteric window. The thickness of the colon is measured using an Endo-Gauge and the correct-sized cartridge is selected. The stapling device is applied across the bowel and then fired (Fig. 5.12). Finally, the staple lines are checked for haemostasis. The mesosigmoid is then divided with the Endo-GIA stapling device or electrocautery scissors and clips. The former method is speedy though expensive whilst the latter involves isolating, clipping and cutting individual vessels and can be time consuming particularly in the obese patient.

Figure 5.12
Transection of the proximal colon.

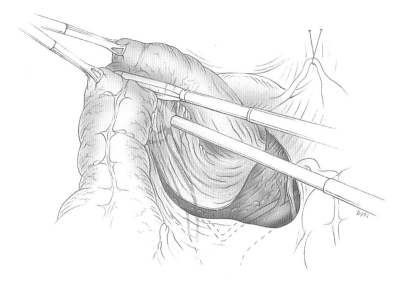

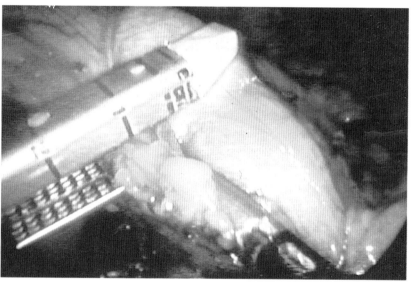

The perineal stage

The approach to this phase of the operation is identical to that required for the conventional open approach and is shown in Fig. 5.13; however, the extent of pelvic dissection that remains to be completed from below will depend upon the laparoscopic experience of the abdominal surgeon and the technical difficulty of the case.

A circumferential skin incision is made around the anus, grasping the edges of the perianal skin with Kocher's clamps. The incision is then continued through the subcutaneous fat into the ischiorectal fossa, ligating and dividing the inferior haemorrhoidal vessels, and exposing the anococcygeal ligament, which is divided. A finger is then passed into the presacral space. As this finger is swept along the superior border of the levators the mesorectum is freed and the levators are pulled down and divided.

The superficial transverse perineal muscle is next divided (Fig. 5.14) freeing the anterior aspect of the rectum at the posterior border of the deep transverse

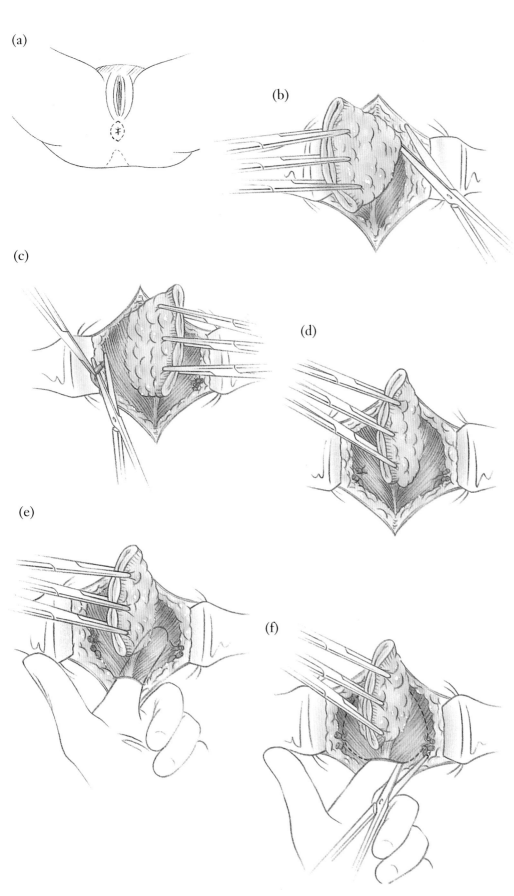

(a)

(b)

(c)

(d)

(e)

(f)

Figure 5.13
Perineal phase (1).
(Reproduced with permission
from United States Surgical
Corporation, Connecticut)

Figure 5.14
*Perineal phase (2).
(Reproduced with permission
from United States Surgical
Corporation, Connecticut)*

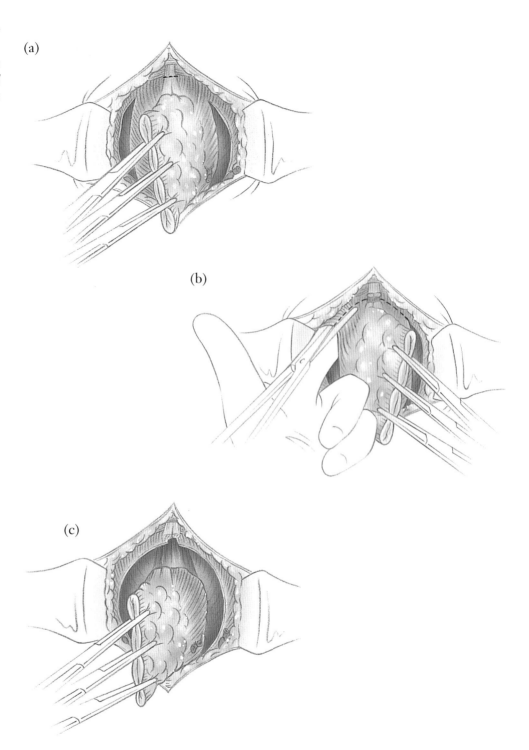

(a)

(b)

(c)

perineal muscle. After dividing the recto-urethralis and puborectalis the perineal surgeon is able to place his or her hand palm upwards behind the rectum into the presacral space. If Waldeyer's fascia was not breached during the laparoscopic phase of the operation it is now tented up by the fingers of the perineal surgeon and divided by the laparoscopist (Fig. 5.15). The bulk of the perineal surgeon's hand provides an almost air-tight seal, which maintains the pneumoperitoneum for some moments, allowing the pelvic dissection to be completed by a

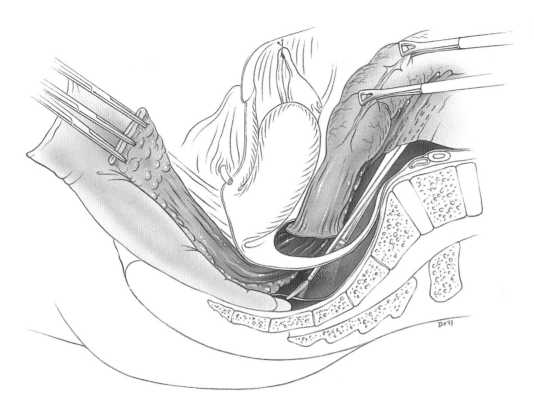

Figure 5.15
Opening Waldeyer's fascia.

combination of sharp laparoscopic dissection and blunt dissection from below. The laparoscopic surgeon must be aware of the position of the ureters at all times since these may be pulled, by traction on the rectum, deep into the pelvis where they are at risk of injury by the perineal surgeon.

With strong traction on the rectum and mesorectum from the perineal surgeon any remaining component of the lateral ligaments is now divided by the laparoscopic surgeon and the middle haemorrhoidal vessels are dealt with.

The final stages of the anterior dissection are now completed by the perineal operator since this is difficult to achieve laparoscopically. First the peritoneal reflection in the rectovesical pouch or the rectovaginal pouch and ideally the fascia of Denonvilliers should be incised by the laparoscopic surgeon. Having divided the lateral ligaments the perineal operator's hand is now easily swept around the front of the rectum completing this blunt dissection. Finally, the staple line on the proximal end of the specimen is grasped by the laparoscopic operator and placed in the hand of the perineal surgeon, who then withdraws his or her hand from the pelvis along the sacrum in order to deliver the specimen. The remaining attachments of the specimen to the posterior vaginal wall, or to the prostate in men, are divided and the specimen delivered. The pneumoperitoneum is rapidly lost during specimen extraction.

Closure

The pelvis is thoroughly irrigated through the perineal wound with warm saline. A close inspection must be made to ensure adequate haemostasis, if necessary restoring the table to a neutral position. We drain the pelvis with two closed non-suction drains, brought out through the abdominal wall. Alternatively, these may be inserted through the levators and brought out through stab wounds in the perineal skin (anterior to a line between the ischial tuberosities in order to avoid damaging the sciatic nerve).

The levators and subcutaneous tissues are apposed with a stout absorbable suture, and the skin is closed by the individual's preferred method. The fascial sheath must be carefully closed at all trocar sites to guard against the troublesome complication of port site herniation. We close the skin at these sites with tissue adhesive or an absorbable subcuticular suture.

Constructing the colostomy

Before the bowel is transected, and with a full pneumoperitoneum, the mobilized colon is grasped with a Babcock and brought up to the abdominal wall (Fig. 5.16). Provided this is easily achieved the colon can be divided safely in the knowledge that a tension-free end colostomy can be constructed once the abdomen has been deflated. After transection of the bowel it is our practice to leave a Babcock attached to the blind stapled proximal end. This can then be brought out to a left iliac fossa port site at the end of the procedure. The port site is first enlarged by excising a disc of skin and subcutaneous fat down to the rectus sheath, which is also enlarged. After the perineal and abdominal wounds are closed and dressed the staple line is opened and the colostomy sutured in the standard manner (Fig. 5.17).

Figure 5.16
Bowel mobilized prior to colostomy formation.

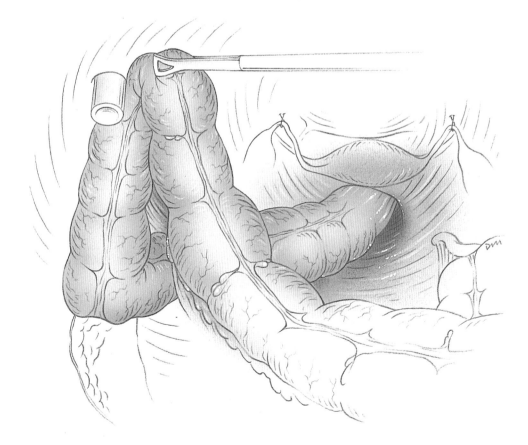

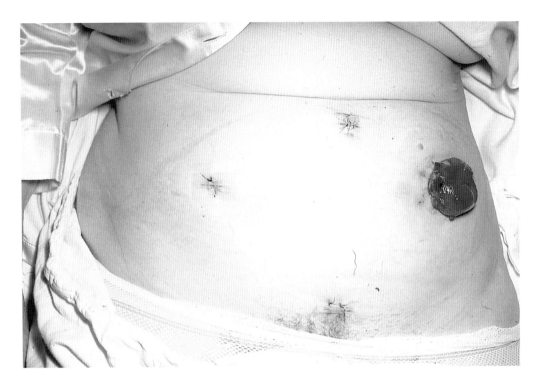

Figure 5.17
End colostomy following laparoscopic abdominoperineal resection.

Postoperative care

The postoperative management of patients who have undergone laparoscopic abdominoperineal resection is, in essence, identical to that of patients who have been subjected to open colorectal surgery. Thus antibiotic prophylaxis is administered. The nasogastric tube is removed on the first postoperative day and oral fluids are commenced at the first sign of resolution of the ileus. The intravenous cannulae are removed as soon as this oral intake is adequate and a light diet is then instituted.

Chest physiotherapy should be routine and the patient is mobilized as soon as possible. Thromboembolic prophylaxis must be continued until the patient is fully mobile. The patient is discharged when he or she is tolerating a normal diet and managing the colostomy; in our experience this is usually the case at about 10 or 11 days after surgery.

Results

We have, to date, successfully performed laparoscopic abdominoperineal resection for malignancy in 14 patients [23,24]. All procedures were performed with the intention of cure and all patients underwent preliminary examination under anaesthesia to confirm the necessity for abdominoperineal excision. Our assessment of the morbidity and mortality rates consequent upon the laparoscopic approach was made by comparison with the last 16 patients to undergo conventional abdominoperineal resection under our care. The results of this analysis are presented in Tables 5.1 and 5.2.

The operating time required for laparoscopic abdominoperineal resection has been invariably longer than for the conventional approach. However, the laparoscopic approach has resulted in a reduction in the length of postoperative

Table 5.1

Comparison of the operating time, duration of ileus and hospital stay for laparoscopic and conventional abdominoperineal resection (APR).

	Laparoscopic APR	Open APR
No. of patients	14	16
Mean age (range)	63.2 (31–91)	67 (48–93)
Male:female	5:9	5:11
Mean operation time (min)	194	104
Mean time for flatus (days)	3.2 (0–6)	5.9 (2–11)
Median postoperative stay (days) (range)	11.2 (5–50)	17.5

Table 5.2

Postoperative complications after laparoscopic and conventional abdominoperineal resection (APR).

	No. of patients	
	Laparoscopic APR	Open APR
Obstruction	1	3
Urinary retention	2	0
Urinary infection	0	1
Urethral injury	1	0
Pulmonary embolus	0	1
Perineal haematoma	2	2
Wound infection	0	2
Death	1	1

ileus as evident by the time to flatus. In addition, reduced postoperative pain and earlier mobility have been striking features to date, resulting in a significant decrease in the length of postoperative hospitalization. We have seen no operative mortality. One patient in each group has required re-operation within 30 days because of mechanical small obstruction. The re-operative findings were in both cases impaction of the small bowel in the pelvis. The recovery of both patients was thereafter unremarkable. In two further cases small bowel obstruction following open resection resolved with conservative management. In one patient haemorrhage within the perineum required re-operation after laparoscopic resection, and in a further patient an incomplete urethral laceration of the urethra, recognized at operation, was managed by an extended period of urinary catherization with good functional result thus far.

Our assessment of the oncological safety of the laparoscopic procedure was made by measurement of the adequacy of tumour excision by laparoscopic and open procedures (see Table 5.3). The Dukes' staging and the Jass score of the resected lesions was similar in both groups and the tumour was not macroscopically fixed in any patient. In all these patients the inferior mesenteric pedicle was taken as close to the aorta as possible. The lymph node yields and radial excision margins achieved using the laparoscopic approach were similar to those obtained by conventional surgical techniques. In addition there were no positive radial excision margins after laparoscopic resection whereas the radial margin was positive in two patients subjected to conventional resection although all margins were macroscopically clear.

	Laparoscopic APR	Open APR
No. of patients	14	16
Mean radial margin (cm) (range)	0.51 (0.1–1.5)	0.9 (0.1–3.6)
Mean no. of lymph nodes (range)	8.1 (6–19)	6.0 (4–14)
Histological margin involvement	0	2

Table 5.3
Assessment of the adequacy of excision of cancer by laparoscopic and conventional abdominoperineal resection (APR).

Conclusion

Cumulative experience to date confirms the technical feasibility of the laparoscopic approach to abdominoperineal excision and this procedure seems certain to play a prominent role in the continuing expansion of laparoscopic colorectal surgery. The operation is particularly attractive for a number of reasons.

Firstly, it provides one of the few examples of a truly laparoscopic procedure, since no significant abdominal incision is required, and therefore ought to provide more reward in terms of reduced morbidity and early postoperative mobility than other laparoscopically assisted procedures. Our experience supports this argument as shorter duration of ileus and earlier discharge from hospital have been striking features. The true rate of complications following laparoscopic abdominoperineal resection is not yet known. However, whilst it seems likely that those complications associated with a major laparotomy wound will be seen to occur less frequently, there seems little reason to expect the incidence of stomal complications and perineal sepsis to be altered.

Secondly, the excision of low rectal cancers during abdominoperineal resection is almost entirely performed by the perineal surgeon, so that the major concern of the uncertain oncological safety of the laparoscopic approach is less of a factor. It is our belief that laparoscopy provides unrivalled views, particularly in the depths of the pelvis, which may allow for a more meticulous dissection under direct vision. Our experience suggests that radical excision of lymph node-bearing tissue is possible using the laparoscopic approach. In addition the radial excision margins achieved laparoscopically have been little different from those achieved at open operation and this is in keeping with the role of the perineal operator. On a more cautionary note, the high proportion of rectal cancer treated by abdominoperineal resection in some laparoscopic series has caused concern [25]. Sphincter preservation must remain one of the primary goals in the treatment of rectal cancer. Inappropriate sphincter removal will only be avoided if the selection criteria outlined above are rigorously applied.

The true efficacy of this new approach to the surgical treatment of low rectal cancer will only be proven by long-term follow-up data. However, there appear to be significant short-term benefits for the patient conferred by this truly minimally invasive procedure. If these are seen to be balanced by oncological safety, as evident by stage-for-stage locoregional recurrence and survival rates, then laparoscopic abdominoperineal resection may be the first of the new wave of laparoscopic colorectal procedures to be wholeheartedly embraced.

References

1 Sackier J, Berci G, Hiatt J, Hartunian S. Laparoscopic abdominoperineal resection of the rectum. *Br J Surg* 1992; **79**: 1207–8.

2 Larach SW, Salomen MC, Williamson PR, Goldstein E. Laparoscopic assisted abdominoperineal resection. *Surg Laparosc Endosc* 1993; **3**: 115–18.

3 Monson J, Darzi A, Carey P, Guillou P. Prospective evaluation of laparoscopic-assisted colectomy in an unselected group of patients. *Lancet* 1992; **340**: 831–3.

4 Nogueras JJ, Wexner SD. Laparoscopic colon resection. *Perspect Colon Rectal Surg* 1992; **5**: 79–97.

5 Jacobs M, Verdeja JC, Goldstein HS. Minimally invasive colon resection (laparoscopic colectomy). *Surg Laparosc Endosc* 1991; **1**: 144–50.

6 Kim LH, Chung KE, AuBuchon P. Laparoscopic-assisted abdominoperineal resection with pull through (sphincter saving). *Surg Laparosc Endosc* 1992; **2**: 237–40.

7 Phillips E, Franklin M, Carroll B, Fallas M, Ramos R, Rosenthal D. Laparoscopic colectomy. *Ann Surg* 1992; **216**: 703–7.

8 Wexner S, Cohen S, Johansen O, Nogueras J, Jagelman D. Laparoscopic colorectal surgery: a prospective assessment and current perspective. *Br J Surg* 1993; **80**: 1602–5.

9 Hoffman G, Baker J, Fitchett C, Vansant J. Laparoscopic-assisted colectomy. Initial experience. *Ann Surg* 1994; **219**: 732–43.

10 Gall FP, Hermanek P. Update of the German experience with local excision of rectal cancer. *Surg Oncol Clin North Am* 1992; **1**: 99–109.

11 Heald RJ, Goligher JC. Anterior resection of the rectum. In: Fielding LP, Goldberg SM (eds) *Rob and Smith's Operative Surgery, Rectum and Anus*. Butterworth-Heinemann, Oxford, 1993: 456–71.

12 Safran DB, Orlando R. Physiologic effects of pneumoperitoneum. *Am J Surg* 1994; **167**: 281–6.

13 McMahon AJ, Baxter JN, Kenny G, O'Dwyer PJ. Ventilatory and blood gas changes during laparoscopic and open cholecystectomy. *Br J Surg* 1993; **80**: 1252–4.

14 Freeny PC, Marks WM, Ryan JA, Bolen JW. Colorectal carcinoma evaluation with CT: preoperative staging and detection of postoperative recurrence. *Radiology* 1986; **158**: 347–53.

15 Balzarini L, Ceglia E, D'lppolito G, Petrillo R, Tess JD, Musuneci R. Local recurrence of rectosigmoid cancer: what about the choice of MRI for diagnosis? *Gastrointest Radiol* 1990; **15**: 338–42.

16 Beynon J, Mortenson NJ McC, Foy DM, Channer JL, Rigby H, Virjee J. The detection and evaluation of locally recurrent rectal cancer with rectal endosonography. *Dis Colon Rectum* 1989; **32**: 509–17.

17 Hasson HM. Open laparoscopy: a report of 150 consecutive cases. *J Reprod Med* 1974; **12**: 234–8.

18 Cuesta MA, Meijer S, Borgstein PJ, Sibinga-Mulder L, Sikkenk AC. Laparoscopic ultrasonography for hepatobiliary and pancreatic malignancy. *Br J Surg* 1993; **80**: 1571–4.

19 Jakimowicz JJ. Review: intraoperative ultrasonography during minimal access surgery. *J R Coll Surg Edinb* 1993; **38**: 231–8.

20 Rothlin M, Largiader F. New mobile-tip ultrasound probe for laparoscopic sonography. *Surg Endosc* 1994; **8**: 805–8.

21 Sackier JM. Visualisation of the ureter during laparoscopic colonic resection. *Br J Surg* 1993; **80**: 1332.

22 MacFarlane J, Ryall R, Heald R. Mesorectal excision for rectal cancer. *Lancet* 1992; **341**: 457–60.

23 Lewis C, Darzi A, Goldin R, Menzies-Gow N, Guillou PJ, Monson JRT. Laparoscopic abdominoperineal resection of the rectum: assessment of adequacy of excision. *Br J Surg* 1993; **80**: S46.

24 Darzi A, Lewis C, Menzies-Gow N, Guillou PJ, Monson JRT. Laparoscopic abdominoperineal excision of the rectum. *Surg Endosc* 1995 (in press).

25 O'Rourke N, Heald R. Laparoscopic surgery for colorectal cancer. *Br J Surg* 1993; **80**: 1229–30.

Chapter 6

Laparoscopic colectomy without pneumoperitoneum

L. Newman III and W.M. Bridges II

Introduction

Laparoscopy is now utilized by surgeons to treat a wide variety of intra-abdominal disorders. The utilization of minimally invasive techniques to perform colorectal surgery has been described by many authors in the United States and other countries. Essentially, all of the laparoscopic colorectal surgery being done at this time involves standard techniques with carbon dioxide (CO_2) insufflation. These techniques are described in detail elsewhere in this text. This chapter describes a different approach to laparoscopic colorectal surgery. Gasless laparoscopic colorectal surgery employs a mechanical lifting device (Laparolift, Origin Medsystems, Menlo Park, CA, USA), which obviates the need for CO_2 and CO_2 pneumoperitoneum and air-tight seals on the laparoscopic ports.

The use of minimally invasive techniques in colorectal surgery is in its infancy. Many surgeons predict that laparoscopically assisted colorectal surgery will be utilized in up to 75% of cases by the year 2000 [1]. Some early results with laparoscopic colectomy have been encouraging [2–4]. Other reports have been less optimistic [5]. Investigators have identified variables such as less postoperative pain, shorter periods in hospital, shortened postoperative ileus, and earlier return to full function as potential benefits of the procedure. The general safety of the procedure is also documented in a number of series [2–4,6].

The very nature of colorectal surgery selects a different patient population than is traditionally seen for gallbladder disease. Ideally the results of laparoscopic colorectal surgery will parallel the results of traditional open colorectal surgery. The oncological safety of laparoscopic colorectal surgery for malignancy has been questioned. It is unclear if the environment created by pneumoperitoneum changes the pattern of local or regional recurrence of carcinoma. Issues such as this mandate further study prior to the widespread acceptance of minimally invasive techniques for colorectal malignancy. Gasless laparoscopic colorectal resection obviates the need for pneumoperitoneum and therefore may provide a safer environment for resectional surgery.

At this time the overwhelming majority of practising surgeons in the United States have been trained in basic laparoscopic techniques. Advanced laparoscopic techniques such as laparoscopic colorectal resection may initially prove more difficult for many surgeons. Gasless laparoscopic surgery has been accepted by a number of investigators as a viable alternative to laparoscopy utilizing pneumoperitoneum [7].

Rationale

The benefits of gasless surgery with pneumoperitoneum include the following.

1 The elimination of problems associated with CO_2 insufflation and maintenance of pneumoperitoneum.
2 A decreased reliance on specialized instrumentation to carry out laparoscopic procedures.

A selected literature review reveals that the creation and maintenance of the pneumoperitoneum environment is responsible for most of the morbidity associated with standard laparoscopic procedures (Table 6.1). Alternatively,

Table 6.1
Laparoscopic literature series.

Reference	Content
Wittgen *et al.* [8]	Haemodynamic and ventilatory effects of pneumoperitoneum during laparoscopic cholecystectomy
Hashimoto *et al.* [9]	Cardiovascular and respiratory changes during pneumoperitoneum
Poulin *et al.* [10]	Evaluation of pulmonary function during laparoscopic cholecystectomy
Liu *et al.* [11]	Prospective analysis of haemodynamics and ventilatory effects of laparoscopic cholecystectomy
Holzman *et al.* [12]	Prospective analysis of hypercarbia during pneumoperitoneum
Root *et al.* [13]	Gas embolism death after laparoscopy with pneumoperitoneum
Dasher *et al.* [14]	Air embolism complicating pneumoperitoneum
Ishak *et al.* [15]	Venous air embolism — a cause for pulmonary oedema
Morrison and Riggs [16]	Cardiovascular collapse in laparoscopy
Ivankovich *et al.* [17]	Cardiovascular collapse in gynaecological laparoscopy
Kelman *et al.* [18]	Cardiac output and arterial blood gas tension during laparoscopy
Newman *et al.* [19]	Laparoscopic herniorrhaphy without pneumoperitoneum
Motew *et al.* [20]	Cardiovascular effects, acid–base and blood gas changes at laparoscopy
Mintz [21]	54 cardiorespiratory accidents and 16 fatalities among 100,000 laparoscopic procedures in France
Baadsgaard *et al.* [22]	Needle insertion pneumoperitoneum as a cause of major vascular laceration
Vilardell [23]	Review of complications in 1455 peritoneoscopy procedures
McQuaide [24]	Air embolism during peritoneoscopy

gasless techniques actually mimic open surgical techniques utilizing much smaller incisions. Several gasless laparoscopic systems are currently in use in the United States, Japan and Europe [25,26]. The authors' experience with gasless laparoscopic surgery has utilized the mechanical lifting arm and disposable laparofans provided by Origin Medsystems.

Complications of pneumoperitoneum

Although laparoscopic surgery utilizing pneumoperitoneum is statistically a safe procedure, morbidity related to insufflation does occur [8,10–12,18,23,27; N. Kathoda, personal communication, 1993]. We described some of the cardiorespiratory changes noted in standard laparoscopic procedures in our first published report of gasless hernia repair [7]. The morbidity associated with pneumoperitoneum includes:

1 subcutaneous and mesenteric emphysema;
2 pneumothorax;
3 shoulder pain;
4 vasovagal reactions;
5 acid–base disturbances;
6 respiratory acidosis with hypercarbia;
7 a decline in the forced expiratory volume and forced vital capacity;
8 a decrease in cardiac output with impairment of venous return;
9 artificial intra-abdominal tamponade;
10 potential for air embolism.

One prevalent objection is that longer procedures, such as colectomy, which utilize CO_2 insufflation create the potential for increasing the risk of CO_2-related morbidity. Morbidity related to CO_2 insufflation is also more prevalent in the aged population. Earlier descriptions of laparoscopic colorectal surgery concluded that advanced techniques would be facilitated with technical modifications and instrument advances. We feel that the gasless technique of colorectal surgery may prove to be a useful alternative to standard laparoscopic techniques by eliminating some of the instrument requirements.

Instrumentation

For our gasless laparoscopic cases we utilize the system devised by Origin Medsystems. The laparolift arm is a reusable mechanical arm that attaches to the side rail of most operating room tables (Fig. 6.1). The laparofan is a disposable device that attaches via a dovetail mechanism on the end of the laparolift arm. The laparofan has variable designs including a 10 cm V-shaped fan, a 15 cm V-shaped fan and quadrant-specific S-shaped and J-shaped fans (Fig. 6.2). The endoscope is generally positioned immediately behind the laparofan after insertion (Fig. 6.3). The draped apparatus is shown in Fig. 6.4 and the planar lifting surface of the quadrant-specific J fan in Fig. 6.5. Mobilization of the lateral peritoneal attachments of the right colon is shown in Fig. 6.6 and visualization of the hepatic flexure during a gasless right hemicolectomy is seen in Fig. 6.7. The extracorporeal anatomosis is completed at the umbilical port (Fig. 6.8). Note that

Figure 6.1
Laparolift fan and arm.

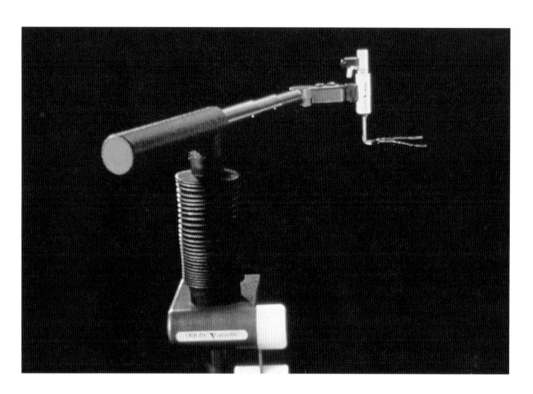

Figure 6.2
'V' shaped fan.

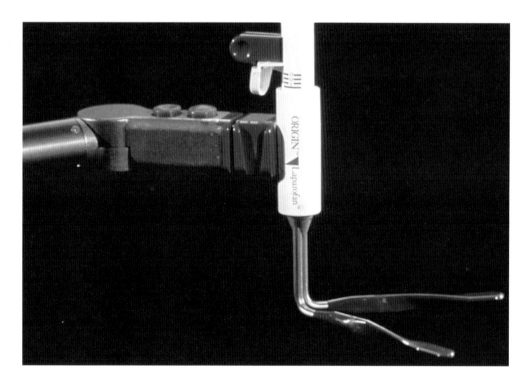

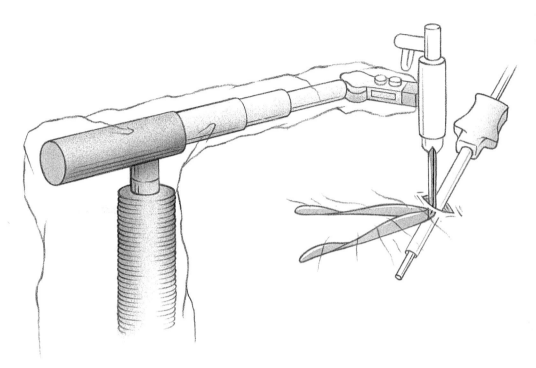

Figure 6.3
Endoscope behind laparofan.

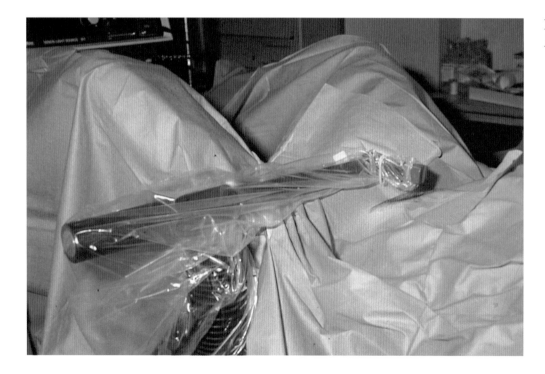

Figure 6.4
Fully draped device in use.

Figure 6.5
Planar lifting surface of the quadrant specific fan.

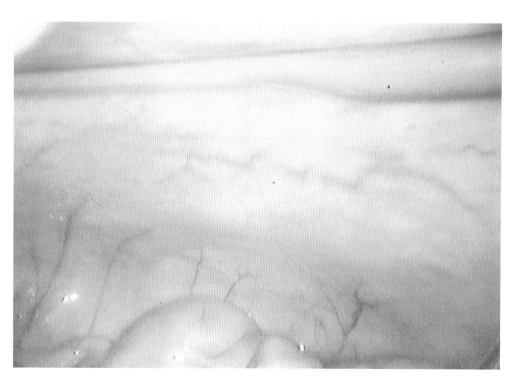

Figure 6.6
Intra-operative dissection of right lateral sidewall.

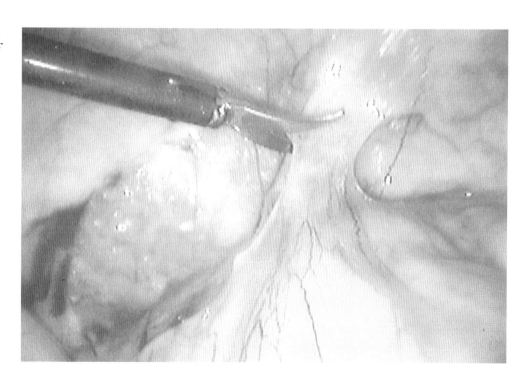

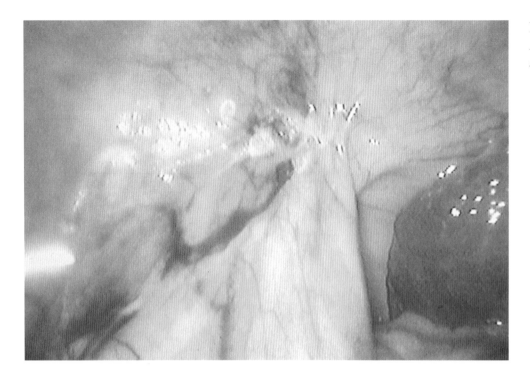

Figure 6.7
Intra-corporeal view of hepatic flexure.

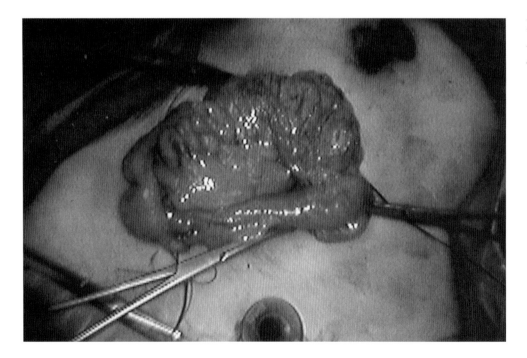

Figure 6.8
Extracorporeal viscera for anastomosis.

only two additional midline 10 mm ports are used during this procedure. In our experience with laparoscopic colectomy the newer quadrant-specific fans have provided superior retraction for laparoscopic colorectal surgery. Additionally, a wide variety of standard tools have been utilized including:

1 suction and irrigation;
2 sponge sticks;
3 right-angle clamps;
4 needle drivers;
5 Kelly clamps;
6 Babcock clamps.

The additional port sites are also simple gasless ports which provide superior tactile feedback during these procedures. The use of valve trocars is unnecessary.

Technique

Patient position

For removal of the right, transverse or descending colon, the patient is placed in the supine position. For resection of the sigmoid colon or abdominoperitoneal resections, the patient is placed in low stirrups or the low lithotomy position. After anaesthesia is initiated an oral gastric tube is placed in position and the urinary bladder is catheterized.

Laparolift placement for right hemicolectomy or transverse colon operations

The abdominal lifting device is placed on the operating room table on the right side of the patient. The surgeon and the assistant usually stand on the left side of the operating table or between the patient's legs. For left-sided lesions the lifting device can be attached to the left side of the operating room table with the surgeon and the assistant standing on the patient's right side. For sigmoid colectomy and abdominal perineal resection the lifting device is placed on the right or left side of the table parallel to the iliac crest.

Trocar placement

Initial abdominal access is obtained through a vertical incision at the base of the umbilicus. After the peritoneal cavity is entered, a finger sweep is used to ascertain the presence or absence of significant intra-abdominal adhesions. The laparofan is placed into the abdomen and attached to the dovetail portion of the laparolift device. The lifting mechanism is engaged and the camera can then be inserted behind the laparofan for abdominal inspection. Additional trocar sites are generally placed in the midline positions under direct visualization. If a temporary or permanent colostomy is anticipated the colostomy site is chosen and created prior to dissection so that additional instrumentation may be used via this wound. With gasless laparoscopic surgery more than one instrument may be used through a single site such as a colostomy wound.

Techniques of resection

Right hemicolectomy

Techniques of resection using gasless laparoscopy are very similar to standard open operating techniques. With the right hemicolectomy the right colon is grasped from the upper midline trocar site with a Babcock and the lower suprapubic port is used for the introduction of dissection scissors. The peritoneal reflection is taken down from the distal ileum along the paracolic gutter and around the hepatic flexure. Occasionally small bleeding points are clipped with the endoclip device. When adequate mobilization is achieved the distal ileum or transverse colon may be brought to the 3–4 cm umbilical wound for assessment. The laparofan is easily removed or replaced during this assessment. We have found that, in properly selected patients, dissection to the base of the mesentery to include the right colic and middle colic vessels is easily achieved. This technique ensures an adequate lymph node harvest. The important manoeuvres of this operation, including major vascular ligation, bowel division and anastomosis are performed at the level of the abdominal wall. Standard suction and irrigation devices may be utilized to access haemostasis and abdominal lavage. This operation is generally carried out in approximately 1 h, which compares favourably to our standard open right hemicolectomy.

Left hemicolectomy

The standard laparoscopic gasless left hemicolectomy is also done in a similar fashion to open left hemicolectomy. Once again, after placement of the laparofan the descending and sigmoid colon is mobilized on its lateral peritoneal reflection. After adequate mobilization the bowel may be divided distally utilizing the Endo-GIA device (Autosuture, Ascot, UK). The proximal division is generally easily performed with the extracorporeal stapling device at the level of the abdominal wall. Once again, vascular ligation is generally performed at the abdominal wall level with standard ligation of the vascular pedicle. The re-anastomosis is generally carried out with the assistance of the end-to-end anastomosis device.

Abdominoperineal resection

Abdominoperineal resection is facilitated by the early creation of the permanent colostomy site. This site facilitates the utilization of extracorporeal instrumentation. A second surgical team may work simultaneously from the perineal side. The site for proximal division colectomy is chosen and matured as a colectomy at skin level after the resected specimen is brought out transrectally.

Experience

Our experience with gasless laparoscopic colorectal surgery includes 20 right hemicolectomies, two segmental transverse colon resections, eight sigmoid and left colectomies, three abdominoperineal resections and three colostomies. Our operative times have been approximately 60–90 min for right and transverse resections, 122–150 min for left and sigmoid resections and 120 min for abdominoperineal resections.

No significant complications secondary to this technique were noted. We have also accumulated a substantial experience with gasless laparoscopic techniques in other surgical procedures prior to this experience. Our experience of cholecystectomy is well over 100 cases. Dr Swanström compared a selected series of his gasless laparoscopic colon procedures with laparoscopic colorectal resection utilizing pneumoperitoneum. In his experience the operative times were significantly less when using gasless techniques [28]. Other postoperative data included comparable lengths of stay of 3–4 days.

Conclusion

Early results with laparoscopic colectomy represent a selected group of patients. While the broad application of these techniques is forthcoming, statistical comparison of these groups is probably uninterpretable. It would seem that laparoscopic colorectal surgery offers significant advantages to some patients. Current techniques may initially be rejected because of the length and difficulty of the procedures. The relative simplicity of gasless laparoscopy allows some surgeons to safely utilize this technique of dissection without dependence upon the numerous devices required for laparoscopic surgery utilizing pneumoperitoneum. Instrumentation specifically designed to assist gasless laparoscopic surgery has recently become available. Ideally, after careful analysis of the data presented in works such as these, surgeons internationally will judge this procedure worthy of their consideration.

References

1   Leahy PF, Furman RH. Laparoscopically-assisted total colectomy. *Surg Endosc* 1992; **6**: 102.
2   Corbitt JD. Preliminary experience with laparoscopic-guided colectomy. *Surg Laparosc Endosc* 1992; **1**: 79–81.
3   Fowler DL, Whites SA. Laparoscopic assisted sigmoid resection. *Surg Laparosc Endosc* 1991; **3**: 183–8.
4   Jacobs M, Verdeja JC, Goldstein HS. Minimally invasive colon resection (laparoscopic colectomy). *Surg Laparosc Endosc* 1991; **1**: 138–43.
5   Wexner S, Johansen OB, Noguerae JJ, Jagelman DC. Laparoscopic total abdominal colectomy. A prospective trial. *Dis Colon Rectum* 1992; **35**: 651–5.
6   Phillips EH, Franklin M, Carroll BJ, Fallas MJ, Ramos P, Rosenthal D. Laparoscopic colectomy. *Ann Surg* 1992; **216**: 703–7.
7   Smith RS, Organ CH. *Gasless Laparoscopy with Conventional Instruments*. Norman Publishing, San Francisco, 1993.
8   Wittgen CH, Andros CH, Fitzgerald SD *et al*. Analysis of hemodynamic and ventilatory effects of laparoscopic cholecystectomy. *Arch Surg* 1991; **126**: 997–1001.
9   Hashimoto S, Munukata Y, Hashikusa Y *et al*. Cardiovascular and respiratory effects of intraperitoneal insufflation with carbon dioxide at laparoscopic cholecystectomy (abstract). *Surg Laparosc Endosc* 1992; **2**: 174.
10 Poulin EC, Mamazza J, Breton G *et al*. Evaluation of pulmonary function in laparoscopic cholecystectomy. *Surg Laparosc Endosc* 1992; **2**: 292–3.
11 Liu SY, Leighton T, David I *et al*. Prospective analysis of cardiopulmonary responses to laparoscopic cholecystectomy. *J Laparoendosc Surg* 1991; **1**(5): 241–6.
12 Holzman M, Sharp K, Richards W. Hypercarbia during carbon dioxide gas insufflation for therapeutic laparoscopy: a note of caution. *Surg Laparosc Endosc* 1992; **2**(1): 11–14.
13 Root B, Levy M, Pollack S. Gas embolism death after laparoscopy delayed by trapping in the portal circulation. *Anesth Analg* 1978; **7**: 232–7.
14 Dasher WA, Black JPM, Weiss W *et al*. Air embolism complicating pneumoperitoneum. *Am Rev Tubercul* 1954; **69**: 396–405.
15 Ishak BA, Seleny FL, Zeheva LN. Venous air embolism: a possible cause of acute pulmonary edema. *Anesthesiology* 1976; **45**: 453–5.
16 Morrison DH, Riggs JRA. Cardiovascular collapse in laparoscopy. *Can Med Assoc J* 1974; **11**: 433–7.
17 Ivankovich AD, Albrecht RF, Zahed B *et al*. Cardiovascular collapse during gynecological laparoscopy. *IMJ Ill Med J* 1974; **145**: 58–61.

18 Kelman GR, Swapp GH, Smith I *et al*. Cardiac output and arterial blood gas tension during laparoscopy. *Br J Anaesth* 1972; **44**: 1155–62.

19 Newman L, Luke JP, Ruben DM, Eubanks WS. Laparoscopic herniorrhaphy without pneumoperitoneum. *Surg Laparosc* 1993; **3**(3): 213–15.

20 Motew M, Ivankovich AD, Bieniarz J *et al*. Cardiovascular effects and acid–base and blood gas changes during laparoscopy. *Am J Gynecol* 1973; **115**: 302–12.

21 Mintz M. Risks and prophylaxis in laparoscopy: a survey of 100,000 cases. *J Reprod Med* 1977; **18**(5): 269–72.

22 Baadsgaard SE, Bille S, Egeblad K. Major vascular injury during gynecologic laparoscopy. Report of a case and reviews of published cases. *Acta Obstet Gynecol Scand* 1989; **68**: 283–5.

23 Vilardell F, Seres I, Marti-Vicente A. Complications of peritoneoscopy; a survey of 1,455 examinations. *Gastrointest Endosc* 1968; **14**: 178–80.

24 McQuaide JR. Air embolism during peritoneoscopy. *S Afr Med J* 1972; **46**: 412–23.

25 Kitano S, Tomikawa M, Iso Y *et al*. A safe and simple method to maintain a clear field of vision during laparoscopic cholecystecomy. *Surg Endosc* 1991; **6**: 197–8.

26 Nagai H, Inaba T, Kemia S *et al*. A new method of laparoscopic cholecystectomy. An abdominal mass lifting technique without pneumoperitoneum (abstract). *Surg Laparosc Endosc* 1991; **1**: 126.

27 Barnett RB, Clement GC, Prizin GS *et al*. Pulmonary changes after laparoscopic cholecystectomy. *Surg Laparosc Endosc* 1992; **2**: 125–7.

28 Swanström LI. Bowel resection. In: Smith RS and Organ CH (eds) *Gasless laparoscopy with conventional instruments: the next phases in minimally invasive surgery*. Norman Publishing, San Francisco, 1993: 73–94.

Chapter 7

Laparoscopic rectopexy for rectal prolapse

A. Darzi and J.R.T. Monson

Introduction

Video-assisted colorectal surgery is one of the latest additions to the range of operations being performed laparoscopically. For colonic resection, in most instances, colonic mobilization and the division of mesenteric vessels and bowel are carried out intracorporeally. A small incision is then made to deliver the specimen and fashion the anastomosis [1]. However, without the need for resection of the bowel, laparoscopic procedures for treating rectal prolapse may constitute some of the best applications for colorectal laparoscopic techniques. Although the condition is benign, rectal prolapse is often debilitating. A technique of laparoscopic rectopexy performed using the endoscopic stapler is described in this chapter.

Operative technique

A nasogastric tube and urinary catheter are passed when the patient is anaesthetized. All procedures are performed with the patient in the Lloyd-Davies position. Pneumoperitoneum is created using a closed technique. A 10 mm 0° telescope is inserted through a subumbilical port and initial laparoscopy is performed. The operator stands on the left side of the patient and a video screen is positioned to the right of the right foot (Fig. 7.1).

Three 12 mm ports are introduced into the abdomen to facilitate the use of laparoscopic stapling instruments (Endo-Hernia, Autosuture, Ascot, UK) (Fig. 7.2). A further 10 mm port is inserted suprapubically. The laparoscope is inserted into the right-sided port, freeing both the umbilical and the left iliac fossa ports for dissecting and grasping instruments.

Initially the patient is placed in a steep Trendelenburg position allowing the small bowel to drop into the peritoneal cavity. To facilitate exposure in the pelvis both round ligaments are elevated and stapled to the peritoneum overlying the pubic ramus exposing the pouch of Douglas (Fig. 7.3). Similarly the uterus is also stapled or sutured to the peritoneum overlying the pubic symphysis (Fig. 7.4). A Babcock grasping instrument is passed through the left iliac fossa port holding the rectosigmoid junction anteriorly and to the left (Fig. 7.5). A second Babcock instrument is passed through the suprapubic port to elevate the middle third of the rectum. This provides tension on the peritoneal reflection on the right side of the rectosigmoid junction.

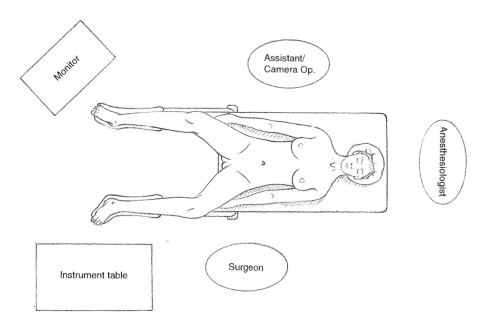

Figure 7.1
Theatre setup.

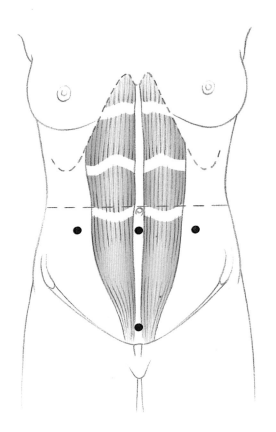

Figure 7.2
Port position.

A small incision is made in the peritoneal reflection just to the right of the rectum overlying the sacral promontory away from the right ureter (Fig. 7.6). This manoeuvre allows carbon dioxide gas into the post-rectal space and assists in identification of the avascular post-rectal plane. By careful dissection the avascular plane between the fascial capsule of the rectum anteriorly and the fascia of Waldeyer posteriorly is dissected under direct vision (Fig. 7.7).

Figure 7.3.
Stapling the right round ligament to the peritoneum to expose the pouch of Douglas.

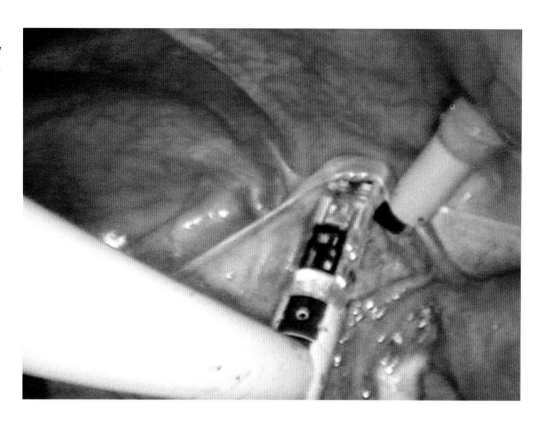

Figure 7.4
The uterine fundus is sutured to the peritoneum overlying the pubic symphysis to expose the pouch of Douglas.

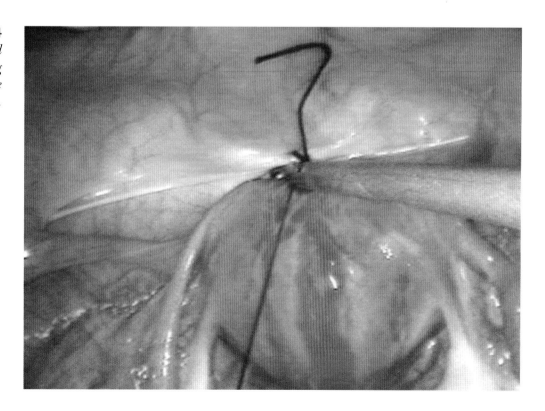

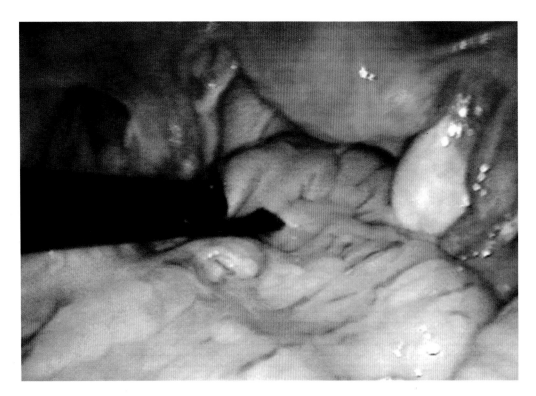

Figure 7.5
The sigmoid colon is pulled out of the pelvis using a Babcock instrument introduced through the left iliac fossa port.

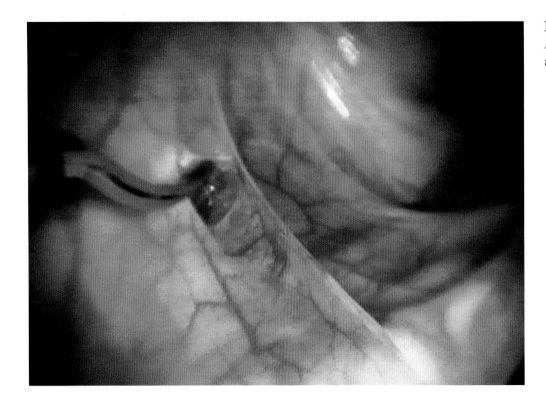

Figure 7.6
Division of the peritoneal reflection.

Figure 7.7
The dissection is continued in the avascular plane between the mesorectum anteriorly and the Waldeyer fascia posteriorly.

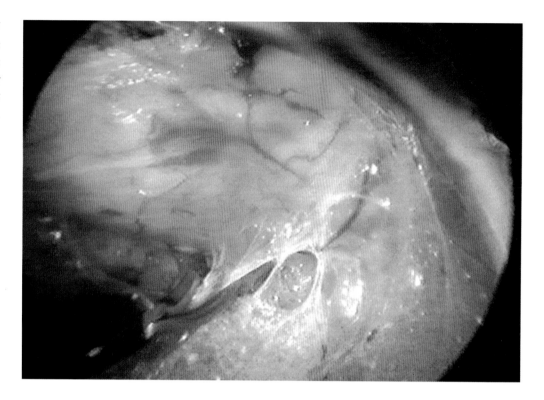

Identification of both ureters is established early in the dissection and the use of diathermy is restricted until the ureters are identified in order to reduce the risk of thermal injury. If there is any difficulty in identifying the ureters, glowing ureteric stents could be inserted transvesically to assist in their identification (Fig. 7.8).

Figure 7.8
Glowing left ureteric stent.

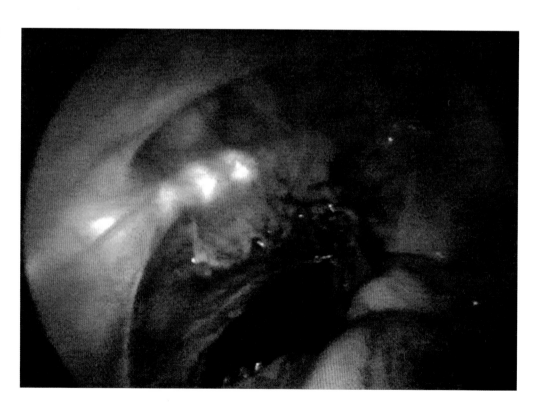

Division of the lateral ligaments is easily performed under direct vision (Fig. 7.9). Posteriorly, the pelvic nerves are identified and preserved. Close and magnified views of the mesorectum ensure that dissection continues within the correct planes with minimal bleeding. In a female, retraction of the pouch of Douglas is facilitated by holding the cervix upwards with a blunt Hulka cervical forceps (Rocket Ltd, Watford, UK) held through the vagina by an assistant. This elevates the cervix and body of the uterus, facilitating completion of the anterior dissection.

Having mobilized the rectum down to the pelvic floor, the surgeon introduced a strip of polypropylene mesh (Surgipro Mesh, Autosuture), approximately 15 × 15 cm, into the abdomen through the subumbilical port for placement in the presacral space (Fig. 7.10). The endoscopic stapler is then introduced through the umbilical port, and the mesh is initially stapled to the sacrococcygeal area. On average three to four staples are then inserted cephalad to the initial staple to fix the mesh to the sacrum and presacral fascia (Fig. 7.11). After fixation of the mesh, the rectum is held on light tension using the laparoscopic Babcock forceps and the right limb of the mesh is sutured to the serosa of the rectum using 2/0 silk on a curved needle. Staples could also be employed to staple the mesh to the side wall of the rectum. The rectum is then retracted to the right, and the left limb of the mesh is brought around the rectum and secured to the rectal wall in a similar fashion at the upper and lower mesh edges. Usually, two or three sutures or staples are required on either side (Fig. 7.12). The Szabo–Berci needle holder and Flamingo (Storz Ltd, Germany) are used to facilitate suture and knot tying.

The stapler is then used to re-approximate the peritoneal edges before the operation is completed. The laparoscopic ports are then removed, followed by closure of the facial defects with interrupted sutures (Fig. 7.13). Peroperative antibiotics are employed in all cases.

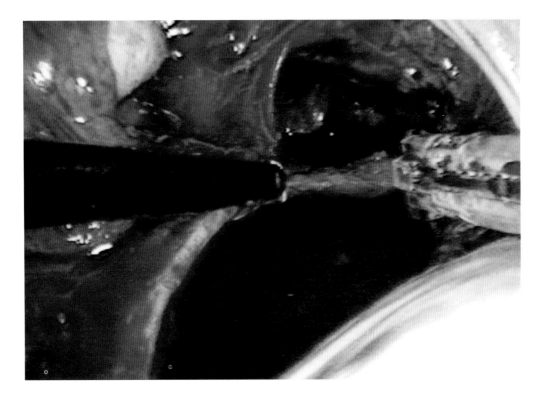

Figure 7.9
The lateral ligaments are clipped and divided.

Figure 7.10
*A piece of Surgipro Mesh
(Autosuture) is inserted into
the post-rectal space.*

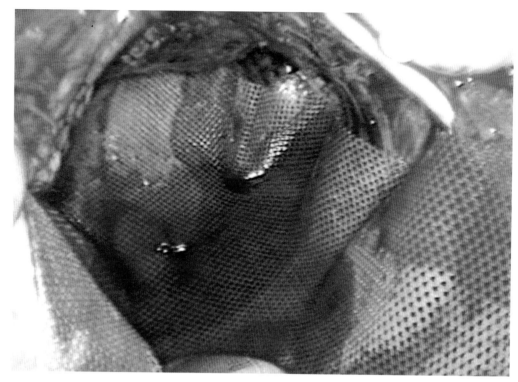

Figure 7.11
*The mesh is stapled to the
presacral fascia using the
Endo-Hernia stapler
(Autosuture).*

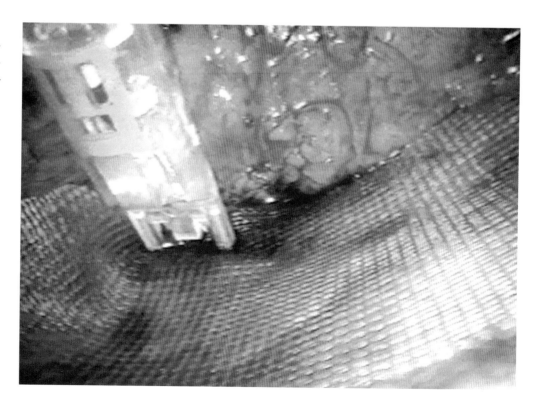

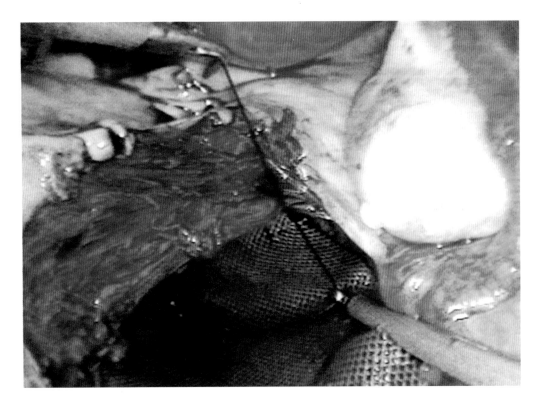

Figure 7.12
The mesh is sutured to the side wall of the rectum with 2/0 silk using the Szabo–Berci needle holder and Flamingo (Storz).

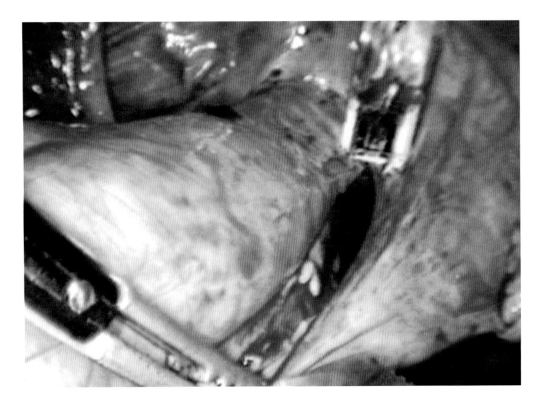

Figure 7.13
The peritoneum is closed with staples on either side of the rectum.

Patients and results

We have carried out this procedure on 48 patients (male : female ratio, 2 : 46) with a mean age of 76 years (range: 52–94 years). Two patients had rectorectal intussusception and an associated solitary rectal ulcer. The remaining patients had a full-thickness rectal prolapse. Patients who were unfit for general anaesthesia were excluded from the study. Nineteen patients had had a hysterectomy in the past. All the procedures were carried out by a single surgeon (AD). In one case the laparoscopic procedure had to be converted to an open procedure due to difficulty in ventilation. The mean operative time was 85 min (range: 45–190 min). The postoperative course has been uneventful, with rapid resumption of normal bowel function. The mean hospital stay was 5 days (range: 4–15 days) and early mobility was a marked feature in these patients. The complications included urinary tract infection (n=1), incisional hernia through a port hole (n=1), a large extraperitoneal haematoma at the site of a port hole (n=1), urinary retention (n=1), prolonged ileus (n=1) and severe constipation (n=10).

The mean follow-up to date is 8 months. One patient developed mucosal prolapse after 3 months which required an injection with phenol in almond oil. One patient developed a full-thickness recurrence 18 months after the operation.

Discussion

As patients presenting with rectal prolapse are frequently old and infirm, many surgeons have tended to favour low-morbidity local operations on the anal canal [2]. Such local procedures include the Thiersch wire or a silastic sling around the anal canal [3]. In contrast, some surgeons advocate radical operations such as anterior resection [4] or combined abdominoperineal pelvic floor repair [5,6] for those patients who are fit to undergo major procedures. Where resection is not undertaken, others have advocated rectal fixation or rectopexy. Graham [7] was the first to mobilize the rectum down to the levator muscles, a manoeuvre which is still considered the most important element required for a successful outcome. Most currently preferred operative techniques represent a modification of Graham's approach in which fixation procedures of the entire mobilized rectum are used. Originally these procedures relied on a polyvinyl alcohol sponge inserted in the presacral space to fix the rectum to the sacrum [8] or on suturing an inert sling to fix the mobilized rectum to the sacral promontory. The irritant properties of the polyvinyl alcohol sponge helped to fix the rectum firmly but also predisposed the patient to infection and rejection. Fixation of an inert polypropylene mesh in front of the rectum was described by Ripstein but has been associated with acute kinking of the bowel or, if too tight, with intestinal obstruction [9]. Early experience with these complications led us to adopt a modification of the procedure whereby the inert polypropylene mesh is inserted behind the rectum and is attached to the sacrum to achieve posterior fixation.

Our own preliminary experience with laparoscopic rectopexy has been encouraging. Early mobilization and discharge from hospital has been a marked feature. Although follow-up is short the functional results have been excellent.

Laparoscopic colonic surgery has the same potential benefits as laparoscopic cholecystectomy with potentially a shorter postoperative stay and less postoperative pain [1]. The recent introduction of a commercially available endoscopic stapler for use in laparoscopic hernia repair and a specifically designed needle holder has provided us with the tools necessary for laparoscopic rectopexy. Initial concerns of haemorrhage resulting from the application of staples to the sacrum and presacral fascia were averted by avoiding stapling in the midline and by using short staples. In addition Hill *et al.* [10] have reported the use of the endoscopic hernia stapler to control presacral haemorrhage in open rectal surgery. Berman described a similar technique employing a laparoscopic sacral tacker and laparoscopic staplers to fix the mesh to the sacrum and rectum [11]. Laparoscopic sacral tackers have the obvious advantage of being haemostatic; however, we feel the mesh is best sutured to the side wall of the rectum.

Patients with normal bowel habits (or diarrhoea) and no history of constipation or obstructed defaecation are probably ideal candidates for laparoscopic rectopexy without resection, especially if there is no significant redundancy of the sigmoid colon. In patients with massive procidentia, the presence of a large mesorectum and redundant sigmoid will probably mandate a resective procedure, and simple rectopexy should be avoided. As laparoscopic experience increases it may be that those patients requiring resection for rectal prolapse may undergo this procedure laparoscopically. In benign disease such as this, concerns over adequacy of colonic resection margins are not an issue and simple transanal delivery of the specimen with subsequent intracorporeal anastomosis may be a suitable option.

Our preliminary experience leads us to suggest that, as laparoscopic technology advances and surgical expertise is gained, this minimally invasive approach will soon have a major impact on the practice of colorectal surgery. The benefit of such a minimally invasive approach to rectal prolapse becomes especially obvious in the elderly or physiologically disabled patient with prolapse.

References

1   Monson JRT, Darzi A. Carey PD, Guillou PJ. Prospective evaluation of laparoscopic assisted colectomy in an unselected group of patients. *Lancet* 1992; **340**: 831–3.
2   Goligher JC. *Surgery of the Colon, Anus and Rectum*, 4th edn. Bailliere Tindall, London, 1980.
3   Jackman FR, Francis JN, Hopkinson BR. Silicon rubber band treatment of rectal prolapse. *Ann R Coll Surg Engl* 198; **62**: 386–7.
4   Porter NH. Collective results of operations for rectal prolapse. *Ann R Coll Surg Engl* 1980; **62**: 386–7.
5   Goligher JC. The treatment of complete prolapse of the rectum by the Roscoe Graham operation. *Br J Surg* 1957; **45**: 323–33.
6   Hughes ESR, Gleadell LW. Abdominoperineal repair of complete prolapse of the rectum. *Proc R Soc Med* 1962; **55**: 1077–80.
7   Henry MM. Rectal prolapse. *Br J Hosp Med* 1980; **24**: 302–7.
8   Wells CA. Polyvinyl-alcohol sponge. An inert plastic for use as a prosthesis in the repair of large hernias. *Br J Surg* 1955; **42**: 618.
9   Miller RL. Ripstein procedure for rectal prolapse. *Am Surg* 1979; **45**: 531–4.
10 Hill ADK, Menzies-Gow N, Darzi A. Methods of controlling presacral bleeding. *J Am Coll Surgeons* 1994; **178**: 183–4.
11 Berman IR. Sutureless laparoscopic rectopexy for procidentia. Technique and implications. *Dis Colon Rectum* 1992; **35**: 689–93.

Chapter 8

Laparoscopic colorectal surgery — a provocative critique

S.D. Wexner and P. Reissman

Introduction

A growing number of reports have been published concerning laparoscopic surgery for colorectal disorders [1–9]. The advantages of other laparoscopic procedures, the continuous advancement in technology and instrumentation, and patient demand all led to extensive enthusiasm, long before some crucial unresolved issues were addressed. In many cases, surgeons sought to perform the procedures before anyone else or even to the exclusion of performing open procedures. The surgical and technical challenges, and the absence of scientifically valid results, often outweighed all other considerations including some serious early and late complications.

In many cases demands by biomedical technology companies and by patients seem to have obfuscated all other considerations. Although a 'learning curve' is a well-known facet of any procedure, its degree of ascent and its length are variable. Specifically, the continent ileostomy and the ileo-anal reservoir were well documented as having steep learning curves. However, unlike laparoscopic colectomy, the vast majority of surgeons chose to assiduously avoid the problems associated with these procedures by not performing them. Only a few surgeons in high-volume inflammatory bowel disease practices chose to undertake pouch surgery [10]. More than 10 years of experience in these centres led to technical refinements which enabled simplication of the procedure to the point that ileo-anal reservoirs are now undertaken in moderate-volume practices as well. Despite their improvement, however, even recent reports have shown that a learning curve still exists and that it is the patient who suffers the most while the surgeon is learning the technique [11–15].

Unlike pouch surgery, laparoscopic colorectal surgery immediately became familiar to all surgeons. The responses ranged from refusal (mainly by older surgeons), to laboratory training followed by refusal, to selective application to universal application. Proponents of laparoscopic colorectal surgery claim that universal application is appropriate because surgeons are already familiar with other laparoscopic procedures. It is therefore important to highlight several fundamental differences between laparoscopic colorectal surgery and all other intra-abdominal laparoscopic procedures.

1 The procedure often involves more than one anatomical region and therefore relocation of instruments, monitors and even personnel is needed; working in multiple regions may also increase the length of the procedure and the intraoperative complication rate.

2 Removing a small organ through a small port or suturing a defect without any organ removed allows the entire procedure to be performed through small (5–12 mm) ports. Most colorectal procedures require specimen retrieval and therefore necessitate the use of larger calibre trocars or an incision.

3 While the requisite skills to remove a gallbladder or repair a hernia defect are no doubt formidable, once the end organ is extirpated or the defect is repaired the procedure is concluded. However, at this point in a laparoscopic colectomy the challenging part begins: a well-vascularized tension-free circumferentially intact anastomosis must be fashioned.

4 A large number of mesenteric vessels are divided during the procedure. Again, division of a single small vessel such as during a cholecystectomy or appendicectomy can be rapidly, inexpensively and safely effected. However, ensuring safe vascular control of the entire colonic mesentery is a more challenging and time-consuming procedure. Moreover, efforts to expedite this phase of the procedure, mainly vascular stapling, achieve their goal only at a high financial cost. Such concerns do not have to be considered in procedures such as herniorrhaphy and fundoplication.

5 None of the other laparoscopic procedures are performed for cure of malignancy and therefore issues like local or distant recurrence and long-term survival are irrelevant.

Not surprisingly, therefore, an initial large number of complications uncommon in the open surgery setting including recognized and unrecognized enterotomies, ureteric injuries, epigastric and intra-abdominal major vessel injures, port site hernias and removal of the wrong bowel segment have been reported [1–8,16–19]. Physiological derangement due to the adverse effect of prolonged intra-abdominal pressure and high carbon dioxide content are still a cause for concern. [20]. Again, pioneer laparoscopic surgeons have regaled us with tales of injury to virtually every organ as well as Herculean 6–8 h long colectomies followed by venous thrombosis, pulmonary embolus and even death.

Although many of these complications may have been related to the beginning of the learning curve, the cost–benefit for many laparoscopic colorectal procedures should be questioned. Adequate training and credentialing of residents as well as experienced general and colorectal surgeons should be mandatory [21,22].

Colorectal cancer is the third most common malignancy in the United States, Canada, United Kingdom and most other western countries [23]. The potential use of laparoscopic surgery for curative treatment of this cancer is therefore inevitable. Considering the risk of inadequate surgery when treating a curable cancer even by laparotomy, laparoscopic colorectal surgery should be carefully assessed and critically evaluated before it is widely applied in the treatment of such lesions. Particularly in the case of rectal cancer, surgeon variability is tremendous and directly impacts upon recurrence and survival [24–26]. Again, in the wave of enthusiasm to become the first laparoscopic surgeon in a given geographical area, many surgeons have abandoned fundamental precepts and tenets to facilitate the (often inadequate) early technology. Although the laparoscope has not yet made technically inept surgeons facile, it has sadly clouded the judgement of many good surgeons. This problem has even been discussed in the lay press [27,28].

It is important at this juncture to review some results to date. Unfortunately, none of the series which have compared open and laparoscopic colon resections have been prospective randomized studies and obviously none have included long-term outcome. Dodson and colleagues reported three abdominoperineal resections having been performed [29]. Their 33% reported mortality rate seems a high price for a mean of 4.2 lymph nodes harvested. Larach and co-workers reported having attempted laparoscopic colectomy in 18 patients and having successfully completed it in 11 [6]. The length of surgery ranged up to 8.5 h and the mean length of hospitalization was 8.4 days. Moreover, because of the lack of tactile sensation the wrong segment of colon was removed in one patient necessitating conversion to laparotomy and an additional resection.

Larach *et al.* highlight two fundamental issues. The first, resection of the wrong segment of bowel, has also been noted by Monson and co-authors [8]. Methods exist to limit this problem including colonoscopic injection of a variety of compounds including indian ink, methylene blue, indocyanine green and indigo carmine. Other surgeons have recommended routine use of preoperative air contrast barium enemas or intraoperative colonoscopy. In a recent survey of the members of the American Society of Colon and Rectal Surgeons, 12 additional wrong segment removals were reported. Furthermore, 69% of the responders advocated a routine addition of one or more of the aforementioned manoeuvres to limit the occurrence of this problem [16]. However, it is difficult to justify a procedure if its execution demands additional costly or invasive procedures which would not be done in the equivalent 'open' setting.

The second facet of the study of Larach *et al.* that is worth discussion is the use of the term 'conversion'. Conversion, and not failure, should be used to describe the creation of an incision longer than that initially planned or premature termination of the laparoscopic phase of the procedure. Failure should be restricted to describing the inability to confer upon the patient the optimal results. Failure should not be used to describe inadequate ego satisfaction to the surgeon. Termination of the laparoscopic procedure should represent sound surgical judgement. Specifically, postulate that a patient undergoes a completely laparoscopic sigmoid colectomy through four 10 mm ports as an outpatient procedure, has no ileus, takes only acetaminophen for pain, and returns to work the same day. That patient might be considered to have had a 'successful' laparoscopic procedure. However, assume that the patient underwent the colectomy for cure of a Dukes' B lesion and develops a local recurrence 3 months later. That patient, in fact, should be reported as a 'failure' of laparoscopy (or as a failure of the laparoscopist's judgement). Conversely, postulate a patient in whom the laparoscopy is converted to a laparotomy because the left ureter could not be visualized prior to inferior mesenteric vessel ligation. During the open phase the ureter is easily seen and the procedure is safely completed. In this latter scenario a successful outcome is ensured after conversion. The stout refusal to compromise surgical principles, even at the expense of ego erosion, is fundamental to safe laparoscopic surgery.

The issue of conversion is not uniformly agreed upon. Senagore and associates [30] reported a 32% conversion rate very similar to the 38% rate of Larach. However, the definition of conversion varies as Senagore *et al.* consider a

10 cm incision as 'small' and one through which a successful laparoscopic procedure was performed.

There is also much subjectivity related to blood loss. Specifically Senagore and associates reported a mean blood loss laparoscopically of 157 cm^3. They claimed that this loss was lower than the mean 687 cm^3 loss noted during similar open cases. Conversely the objective data reported by Peters and Bartels [31] indicate a greater decline in postoperative haemoglobin after laparoscopic than after open surgery.

One must also be assured of comparing similar groups for data analysis. Specifically the mean length of hospitalization in a total of 486 patients reported in 17 series was 6.6 days with a range of 1–40 days (Table 8.1) [2,6–8,30,32–42]. Longer hospitalizations may reflect patients who underwent total abdominal colectomy or who had a stoma constructed and required predischarge enterostomal therapy education. Conversely, shorter hospitalization may reflect patients who underwent segmental or wedge resections. The latter operation is mentioned only to be condemned as it plays no role in the appropriate resection of a lesion which may harbour malignancy. The wedge resection was abandoned 70 years ago due to an unacceptably high rate of tumour implantation in the small wounds [43,44]. Nonetheless, it has recently enjoyed a resurgence because of its technical ease [45]. Several authors have performed this procedure laparoscopically for a 'benign' polyp. However, despite preoperative biopsies, as many as 40% of 'benign' neoplasms may harbour an invasive carcinoma [46]. Again, one should never forsake basic tenets to facilitate the procedure.

Table 8.1
Length of hospitalization.

Reference	No. of patients	Length of hospitalization (days)	
		Mean	Range
Lointier et al. [32]	6	10	7–16
Milsom et al. [33]	9	7	5–12
Tate et al. [34]	11	12.3	NS
Van Ye et al. [35]	14	9.1	4–29
Corbitt [36]	18	4.0	3–6
Larach et al. [6]	18	8.4	4–25
Franklin et al. [37]	19	7.4	NS
Quattlebaum et al. [38]	20	4.4	2–12
Scoggin et al. [39]	20	5	2–31
Peters and Bartels [31]	24	4.8	NS
Musser et al. [40]	24	8.5	NS
Etienne et al. [41]	35	9	5–23
Senagore et al. [30]	38	7	NS
Monson et al. [8]	40	8	NS
Phillips et al. [2]	51	4.6	1–30
Zucker et al. [42]	65	4.4	3–8
Wexner et al. [7]	74	7	2–40
Total	486	6.6	1–40

NS, not stated.

The problems of wound implantation and of laparoscopic resection of malignancy are very crucial ones. To date there has been no prospective randomized study to prove the superiority or even the equivalence of laparoscopic procedures to open colectomy for cure of colon cancer [47,48]. The validity of another argument of the laparoscopic advocate concerning basic oncological principles of colon cancer resection is that the number of lymph nodes harvested is equivalent to that harvested during open surgery. However, this logic is fallacious as the number of lymph nodes in the specimen has not been shown to affect survival [49,50]. Although identical resection margins and a similar number of lymph nodes may be achieved in laparoscopic and open colectomy, the value of such comparisons is doubtful.

Firstly, there exists tremendous variability in terms of the number of nodes harvested even after standard colectomy [51]. Secondly, the number of nodes reported reflects not only the surgeon's prowess, but also the pathologist's enthusiasm. A pathologist trying to help a surgical colleague prove the oncological wisdom of laparoscopic colectomy may persevere to find extra nodes. Unfortunately the process is highly subjective. Thirdly, the number of nodes may reflect the number of paracolic nodes, the prognostic significance of which is different from that associated with apical nodes. Thus, a long sleeve resection may yield as many nodes as a more traditional segmental resection with high ligation. These variations are not generally addressed in most laparoscopic manuscripts. Furthermore, Table 8.2 shows that the number of nodes harvested despite being called 'adequate', 'large', 'sufficient' or 'equivalent to that noted after open surgery' may be questionable. Specifically, although the maximum reported yield was 84 nodes, between as few as 0 and 2 nodes were also noted at the minimum end of the range [6,7,29,34,35,37,40,42]. It is difficult to explain to a patient in whom only two lymph nodes were removed that adequate staging is possible.

Lack of equivalent patient groups seems to be the hallmark of laparoscopic publications. Tate and co-workers claimed that laparoscopy is appropriate for the cure of rectal carcinoma [34]. They drew this conclusion even though the distal resection margin was as little as 0.5 cm in the laparoscopic group. Again, although the mean resection margin reported was 2.0 cm, it would seem difficult to explain to the patients with the 0.5 cm margin that because the group mean

Table 8.2
Laparoscopic colectomy lymph node harvest.

Reference	No. of patients	No. of nodes	
		Mean	Range
Dodson et al. [29]	3	4.2	NS
Zucker et al. [42]	8	7.7	5–11
Larach et al. [6]	13	9.8	0–22
Van Ye et al. [35]	14	10.5	0–32
Tate et al. [34]	11	10	2–14
Musser et al. [40]	15	10.6	NS
Franklin et al. [37]	24	14	8–22
Wexner et al. [7]	12	19	3–84

NS, not stated.

was adequate their laparoscopic operation was successful and oncologically curative. Further reading reveals that selection criteria for laparoscopic surgery included an age of more than 65 years and/or unresectable or metastatic disease with availability of 'sufficient operating room time'. Conversely, selection criteria for open surgery included younger patients with curable lesions.

Regardless of the importance or lack thereof of lymph node clearance or distal margins, a further more critical and mysterious complication has been recently observed after laparoscopic 'curative' colon cancer resection — early recurrence of cancer at the trocar sites. The first case was reported by Alexander *et al.* [52]. This patient was a 67-year-old female who developed a port site recurrence 3 months after a laparoscopically assisted right hemicolectomy for a Dukes' C lesion [52]. Subsequently, O'Rourke *et al.* reported an 82-year-old woman with two port sites recurrences 10 weeks after a similar procedure for a Dukes' B lesion [53]. Similar cases have been noted [54,55; G. Gionnore, personal communication]. At least 11 additional reports of trocar site recurrences of colorectal cancer have been reported [56–58; R. Gould, personal communication]. Interestingly, several reports of port site implantation of other malignancies have been reported including: cholangiocarcinoma [59; L. Hultén, personal communication], ovarian malignancy [60] and gastric and pancreatic cancer [61,62]. The exact cause of this bizarre phenomenon is still obscure, but must be related to the laparoscopic technique since incisional recurrence after curative abdominal cancer excision is virtually unpublished. In fact, *Index Medicus*, textbook and citation index searches revealed only a single reference to this exceedingly rare complication [63]. Thus, the number of reported cases in only 3 years of laparoscopic colectomy has vastly exceeded that of centuries of standard colectomy.

This unexpected alarming complication of laparoscopic colorectal surgery is particularly concerning for several reasons. Firstly, not all the recurrences were noted in the ports through which the specimen was removed and, therefore, may not be related to malignant cell contamination and thus cannot be prevented by using specimen bags. Secondly, the phenomenon is not limited to advanced lesions as localized curable lesions have also implanted tumour cells at port sites. Lastly, the fact that this complication occurred after a variety of laparoscopic procedures may implicate some basic underlying problem associated with the laparoscopic technique.

The initially promising advantage of laparoscopic colectomy was saving money through shorter hospitalization. Several authors have demonstrated shorter hospitalizations in prospective or retrospective non-randomized studies. However, to date no study has shown a statistically significant cost saving [30,47,64,65].

Despite all of the scepticism and admonitions within this chapter, laparoscopic colectomy has benefited patients. Specifically, it has taught us to question the need for denying oral intake immediately after bowel resection or for hospitalization until full bowel function is resumed. After a careful analysis of the studies that showed some of the earlier mentioned benefits, it was obvious that patients after laparoscopic colon resection underwent aggressive postoperative care including early oral feeding or discharge home on a liquid diet, while none of these criteria were applied in the open surgery cases [3,66]. Ironically, these measures have recently been successfully applied to patients who have undergone standard open colectomy with equally good results [67,68]. Specifically, in two prospective randomized trials, patients after elective open colorectal procedures were shown to safely tolerate early oral feeding, early mobilization and shorter hospitalization without increased morbidity. In fact the mean hospital stay after early oral feeding following open colectomy was 6 days, fewer than the mean of 7.1 days noted in the 486 patients in Table 8.1.

In conclusion, the feasibility and capability to perform laparoscopic colorectal surgery has been well established; however, does it justify a routine universal use of this relatively new technique? The answer is obvious 'no'. Although its superiority has yet to be confirmed, laparoscopic colorectal surgery may presently have a role in the management of benign colorectal disorders and palliative resections for cancer. These procedures should be performed by an adequately trained team, in a proper setting where prospective analysis of the patient's outcome will be available. It is crucial, however, that the issue of laparoscopic colorectal surgery for cure of cancer is separately addressed and only performed as part of a controlled prospective randomized long-term study.

References

1   Wexner SD, Johansen OB, Nogueras JJ, Jagelman DG. Laparoscopic total abdominal colectomy: a prospective assessment. *Dis Colon Rectum* 1992; **35**: 651–5.
2   Phillips EH, Franklin M, Carroll BJ *et al*. Laparoscopic colectomy. *Ann Surg* 1992; **216**: 703–7.
3   Jacobs M, Verdeja GD, Goldstein DS. Minimally invasive colon resection (laparoscopic colectomy). *Surg Laparosc Endosc* 1992; **1**: 144–50.
4   Nogueras JJ, Wexner SD. Laparoscopic colon resection. *Perspect Colon Rectal Surg* 1992; **5**: 79–97.
5   Wexner SD, Johansen OB. Laparoscopic bowel resection: advantages and limitations. *Ann Med* 1992; **24**: 105–10.
6   Larach SW, Salomon MC, Williamson PR *et al*. Laparoscopic assisted colectomy: experience during the learning curve. *Coloproctology* 1993; **1**: 38-41.
7   Wexner SD, Cohen SM, Johansen OB *et al*. Laparoscopic colorectal surgery: a prospective assessment and current perspective. *Br J Surg* 1993; **80**: 1602–5.
8   Monson JRT, Darzi A, Carey PD, Guillou PJ. Prospective evaluation of laparoscopic-assisted colectomy in an unselected group of patients. *Lancet* 1992; **340**: 831–3.
9   Schmitt SL, Cohen SM, Wexner SD *et al*. Does laparoscopic assisted ileal pouch anal anastomosis reduce the length of hospitalization? *Int J Colorectal Dis* (in press).
10 Parks AG, Nicholls RJ, Belliveau P. Proctocolectomy with ileoanal reservoir and anal anastomosis. *Br J Surg* 1980; **67**: 533–8.
11 Becker JM. Ileal pouch anal anastomosis: current status and controversies. *Surgery* 1993; **113**: 599–602.
12 Poggioly G, Marchetti F, Selleri S *et al*. Redo pouches: salvaging of failed ileal pouch–anal anastomoses. *Dis Colon Rectum* 1993; **36**: 492–6.
13 Nicholls RJ. Restorative proctocolectomy with ileal reservoir: indications and results. *Schweiz Med Wochenschr* 1990; **120**: 485–8.
14 Motta JC, Ricketts RR. The J pouch Swenson procedure for ulcerative colitis and familial polyposis. *Am Surg* 1992; **58**: 613–17.
15 Keighley MRB, Winslet MC, Flinn R, Kmiot W. Multivariate analysis of factors influencing the results of restorative proctocolectomy. *Br J Surg* 1989; **76**: 740–4.
16 Cohen SM, Wexner SD. Laparoscopic colorectal surgery: are we being honest with out patients? Presented at the annual meeting of the American Society of Colon and Rectal Surgeons 1994, Orlando, Florida, USA.
17 Hass BE, Schrager RE. Small bowel obstruction due to Richter's hernia after laparoscopic procedures. *J Laparosc Surg* 1993; **3**: 421–3.
18 Reissman P, Shiloni E, Gofrit O *et al*. Incarcerated hernia in a lateral trocar site — an unusual early postoperative complication of laparoscopic surgery. *Eur J Surg* (in press).
19 Colver RM. Laparoscopy: basic techniques, instrumentation, and complications. *Surg Laparosc Endosc* 1992; **2**: 35–40.
20 Holzman M, Sharp K, Richards W. Hypercarbia during carbon dioxide insufflation for therapeutic laparoscopy: a note of caution. *Surg Laparosc Endosc* 1992; **2**: 11–14.
21 Weiss EG, Wexner SD. Training and preparing for laparoscopic colectomy. *Semin Colon Rectal Surg* (in press).

22 Dent TL. Training credentialing and evaluation in laparoscopic surgery. *Surg Clin North Am* 1992; **72**: 1003–11.

23 Mettlin C, Natarajan N, Mittelman A *et al*. Management and survival of adenocarcinoma of the rectum in the United States: results of a national survey by the American College of Surgeons. *Oncology* 1987; **39**: 265–87.

24 Heald R, Ryall R. Recurrence and survival after total mesorectal excision for rectal cancer. *Lancet* 1986; **1**: 1497–82.

25 Fielding LP. Colorectal carcinoma: mesorectal excision for rectal cancer. *Lancet* 1993; **341**: 471–2.

26 Fielding LP, Stewart-Brown S, Dudley HA. Surgeon related variables and the clinical trial. *Lancet* 1979; **2**: 778–81.

27 Altman LK. Surgical injuries lead to new rules. *New York Times* 14 June 1992.

28 Altman LK. Standard training in laparoscopy found inadequate. *New York Times* 14 December 1993.

29 Dodson RW, Cullado MJ, Tangen LE *et al*. Laparoscopic assisted abdominoperineal resection. *Contemp Surg* 1993; **42**: 42–4.

30 Senagore AJ, Luchtefeld MA, Macheigan JM *et al*. Open colectomy versus laparoscopic colectomy: are there differences? *Am Surg* 1993; **59**: 549–54.

31 Peters WR, Bartels T. Minimally invasive colectomy: are the potential benefits realized? *Dis Colon Rectum* 1993; **36**: 751–6.

32 Lointier PH, Lautard M, Massoni C *et al*. Laparoscopically assisted subtotal colectomy. *J Laparoendosc Surg* 1993; **3**: 439–453.

33 Milsom JW, Lavery IC, Böhm B, Fazio VW. Laparoscopically assisted ileocolectomy in Crohn's disease. *Surg Laparosc Endosc* 1993; **3**: 77–80.

34 Tate JJT, Kwok S, Dawson JW *et al*. Prospective comparison of laparoscopic and conventional anterior resection. *Br J Surg* 1993; **80**: 1396–8.

35 Van Ye TM, Cattery RP, Henry LG. Laparoscopically assisted colon resections compare favorably with open technique. *Surg Laparosc Endosc* 1994; **4**: 25–31.

36 Corbitt JD Jr. Preliminary experience with laparoscopic guided colectomy. *Surg Laparosc Endosc* 1992; **2**: 79–81.

37 Franklin ME, Ramos R, Rosenthal D, Schuessler W. Laparoscopic colonic procedures. *World J Surg* 1993; **17**: 51–6.

38 Quattlebaum JK Jr, Flanders D, Usher CH III. Laparoscopically assisted colectomy. *Surg Laparosc Endosc* 1993; **3**: 81–7.

39 Scoggin SD, Frazee RC, Snyder SK *et al*. Laparoscopic assisted bowel surgery. *Dis Colon Rectum* 1993; **36**: 747–50.

40 Musser DJ, Boorse RC, Madera F, Reed JF III. Laparoscopic colectomy: at what cost? *Surg Laparosc Endosc* 1994; **4**: 1–5.

41 Etienne J, Jehaes C, Kartheuser A *et al*. Laparoscopic surgery for benign colorectal disease: a multicentric prospective study (abstract). *Br J Surg* 1993; **80**: S45.

42 Zucker KA, Pitcher DE, Martin DT, Ford RS. Laparoscopic assisted colon resection. *Surg Endosc* 1994; **8**: 12–18.

43 Paul FT. Personal experiences in surgery of the large bowel. *Lancet* 1912; **2**: 217–26.

44 Sistrunk WE. The Mikulicz operation for resection of the colon. Its advantages and dangers. *Ann Surg* 1928; **88**: 597–606.

45 Shallman RW, Shaw TJ, Roach JM. Colonoscopically assisted intracorporeal laparoscopic wedge resection of a benign right colon lesion. *Surg Laparosc Endosc* 1993; **3**: 482–4.

46 Harford FJ. Other rectal neoplasms. In: Beck DE, Wexner SD (eds) *Fundamentals of Anorectal Surgery*. McGraw-Hill, New York, 1992: 370–9.

47 Falk PM, Beart RW, Wexner SD *et al*. Laparoscopic colectomy: a critical appraisal. *Dis Colon Rectum* 1993; **36**: 28–34.

48 Cohen SM, Wexner SD. Laparoscopic colorectal resection for cancer: the Cleveland Clinic Florida experience. *Surg Oncol* 1993; **2**: 35–42.

49 Shida J, Ban K, Matsumoto M *et al*. Prognostic significance of location of lymph nodal metastases in colorectal cancer. *Dis Colon Rectum* 1992; **35**: 1046–50.

50 Harnsberger JR, Vernava AM, Longo WE. Radical abdominopelvic lymphadenectomy: historic perspective and current role in the surgical management of rectal cancer. *Dis Colon Rectum* 1994; **37**: 73–87.

51 Cohen SM, Wexner SD, Schmitt SL *et al*. Does xylene mesenteric fat clearance improve lymph node harvest after colon resection? *Eur J Surg* (in press).

52 Alexander RJT, Jaques BC, Mitchell KG. Laparoscopically assisted colectomy and wound recurrence (letter). *Lancet* 1993; **341**: 249–50.

53 O'Rourke N, Price PM, Kelly S, Sikora K. Tumor inoculation during laparoscopy (letter). *Lancet* 1993; **342**: 368.

54 Fusco MA, Paluzzi MW. Abdominal wall recurrence after laparoscopic assisted colectomy for adenocarcinoma of the colon. *Dis Colon Rectum* 1993; **36**: 858–61.

55 Guillou P, Darzi A, Monson JRT. Experience with laparoscopic colorectal surgery for malignant disease. *Surg Oncol* 1993; **2**: 43–50.

56 Goh P. Laparoscopic colon resection — the Singapore experience. Presented at the Tripartite Colorectal Meeting 1993, Sidney, Australia.

57 Stitz R. Presented at the Tripartite Colorectal Meeting 1993, Sidney, Australia.

58 Franklin M. *Laparoscopic Colectomy*. International Symposium on Advances in Laparoscopic Colectomy 1993, Indianapolis, Indiana, USA.

59 Fong Y, Brennan MF, Turnbull A *et al*. Gallbladder cancer discovered during laparoscopic surgery. Potential for iatrogenic tumor dissemination. *Arch Surg* 1993; **128**: 1054–6.

60 Gleeson NC, Nicosia SV, Mark JE *et al*. Abdominal wall metastases from ovarian cancer after laparoscopy. *Am J Obstet Gynecol* 1993; **169**: 522–3.

61 Cava A, Roman J, Quintela AG *et al*. Subcutaneous metastasis following laparoscopy in gastric adenocarcinoma. *Eur J Surg Oncol* 1990; **16**: 63–7.

62 Siriwardena A, Samarji WN. Cutaneous tumor seeding from a previous undiagnosed pancreatic carcinoma after laparoscopic cholecystectomy. *Ann R Coll Surg Engl* 1993; **75**: 199–200.

63 Hughes ES, McDermott FT, Proliglase AI, Johnson WR. Tumor recurrence in the abdominal wall scar after large bowel cancer surgery. *Dis Colon Rectum* 1983; **26**: 571–2.

64 Larach SW. Presented at the Tripartite Colorectal Meeting 1993, Sidney, Australia.

65 Reiver D, Kmiot W, Cohen SM *et al*. Presented at the Annual Meeting of the American Society of Colon and Rectal Surgeons 1994, Orlando, Florida, USA.

66 Uddo J. Laparoscopic colectomy. Presented at the University of Minnesota Postgraduate Course 1992, Minneapolis, Minnesota, USA.

67 Binderow SR, Cohen SM, Wexner SD *et al*. Must early postoperative oral intake be limited to laparoscopy? *Dis Colon Rectum* (in press).

68 Reissman P, Teoh TA, Weiss EG *et al*. Is early oral feeding safe after elective colorectal surgery? Presented at the Annual Meeting of the American Society of Colon and Rectal Surgeons 1994, Orlando, Florida, USA.

Chapter 9
Anaesthesia for laparoscopic colorectal surgery

A.H.S. Saleh

Introduction

Laparoscopy and laparoscopic surgery are not new but have a long history. As early as 1910, Jacobeus in Stockholm discussed the application of endoscopy and pneumoperitoneum to inspect the peritoneum, pleura and pericardium. Although most general surgeons have discovered this technology only recently with the advent of video laparoscopy, extensive diagnostic and therapeutic laparoscopy has been accomplished throughout the twentieth century (especially in Europe) [1]. During the 1950s and 1960s, hospitals acquired the relatively inexpensive basic laparoscopic instrumentation, and education for physicians learning the techniques was done mostly by academic teaching centres [2]. Interest in expansion of laparoscopic procedures was slight until the mid-1980s when operative laparoscopic management of ectopic pregnancies began to spread. Major technological developments in instrumentation including video laparoscopy greatly simplified the endoscopic procedures and provided the first thrust for an explosive growth of operative laparoscopic applications in surgery.

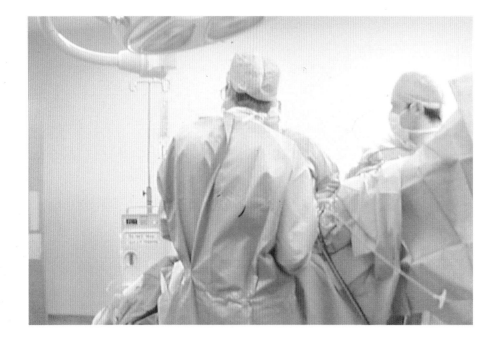

Figure 9.1
Operating theatre setup for laparoscopic colorectal surgery.

Surgeons have developed and refined the operative principles and techniques of laparoscopic surgery, extending its application to cholecystectomy, nephrectomy, appendicectomy, inguinal hernia repair, splenectomy and colorectal resection [3–6].

Laparoscopic surgery minimizes postoperative morbidity. Patient benefits include reduction in postoperative pain, a better cosmetic result, a quicker return to normal activities and a shorter hospital stay resulting in a reduction of the overall medical cost. The intraoperative requirements of laparoscopic surgery, however, can lead to serious physiological changes and complications. While there is a low but definite perioperative mortality rate associated with minor gynaecological laparoscopic procedures, laparoscopy for lengthy general surgical procedures is performed on older patients and patients with acute surgical conditions and is likely to be associated with a higher incidence of perioperative complications. Understanding the nature of the physiological disturbances and complications that might occur during these procedures is essential for optimal anaesthetic care of patients undergoing laparoscopic surgery and helps the anaesthetist in dealing with them and avoiding serious consequences.

The major problems during laparoscopic surgery are related to the cardiopulmonary effects of pneumoperitoneum, systemic carbon dioxide (CO_2) absorption, extraperitoneal gas insufflation, venous gas embolism and unintentional injuries to intra-abdominal structures.

Surgical technique

The surgical technique involves the intraperitoneal insufflation of CO_2 through a Veress needle inserted into the infra-umbilical region with the patient in a 15–20° Trendelenburg position. The electronic variable-flow insufflator terminates flow when a preset intra-abdominal pressure of 12–15 mmHg has been reached. A cannula is then inserted in place of the needle to provide and maintain adequate insufflation during surgery. The laparoscope is then inserted through the cannula and the operative field is visualized by television camera and monitor systems. The surgery is then started and the patient is usually put in a variety of positions including a very steep Trendelenburg position.

Trendelenburg position

Friedrich Trendelenburg, a German urologist, popularized this position in the 1860s for his operations. In laparoscopic surgery, the position of a 10–20° head-down tilt is adopted to keep the small bowel and colon away from the pelvis during blind trocar insertion to minimize complications associated with the insertion. During colorectal surgery various degrees of head-down tilt including steep head-down tilt are adopted. The Trendelenburg position has several cardiovascular and respiratory effects.

Cardiovascular effects
The cardiovascular changes associated with the Trendelenburg position are influenced by several factors, which include:

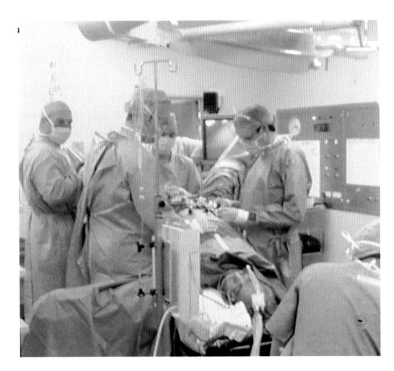

Figure 9.2
Patient in steep Trendelenburg position during laparoscopic colorectal surgery.

1 intravascular volume;
2 extent of head-down position;
3 associated cardiovascular disease;
4 patient's age;
5 ventilatory mode;
6 anaesthetic drugs and technique.

Gravity plays an important role in the cardiovascular and pulmonary systems. The head-up position improves respiratory status (diaphragmatic function) whereas the head-down position increases the venous return and so increases the cardiac output (CO). In a study done by Bivins *et al.* [7] using a non-invasive technique in healthy normovolaemic subjects, it was demonstrated that a 15° head-down tilt caused a 1.8% central shift of blood volume, which is not enough to cause significant haemodynamic changes. Pricolo *et al.* [8] reported a small (10%), but significant, increase in cardiac index without elevation of central venous pressure (CVP), pulmonary wedge pressure, heart rate or systemic vascular resistance in normotensive patients placed in a 10° head-down position. The combination of pneumoperitoneum and head-up tilt causes increased afterload and reduction in CO whereas the combination of pneumoperitoneum and head-down tilt causes increased preload and CO [9,10].

Respiratory effects
The Trendelenburg position causes a decrease in the vital capacity (VC) [11], functional residual capacity (FRC), total lung volume and lung compliance because of the increased weight of the abdominal contents on the diaphragm. The changes are more marked in obese, elderly and debilitated patients. These changes usually have no adverse effects in patients with normal lung function but patients with chronic obstructive airways disease could be severely compromised.

Endobronchial intubation

The potential of inadvertent right main bronchus intubation was first highlighted by Wilcox and Vandam in 1988 [12]. The endotracheal tube, which is firmly secured at its proximal end to the mandible, does not always travel along with the trachea as the diaphragm displaces the lung and carina upward.

Pneumoperitoneum

The most frequent surgical complications are associated with the creation of the initial pneumoperitoneum. These include pneumomentum subcutaneous emphysema, mediastinal emphysema, pneumothorax, hypoxaemia, hypotension, cardiovascular collapse, CO_2 embolism and cardiac dysrhythmias. A thorough understanding of the physiological repercussions of the pneumoperitoneum is essential in order to properly grasp the safety rules governing anaesthesia for laparoscopic surgery.

Pneumoperitoneum is created by intraperitoneal insufflation of CO_2 through a Veress needle with the patient in a 15–20° head-down position during which technical difficulties may be encountered. Results of technical difficulties include extensive surgical emphysema involving the neck, chest, abdomen and extending down to the groin [13] have been reported. Volumes of up to 50 litres of CO_2 can be insufflated during laparoscopic procedures.

Cardiovascular effects

Simple clinical measurement of blood pressure and heart rate may give a misleading impression of the cardiovascular stability. Cardiovascular and respiratory changes associated with pneumoperitoneums have been studied extensively in experimental and clinical investigations. The extent of these changes depends on the intra-abdominal pressure, volume of CO_2 absorbed, intravascular volume, ventilatory technique, surgical conditions and anaesthetic technique.

Modern laparoscopic equipment have an electronic variable-flow insufflator, which automatically terminates the flow when the preset intra-abdominal pressure (12–15 mmHg) is reached. Several studies looked into the haemodynamic effects of pneumoperitoneum [9,10,14–19]. Marshall *et al.* [14] reported no significant changes in CO in a series of anaesthetized patients who were spontaneously ventilating and whose intra-abdominal pressure was 15–20 cmH_2O (11–15 mmHg). Liu *et al.* [15] noted no significant CO changes despite an increase in mean arterial pressure and end-tidal CO_2 during the creation of the pneumoperitoneum. Other studies have looked into the cardiovascular effects of stepwise increases in intra-abdominal pressure up to a maximum of 25 cmH_2O in anaesthetized, mechanically ventilated patients [16]. When the intra-abdominal pressure was 25 cmH_2O, increases in airway pressure, CVP, intrathoracic pressure and femoral venous pressure were accompanied by hypertension, tachycardia and increased end-tidal CO_2. The same group [17] claimed that a moderate increase in intra-abdominal pressure (of up to 25 cmH_2O) may be accompanied by an increased effective cardiac filling pressure and an increased CO. When intra-abdominal pressure was further raised to 40 cmH_2O, tachycardia, hypotension, reduced CVP and decreased CO were observed. These changes were most marked when the patients were in a level position, compared with the head-down tilt position.

So the increase in intra-abdominal pressure has two effects on the cardiovascular system: it forces the blood out of the abdominal organs and the inferior vena cava into the central venous reservoir, while at the same time it increases the peripheral blood pooling and thus decreases the central blood volume. Ivankovich *et al.* reported a reduction in the inferior vena caval bloodflow and CO of more than 60% when the intra-abdominal pressure exceeded 40 mmHg [18].

The relative roles of the factors which contribute to changes in CO may be difficult to separate from each other. The increase in CO at a lower intra-abdominal pressure may result from increased cardiac filling pressures, due partly to mechanical factors, and partly to sympathetically mediated vasoconstriction of the capacitance vessels and hypercarbia-induced effects on cardiac efferent sympathetic activity.

Respiratory effects

Pneumoperitoneum affects the respiratory function as the insufflated CO_2 has to be excreted through the respiratory system. Wittgen *et al.* [20] compared the ventilatory effects of laparoscopic cholecystectomy in 20 patients with normal cardiopulmonary systems to the ventilatory effects in 10 patients with documented cardiopulmonary disease. The patients without cardiopulmonary disease had minor and insignificant increases in the end-tidal and arterial P_{CO_2} and decreases in the arterial pH values following CO_2 insufflation. In contrast, the patients with cardiopulmonary disease had a significant decrease in pH (acidosis) and hypercarbia after CO_2 insufflation. In addition to the potential induction of hypercarbia and respiratory acidosis, hypoxaemia may also occur, especially in patients with documented chronic lung disease. Intraoperative hypoxaemia can be caused by a reduction in alveolar oxygen tension (PaO_2), an increased alveolar–arterial O_2 tension difference or a reduction in CO. Pneumothorax has also been reported during laparoscopic surgery following trocar insertion and intraperitoneal CO_2 insufflation [21]. Finally, a reduction in the FRC relative to the closing volume may be associated with the development of intraoperative atelectasis and intrapulmonary shunting.

Renal effects

Pneumoperitoneum can cause a decrease in renal blood flow, especially if accompanied by a decreased intravascular volume. In animal studies [22], an increase of intra-abdominal pressure of up to 2.7 kPa (20 mmHg) can reduce renal blood flow to less than 25% of the baseline, an effect which is secondary to renal vein compression rather than CO.

Carbon dioxide

Peritoneal gas insufflation is essential for laparoscopic surgery in order to enable exposure, visualization and manipulation of the intra-abdominal contents. Up to 50 litres could be insufflated during a laparoscopic procedure in order to compensate for the gas escaping from around the holes and from absorption.

The properties of the insufflation gas should be that it is colourless, inexplosive in the presence of cautery and laser coagulation, physiologically inert and capable of being excreted through the lungs. Nitrous oxide and room air have been tried and used for diagnostic gynaecologial laparoscopy, but they are unsuitable when cautery is required. CO_2 became the gas of choice for insufflation in laparoscopic surgery because it is readily available, cheap, easily excreted from the lungs and inexplosive. However, CO_2 is not totally innocent and without problems. Cardiac arrhythmias have been reported with elevated $PaCO_2$ in spontaneously breathing patients with halothane [23]. In other studies [24], $PaCO_2$ was highest after completion of the surgical procedure, once the intra-abdominal pressure has been released, suggesting that patients may be at most risk of cardiac dysrhythmias after completion of the procedure independent of the technique of ventilation used.

Rasmussen *et al.* [25] looked into the haemodynamic changes associated with intraoperative hypercarbia in a study of 12 patients with ischaemic heart disease in whom $PaCO_2$ levels exceeded normal values and reached 55–65 mmHg. They reported a significant increase in systolic blood pressure, heart rate and CO, and there was a shortening of the pre-ejection period (PEP) and left ventricular ejection time (LVET) and a decrease in the PEP:LVET ratio, suggesting increased mechanical cardiac activity. It was suggested that hypercarbia caused sympathetic nervous system stimulation as demonstrated by a two to threefold increase in plasma catecholamine concentration.

Complications

Surgical complications

Injuries have been reported as a result of blind insertion of the trocar through the abdominal wall prior to the insertion of the laparoscope. These injuries include bleeding from abdominal wall vessels, gastrointestinal tract perforation, hepatic tears, splenic tears, major vascular injuries, omental disruption and herniation at the trocar insertion site.

Non-surgical complications

The most frequent complications are associated with the introduction of the initial pneumoperitoneum. These include subcutaneous emphysema, pneumothroax [21], hypoxaemia, hypotension, cardiovascular collapse, CO_2 embolism and cardiac dysrhythmias. Other complications include malfunctioning oximeters, pulmonary oedema, endobronchial intubation and the patient falling from the table during position change in the surgical procedure [26].

Cardiac dysrhythmias
The commonest dysrhythmia is bradycardia, which is presumed to be vagally mediated [27,28]. Reasons for bradycardia occurring during laparoscopic surgery include:

1 peritoneal stretch during insufflation;
2 secondary to pelvic manipulations;

3 some anaesthetic drugs like fentanyl, which have a centrally mediated vagal effect, could exacerbate this bradycardia. The use of anaesthetic drugs which have no vagolytic effect make this bradycardia a more frequent problem.

If bradycardia becomes a concern, it will respond to a vagolytic agent such as glycopyrrolate or atropine.

Tachycardia is usually due to inadequate analgesia, hypercarbia and/or hypovolaemia due to blood loss.

Hypotension

The most common cause of hypotension during laparoscopic surgery is the pneumoperitoneum, which diminishes venous return. Other causes of hypotension during laparoscopic surgery include:

1 inappropriate dose of anaesthetic agent;
2 mechanical hyperventilation leading to diminished venous return;
3 hypoxia;
4 bradycardia and other cardiac dysrhythmias causing decreased CO;
5 bleeding;
6 pneumothorax;
7 embolism.

Hypertension

Hypercarbia following CO_2 absorption from the peritoneal cavity and light anaesthesia with inadequate analgesia can both cause hypertension.

Hypoxaemia

Hypoxaemia may occur during laparoscopy especially in patients with documented chronic lung disease. Intraoperative hypoxaemia can be caused by a reduction in alveolar oxygen tension, an increased alveolar-arterial O_2 tension difference or a reduction in cardiac output. Other causes include endobroncheal intubation, pneumothorax [21] and excessive intravenous fluids. A reduction in the functional residual capacity relative to the closing volume as a result of the Trendelenburg position combined with the pneumoperitoneum may be associated with the development of intraoperative atelectasis and intrapulmonary shunting. The Trendelenburg position causes a decrease in the vital capacity (VC) [11], FRC, total lung volume and lung compliance because of the increased weight of the abdominal contents on the diaphragm.

Hypoxaemia is usually more marked in obese patients and patients with COAD.

Anaesthetic considerations

The anaesthetist's goals during laparoscopic surgery are to provide haemodynamic and respiratory stability, appropriate muscle relaxation, control of diaphragmatic excursion, intraoperative and postoperative patient analgesia, and a quick post-anaesthesia recovery. One must also consider that 3–5% of all laparoscopic procedures require conversion to an open laparotomy [29]. Whatever the choice of anaesthetic technique, it is important to maintain cooperation and communication with surgical colleagues in order to ensure a successful patient outcome.

General anaesthesia is the method of choice for laparoscopic colorectal surgery due to the length of time required to perform the surgery, the discomfort to the patient associated with the introduction and maintenance of the pneumoperitoneum, and the extent of the position changes associated with the surgical procedure. Balanced anaesthesia or total intravenous anaesthesia is preferred, and the drugs employed should have rapid elimination kinetics with a short recovery time as wound closure time is drastically reduced. Inhalational anaesthesia alone may inhibit hypoxic pulmonary vasoconstriction, thereby unduly increasing oxygen desaturation. The muscle relaxation is important to minimize the effect of the pneumoperitoneum and make instrumentation easier.

Controlled ventilation with a cuffed endotracheal tube is mandatory in order to decrease the risk of gastric contents aspiration should reflux occur and because of the respiratory changes that might happen, especially the hypercarbia, which may be caused by several factors, including:

1 respiratory depression by anaesthetic agents;
2 mechanical impairment of ventilation by the Trendelenburg position;
3 mechanical impairment of ventilation due to the pneumoperitoneum;
4 CO_2 absorption from the peritoneal cavity.

Use of nitrous oxide

Although there is no conclusive evidence, the use of nitrous oxide (N_2O) during laparoscopy is controversial because of concern regarding its ability to produce bowel distension during surgery and to increase the postoperative incidence of nausea and vomiting. Nitrous oxide may have a clinically significant effect on surgical conditions during laparoscopic surgery; however, most of the surgical procedures reviewed so far are of shorter duration than colorectal surgery.

Nitrous oxide is 31 times more soluble than nitrogen and so a closed air-containing space may increase in size as it may accumulate N_2O more rapidly than it can eliminate the nitrogen. Eger and Saidman [30] observed an increase of more than 200% in intestinal lumen size after 4 h of breathing N_2O.

Lonie and Harper [31] reported a reduction in postoperative vomiting from 49% to 17% when N_2O was omitted in a prospective randomized study of 87 patients presenting for gynaecological laparoscopies. Scheinin et al. [32] reported significantly less intraoperative bowel distension, earlier return of postoperative bowel function and a shorter postoperative hospital stay in a group of patients randomly selected to receive air compared with those receiving N_2O during elective surgery. In contrast, Muir et al. [33], in an extensive randomized and blind study involving 780 patients, found no association between the use of N_2O and the subsequent development of postoperative nausea and vomiting.

Preoperative assessment

Patients presenting for colorectal surgery are of an older age group than those presenting for other laparoscopic surgery procedures and so by nature have a higher incidence of coexisting cardiac, respiratory and other disorders. A careful and thorough assessment, especially of the cardiovascular and respiratory systems, is essential as they are greatly affected by the surgical technique either through the change in position (the Trendelenburg position) or the creation of a pneumoperitoneum or both. All patients should be in optimum condition for surgery. Chronic cardiorespiratory diseases should be optimized before surgery. The presence of significant lung disease has to be considered carefully as there are studies [20,34], as well as our own data, that document profound intraoperative hypoxaemia and respiratory acidosis in patients with chronic obstructive and restrictive lung diseases.

Routine preoperative investigations are required according to the patient's medical fitness. As a part of the preoperative visit, the anaesthetist will explain to the patient the procedures related to the anaesthetic technique and the choice of postoperative analgesia.

Orally administered anxiolytics such as lorazepam or temazepam, given 1–2 h before surgery, should be sufficient as a premedication. Whenever possible, regular medication should not be interrupted. Patients who are on medication for asthma, hypertension, ischaemic heart disease, heart failure or epilepsy should continue with their medication throughout the day of surgery. Patients with diabetes mellitus should have their diabetic medication regimen assessed and modified for the perioperative period.

Anaesthetic technique

Appropriate anaesthetic techniques and monitoring facilitate surgery and allow early detection and reduction of complications.

Monitoring

Patients should be monitored carefully intraoperatively. Standard monitoring should include:

- continuous electrocardiogram;
- non-invasive blood pressure;
- pulse oximetry;
- end-tidal CO_2;
- inspired oxygen concentration;
- neuromuscular blockade monitoring;
- airway pressure;
- temperature;
- central venous pressure;
- breath sounds, especially during pneumoperitoneum, for detection of pneumothorax [21] and gas embolism;
- urine output;
- invasive arterial monitoring in high-risk patients.

Patients with significant cardiac and/or respiratory diseases should have an invasive arterial monitoring device for continuous blood pressure monitoring and for frequent blood gas analyses. It is assumed that end-tidal CO_2 and arterial CO_2 partial pressure are equal in patients with normal cardiorespiratory function, but in patients with cardiorespiratory diseases this is not the case; in addition, the

Figure 9.3
*Anaesthetic monitoring
equipment.*

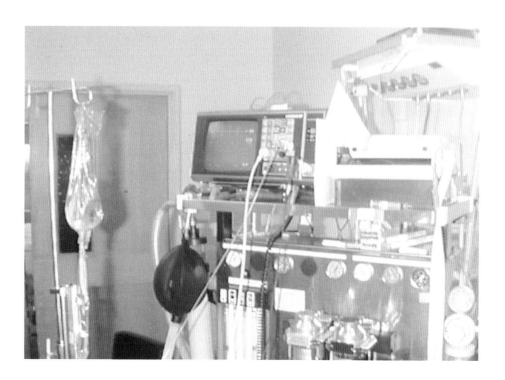

ventilation–perfusion mismatch that occurs due to the Trendelenburg position and the pneumoperitoneum makes repeated arterial blood gas analyses essential.

Induction and maintenance

Once the patient is in the anaesthetic room, a wide bore intravenous cannula should be sited and properly secured in case of severe blood loss. After the patient has been connected to the monitors and the initial readings have been noted, pre-oxygenation followed by induction of anaesthesia commences.

Anaesthesia is induced with fentanyl, propofol and atracurium and the patient is ventilated with oxygen in air. After the patient is asleep, the eyes are taped shut for protection, a nasogastric tube is placed in position and the CVP line is inserted. Anaesthesia is maintained using total intravenous anaesthesia with propofol and atracurium infusions and intermittent doses of fentanyl. The atracurium infusion is usually stopped about 5–10 min before the surgery finishes.

Colorectal surgery is usually a lengthy procedure and measures should therefore be taken to minimize heat loss. Ventilatory settings should be reviewed and adjusted frequently, using end-tidal CO_2 or $PaCO_2$ measurements if an arterial line is *in situ*, in order to prevent hypercarbia. Urine output should be monitored and, if decreased, should be encouraged. Patients should be monitored carefully and anaesthetists should communicate with the surgeons and should not hesitate to recommend continuing the procedure as an open one if haemodynamics or ventilatory difficulties arise at any time.

Once the patient is in the recovery room, routine monitoring of blood pressure, oxygen saturation and heart rate is performed. If the patient is hypothermic, measures are taken to warm the patient and to prevent further heat loss. Postoperative analgesia is instituted immediately once the patient is in the recovery room.

Postoperative analgesia

Postoperative pain relief is a very important issue in colorectal surgery as it is major surgery. Although the incision used to deliver the resected segment is considerably smaller than a formal laparotomy incision, pain is still present and is an issue that needs addressing. Patients who undergo laparoscopic colorectal surgery without perineal involvement are usually given intravenous morphine delivered through patient-controlled analgesia (PCA) machines. Those who have perineal involvement or those who cannot be given PCA are best given epidural analgesia. In our unit we use fentanyl 10 μg/ml in 0.1% bupivacaine for our epidural infusion and it is given either as an infusion only or as PCA with background infusion.

Postoperative respiratory function

Laparoscopic surgery has a less profound effect on respiratory function than conventional abdominal surgery (laparotomy), especially when involving upper abdominal surgery. Forced expiratory volume (FEV_1) and forced VC are markedly reduced after upper abdominal surgery, by up to 50% in the first 24 h [35,36], and a reduction of more than 20% is still present on the third postoperative day. Reduction in forced VC and FEV_1 after laparoscopic cholecystectomy is much less marked in the first 24 h and by the third postoperative day respiratory function has almost returned to normal [37].

Management of intraoperative complications

Gas embolism

Gas embolism can occur during insufflation through a misplaced Veress needle. Death from gas embolism has been reported [38–40] and is a well recognized cause of cardiovascular collapse during laparoscopy. The clinical features of gas embolism are due to the reduction in CO and the ventilation perfusion mismatch that follows and includes a splashing millwheel murmur, hypotension, a progressive drop in end-tidal CO_2, cyanosis and eventually cardiovascular collapse causing death if the gas embolism is big enough to produce cessation of CO. Management of a clinically significant gas embolism is to stop gas insufflation immediately, administer 100% oxygen and position the patient in a steep left lateral Trendelenburg position in order to keep the gas embolus in the right atrium, and aspirate the gas through the CVP. Cardiac resuscitation including cardiac massage may be required for restoration of cardiac rhythm and output.

Pneumothorax

Pneumothorax has been associated with laparoscopic surgery [21,41–44]. It can occur after the pneumoperitoneum because of passage of gas through weak points or defects in the diaphragm [21] or through a puncture hole in the mesentery or falciform ligament [42,43]. Breath sounds should be monitored carefully during laparoscopic surgery. An anaesthetic gas analyser and capnometer are useful in confirming the cause of the pneumothorax. Clinical signs may include a drop in oxygen saturation, diminished breath sounds, increased airways pressure, hypotension, tachycardia or bradycardia. If the patient is haemodynamically stable, then this pneumothorax can be treated conservatively as CO_2 is rapidly absorbed and once the pneumoperitoneum is released it should not recur. However if the patient is haemodynamically unstable, aspiration of the gas rather than a formal chest drain is acceptable.

Hypotension

Hypotension may happen as a result of blood loss, pneumoperitoneum or cardiac arrhythmias. Whether the hypotension is due to pneumoperitoneum or blood loss, the administration of intravenous fluids will increase the preload and should be enough to restore the blood pressure. If hypotension is due to cardiac arrhythmias, then it should be treated appropriately. If hypotension is severe and not responding to simple measures like intravenous fluids and the Trendelenburg position, the possibility of gas embolism occurring should be considered.

Bradycardia

Bradycardia is usually due to vagal stimulation and responds well to small doses of either glycopyrrolate (0.2–0.6 mg) or atropine (0.3–0.6 mg). Other causes of bradycardia should be first eliminated (e.g. hypoxia).

Hypoxaemia

Hypoxaemia may occur during laparoscopy. Intraoperative hypoxaemia can be caused by a reduction in alveolar oxygen tension, an increased alveolar-arterial O_2 tension difference, a reduction in cardiac output, endobroncheal intubation, pneumothorax [21], excesive intravenous fluids and a reduction in the functional residual capacity relative to the closing volume as a result of the Trendelenburg position combined with the pneumoperitoneum.

Hypoxaemia is usually more marked in obese patients and patients with COAD. Generally treatment is directed towards treating the cause and increasing the inspired oxygen concentration.

Conclusion

Laparoscopic surgery minimizes postoperative morbidity. Patient benefits include reduction in postoperative pain, a better cosmetic result, a quicker return to normal activities and a shorter hospital stay. The intraoperative requirements of laparoscopic surgery, however, can lead to serious physiological changes and complications. Understanding the nature of the physiological disturbances and complications that might happen during these procedures is essential for optimal anaesthetic care of patients undergoing laparoscopic surgery and helps the anaesthetist in dealing with them and avoiding serious consequences. Appropriate anaesthetic techniques and monitoring facilitate surgery and allow early detection and reduction of complications.

References

1   Stellato TA. History of laparoscopic surgery. *Surg Clin North Am* 1992; **72**(5): 997–1002.
2   Rock JA, Warshaw JR. The history and future of operative laparoscopy. *Am J Obstet Gynecol* 1994; **170**(1): 7–11.

3   McKiernan J, Saye W. Laparoscopic general surgery. *J Med Assoc Georgia* 1990; **79**: 148.

4   Semm K. Endoscopic appendectomy. *Endoscopy* 1983; **15**: 59–64.

5   Whitworth CM, Whitworth PW, Sanfillipo J, Polk HC Jr. Value of diagnostic laparoscopy in young women with possible appendicitis. *Surg Gynecol Obstet* 1988; **167**: 187–90.

6   Schlinkert RT. Laparoscopic assisted right hemicolectomy. *Dis Colon Rectum* 1991; **34**: 1030–1.

7   Bivins HG, Knopp R, dos Santos PA. Blood volume distribution in the Trendelenburg position. *Ann Emerg Med* 1985; **14**: 641–3.

8   Pricolo VE, Burchard KW, Singh AK, Moran JM, Gann DS. Trendelenburg versus PASG application — haemodynamic response in man. *J Trauma* 1986; **26**: 718–26.

9   Odeberg S, Ljungqvist O, Svenberg T *et al.* Haemodynamic effects of pneumoperitoneum and the influence of posture during anaesthesia for laparoscopic surgery. *Acta Anaesthesiol Scand* 1994; **38**(3): 276–83.

10 Joris JL, Noirot DP, Legrand MJ, Jacquet NJ, Lamy ML. Hemodynamic changes during laparoscopic cholecystectomy. *Anesth Analg* 1993; **76**(5): 1067–71.

11 Case EH, Stiles JA. The effects of various surgical positions on vital capacity. *Anesthesiology* 1946; **7**: 29–31.

12 Wilcox S, Vandam LD. Alas, poor Trendelenburg and his position! A critique of its uses and effectiveness. *Anesth Analg* 1988; **67**: 574–8.

13 Lew JKL, Gin T, Oh TE. Anaesthetic problems during laparoscopic cholecystectomy. *Anaesth Intensive Care* 1992; **20**: 91–2.

14 Marshall RL, Jebson PJR, Davie IT, Scott DB. Circulatory effects of carbon dioxide insufflation of the peritoneal cavity for laparoscopy. *Br J Anaesth* 1972; **44**: 680–4.

15 Liu SY, Leighton T, Davis I, Klein S, Lippmann M, Bongard F. Prospective analyses of cardiopulmonary responses to laparoscopic cholecystectomy. *J Laparoendosc Surg* 1991; **1**: 241–6.

16 Smith I, Benzie RJ, Gordon NLM, Kelman GR, Swapp GH. Cardiovascular effects of peritoneal insufflation of carbon dioxide for laparoscopy. *BMJ* 1971; **3**: 410–1.

17 Kelman GR, Swapp GH, Smith I, Benzie RJ, Gordon NLM. Cardiac output and arterial blood gas tension during laparoscopy. *Br J Anaesth* 1972; **44**: 1155–62.

18 Ivankovich AD, Miletich DJ, Albrecht RF *et al.* Cardiovascular effects of intraperitoneal insufflation with carbon dioxide and nitrous oxide in the dog. *Anesthesiology* 1975; **42**: 281–7.

19 Schoeffler P, Bazin JE, Fourgeaud L. Anesthesia for laparoscopic surgery. *Ther Umsch* 1993; **50**(8): 559–63.

20 Wittgen CM, Andrus CH, Fitzgerald SD *et al.* Analysis of hemodynamic and ventilatory effects of laparoscopic cholecystectomy. *Arch Surg* 1991; **126**: 997–1001.

21 Miyamoto Y, Higuchi A, Kamitani K, Shakunaga K. Pneumothorax during laparoscopy. *Masui* 1992; **41**(8): 1311–13.

22 Harman PK, Kron IL, McLachlan HD, Freedlender AE, Nolan SP. Elevated intra-abdominal pressure and renal function. *Ann Surg* 1982; **196**: 594–7.

23 Lewis DG, Ryder W, Burn N, Wheldon JT, Tacchi D. Laparoscopy — an investigation during spontaneous ventilation with halothane. *Br J Anaesth* 1972; **44**: 685–91.

24 Desmond J, Gordon RA. Ventilation in patients anaesthetised for laparoscopy. *Can Anaesth Soc J* 1970; **17**: 378–87.

25 Rasmussen JP, Dauchot PJ, DePalma RG *et al.* Cardiac function and hypercarbia. *Arch Surg* 1978; **113**: 1196–200.

26 Shantha TR, Harden J. Laparoscopic cholecystectomy: anesthesia-related complications and guidelines. *Surg Laparosc Endosc* 1991; **1**(3): 173–8.

27 Doyle DJ, Mark PWS. Reflex bradycardia during surgery. *Can J Anaesth* 1990; **37**: 219–22.

28 Melville RJ, Frizis HI, Forsling ML, LeQuesne LP. The stimulus for vasopressin release during laparoscopy. *Surg Gynecol Obstet* 1985; **161**: 253–6.

29 Hanley ES. Anesthesia for laparoscopic surgery. *Surg Clin North Am* 1992; **72**(5): 1013–19.

30 Eger El II, Saidman LJ. Hazards of nitrous oxide anesthesia in bowel obstruction and pneumothorax. *Anesthesiology* 1963; **26**: 61–6.

31 Lonie DS, Harper NJN. Nitrous oxide and anaesthesia: the effect of nitrous oxide anaesthesia on the incidence of vomiting following gynaecological laparoscopy. *Anaesthesia* 1986; **41**: 703–7.

32 Scheinin B, Lindgren L, Scheinin TM. Peroperative nitrous oxide delays bowel function after colonic surgery. *Br J Anaesth* 1990; **64**: 154–8.

33 Muir JJ, Warner MA, Offord KP *et al.* Role of nitrous oxide and other factors in postoperative nausea and vomiting. A randomized and blinded prospective study. *Anesthesiology* 1987; **66**: 513–18.

34 Cunningham AJ, Schlanger M. Intraoperative hypoxemia complicating laparoscopic cholecystectomy in a patient with sickle hemoglobinopathy. *Anesth Analg* 1992; **75**: 838–43.

35 Frazee RC, Roberts JW, Okeson GC *et al.* Open versus laparoscopic cholecystectomy. A comparison of postoperative pulmonary function. *Ann Surg* 1991; **213**: 651–4.

36 Joris J, Cigarini I, Legrand M *et al.* Metabolic and respiratory changes after cholecystectomy performed via laparotomy or laparoscopy. *Br J Anaesth* 1992; **69**: 341–5.

37 Putensen-Himmer G, Putensen C, Lammer H, Lingnau W, Aigner F, Benzer H. Comparison of postoperative respiratory function after laparoscopy or open laparotomy for cholecystectomy. *Anesthesiology* 1992; **77**: 675–80.

38 Root B, Levy MN, Pollack S, Lubert M, Pathak K. Gas embolism death after laparoscopy delayed by 'trapping' in portal circulation. *Anesth Analg* 1978; **57**: 232–7.

39 Yacoub OF, Cardona I, Coveler LA, Dodson MG. Carbon dioxide embolism during laparoscopy. *Anesthesiology* 1982; **57**: 533–5.

40 Clark CC, Weeks DB, Gusdon JP. Venous carbon dioxide embolism during laparoscopy. *Anesth Analg* 1977; **56**: 650–2.

41 Doctor NH, Hussain Z. Bilateral pneumothorax associated with laparoscopy. A case report of a rare hazard and review of literature. *Anaesthesia* 1973; **28**: 75–81.

42 Smiler BG, Falick VS. Complication during anaesthesia and laparoscopy. *JAMA* 1973; **226**: 676.

43 Gabbott DA, Dunkley AB, Roberts FL. Carbon dioxide pneumothorax occurring during laparoscopic cholecystecomy. *Anaesthesia* 1992; **47**: 587–8.

44 Heddle RM, Platt AJ. Tension pneumothorax during laparoscopic cholecystectomy. *Br J Surg* 1992; **79**: 374.

Chapter 10

Anastomosis in laparoscopic colorectal surgery

J.E. Hartley, A. Darzi and J.R.T. Monson

Introduction

The successful restoration of intestinal continuity in conventional colorectal surgery depends upon strict adherence to principles well founded in surgical practice: the anastomosis must be circumferentially intact, constructed without tension and have an adequate blood supply. These basic tenets are of equal importance in laparoscopic colorectal surgery. In the approach to laparoscopic colorectal anastomosis, application of the axiom 'laparoscopic surgical principles are open surgical principles' is thus crucial.

The preliminary steps taken during laparoscopic surgery to permit safe anastomosis are therefore identical to those followed in open surgery. Broad-spectrum antibiotic prophylaxis should be routine, and thorough bowel preparation is considered by most to be requisite for left-sided resection. Adequate mobilization of the colon must be performed in order to allow the construction of the anastomosis without tension, and the vascular supply of the segment of bowel to be resected must be interrupted without compromising the blood supply to the resulting free ends. Finally, bowel resection and anastomosis must be performed with minimal contamination of the peritoneal cavity with intestinal contents. Whether the anastomosis is then constructed intracorporeally or extracorporeally remains largely a matter of personal preference though, as will be evident, this decision is heavily weighted by technical considerations.

With these principles in mind this chapter will review the techniques of intestinal anastomosis available to the laparoscopic colorectal surgeon. Subsequent chapters will present the technical details of the procedures commonly performed and provide illustrations of the application of those methods discussed here.

Which anastomosis?

In theory it is possible to restore intestinal continuity by constructing an intracorporeal or extracorporeal anastomosis. However, in practice, intracorporeal anastomosis is a laborious and relatively expensive venture. The additional expenditure results from the cost of disposable instruments, such as stapling devices, and from the prolonged operating times required. During intracorporeal anastomosis prevention of peritoneal contamination may be difficult. In addition, when performing an extracorporeal anastomosis, dealing with such difficulties as haemorrhage from the anastomotic line, or minor leakage evident on testing the anastomosis, is relatively straightforward. However, all such tasks are correspondingly more difficult to perform intracorporeally, where there is therefore little room for error or subsequent adjustment.

The difficulty with specimen retrieval in laparoscopic colorectal surgery also adds weight to the argument in favour of extracorporeal anastomosis. The dimensions of laparoscopy ports currently available preclude extraction of a typical colectomy specimen through a standard port site. Transanal delivery of the specimen has been advocated. However, for bulky lesions this would require unphysiological dilatation of the anus, and for carcinoma specimens would introduce the risk, as yet ill defined, of tumour seeding throughout the rectum. The authors, therefore, commend this method only for cases of benign left-sided pathology such as diverticular disease or polyps. Transvaginal specimen retrieval may provide a similar alternative for benign right-sided lesions in the female. At present, therefore, most surgeons active in this field elect to perform an abdominal incision, usually by enlarging a convenient port site, in order to retrieve the specimen.

Given the technical problems associated with intracorporeal anastomosis and the requirement for an abdominal incision in the vast majority of laparoscopic colorectal cases, it seems to us sensible to use this access in order to perform an extracorporeal anastomosis as part of a laparoscopically assisted approach to colorectal resection. Nevertheless, intracorporeal anastomoses are commonly performed in certain centres. The various techniques available for intracorporeal anastomosis have no place in our current practice but are included here for the sake of completeness.

Intracorporeal anastomosis

Intracorporeal anastomosis may be used to restore intestinal continuity following right- or left-sided colonic resections. The potential approaches to the construction of an intracorporeal anastomosis are as follows.

Right-sided anastomosis

Side-to-side anastomosis
Multiple applications of a linear stapling device are commonly used at open right hemicolectomy to construct a side-to-side, functional end-to-end anastomosis. Similar devices have been designed specifically for laparoscopic use and are now widely available (Fig. 10.1). These can be used to perform an intracorporeal right-sided anastomosis through a sequence of events identical to that followed at open surgery (Fig. 10.2).

First the bowel is transected with the linear stapler. The two bowel ends are then held with Babcocks in their correct orientation and the antimesenteric corners of each staple line are excised using laparoscopic scissors. A single application of the linear stapler (loaded with the 60 mm cartridge) is then used to create the side-to-side anastomosis. Alternatively two applications of the 30 mm cartridge may be used. The staple line is inspected for haemostasis before closing the enterotomy with a further and final application of the stapler. The mesenteric defect is then closed by either laparoscopic suture or clips.

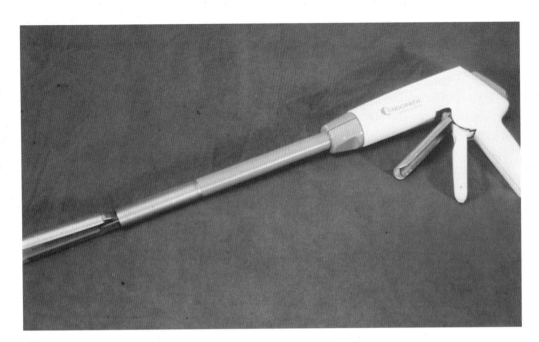

Figure 10.1
A linear stapling device adapted for laparoscopic use.

(a)

(b)

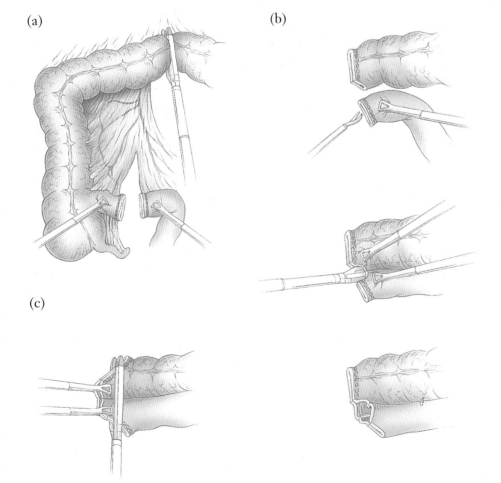

(c)

Figure 10.2
Intracorporeal side-to-side functional end-to-end anastomosis: (a) bowel division; (b) anastomotic creation; (c) enterotomy closure.

End-to-end anastomosis

Whilst the side-to-side technique is generally accepted, if not widely practised, for right-sided colonic work, theoretical alternatives should be considered. Firstly, it may prove possible to construct an end-to-end right-sided anastomosis using a laparoscopic circular stapling device as part of a quadruple stapled intracorporeal technique. Versions of the circular end-to-end anastomosis staple gun have been developed for laparoscopic use, and more specifically for intracorporeal anastomosis. These devices may be introduced via a 33 mm laparoscopy port (Fig. 10.3), but there is little if any experience of their use in right-sided work.

In theory it ought to be possible to fashion an intracorporeal right-sided anastomosis using such a gun as follows. Firstly, the bowel is transected proximally and distally using a linear stapler. The resected specimen is subsequently removed via a small abdominal incision or through the vagina in the female as outlined above. The anvil and shaft of the staple gun are then introduced into the peritoneal cavity via a large laparoscopy port specifically designed for this role (usually 33 mm in diameter), but before doing so a length of 2/0 suture on a curved needle is tied through the eye in the shaft of the anvil, and the needle left attached (Fig. 10.4). The anvil is then detached from the gun and temporarily left free in the peritoneal cavity. Next the staple line on the distal bowel is opened allowing the anvil to be inserted. At this point the needle is passed through the colonic wall 1 or 2 cm proximal to the open end. The needle is left free within the abdomen while the distal bowel is again closed with a further application of the linear stapler. The suture subsequently serves as a pulley to control the shaft of the head of the staple gun. Tension on this suture is used to pull the point of the shaft snug against the colonic wall approximately 1 cm proximal to the staple line. An enterotomy is then made in the tented mucosa to expose the shaft (Fig 10.5). The needle is then removed via one of the 10 mm ports and the staple gun is introduced into the proximal bowel through an enterotomy (Fig. 10.6). The proximal bowel is then grasped by laparoscopic

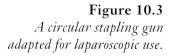

Figure 10.3
A circular stapling gun adapted for laparoscopic use.

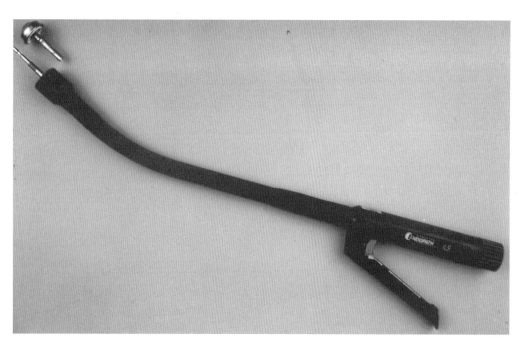

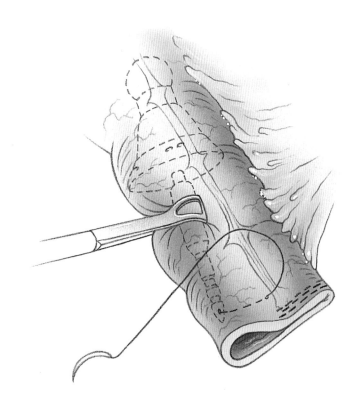

Figure 10.4
The anvil of a staple gun with an attached suture in the distal bowel.

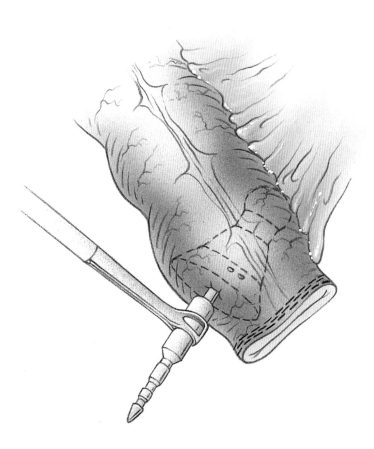

Figure 10.5
The anvil shaft through the distal suture line.

Figure 10.6
Endoluminal stapler being inserted into the proximal bowel.

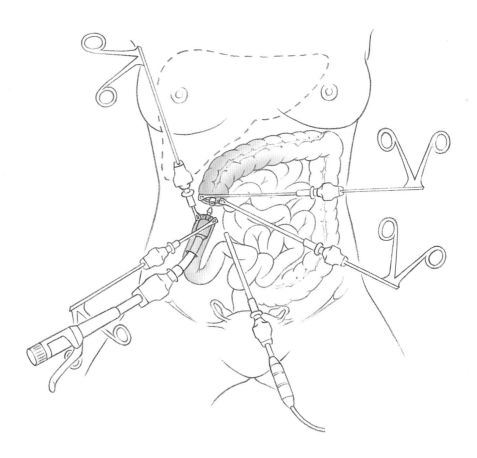

Babcocks whereupon the gun's central spike is advanced through the proximal staple line (Fig. 10.7). The spike is then disconnected and removed through a 10 mm port. The head and shaft of the gun are then engaged (Fig. 10.8), the stapler closed and the gun fired in the traditional manner. After the gun is withdrawn from the proximal bowel the enterotomy is closed by a single application of a linear stapler (Fig. 10.9); alternatively laparoscopic sutures may be used.

The gun is then withdrawn through the port and the 'doughnuts' are checked for completeness. After a final check for bleeding the abdomen is closed without drainage.

Handsewn intracorporeal anastomosis

In theory a handsewn intracorporeal anastomosis can be constructed. This would be performed most readily using a continuous one-layer technique; however, a two-layer or even an interrupted technique could be used. With practice sutures can be tied intracorporeally or extracorporeally. Newer instruments, specifically designed for intracorporeal suturing, are becoming available. However, it is difficult to envisage the construction of a handsewn intracorporeal anastomosis requiring anything other than substantial time and patience, and the associated learning curve is certain to be protracted.

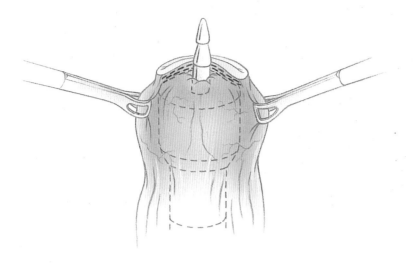

Figure 10.7
The central spike of the staple gun is advanced through the proximal staple line.

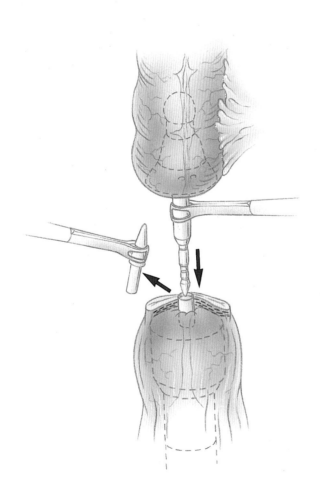

Figure 10.8
The shaft and anvil are engaged.

Figure 10.9
The enterotomy is closed with
a linear stapler.

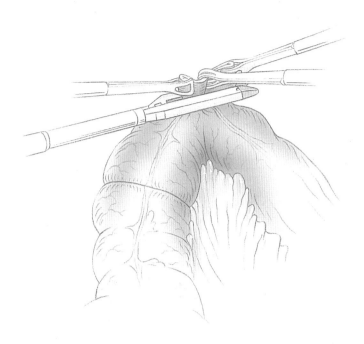

Left-sided anastomosis

There are a variety of techniques by which a left-sided intracorporeal anastomosis can be constructed using one of a range of the circular transanal stapling devices commonly used in open left-sided surgery.

The first of these requires no abdominal incision, and can therefore be considered a true intracorporeal technique. First, the bowel is transected with a linear stapler at the level of the sacral promontory. The proximal colon is then divided leaving the specimen free within the peritoneal cavity. A triple stapled end-to-end anastomosis is then performed as follows. The staple line along the top of the rectum is opened permitting both extraction of the specimen and the introduction of the anvil of the staple gun via the anus. The rectum is then closed once more with the linear stapler. Once again, a suture placed through the eye of the shaft of the anvil serves as a pulley with which to manipulate the anvil (see Fig. 10.4). In this way the shaft of the anvil is brought snug against the proximal staple line whereupon an enterotomy is made in the tented mucosa. The circular staple gun is now introduced via the anus and carefully advanced under laparoscopic guidance until snug against the rectal staple line whereupon the central spike of the staple gun is advanced through the staple line, and then removed. The shaft of the gun is then united with the anvil and the gun is closed and fired producing a circular, triple stapled, end-to-end anastomosis. The integrity of the anastomosis may be tested by examining the 'doughnuts' upon withdrawal of the gun, or by filling the pelvis with saline via the suprapubic port and performing an air insufflation test.

In further modifications of this technique an abdominal incision is made to facilitate specimen retrieval (Fig. 10.10). After delivering the specimen this incision is then closed, the abdomen re-inflated and the anastomosis completed. All these modifications vary in the technique used to deal with the rectal stump

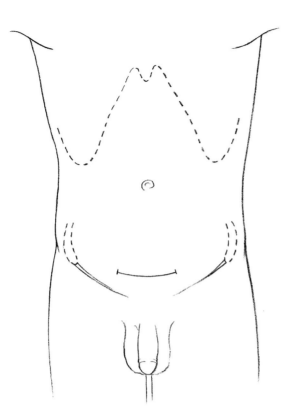

and the means by which the anvil of the staple gun is introduced into the proximal bowel.

Handsewn distal purse-string suture
Here the bowel is transected distally and a purse-string suture is inserted laparoscopically (Fig. 10.11). This is tightened to minimize leakage from the distal stump. A left iliac fossa port site is next enlarged and through this access the bowel is transected proximally and the specimen delivered. The anvil of the staple gun is then introduced into the proximal bowel after a purse-string suture has been inserted (Fig. 10.12). At this point the proximal bowel is returned to the abdomen, the incision closed and the pneumoperitoneum regained. The staple gun is then introduced via the anus and advanced under laparoscopic guidance until snug against the rectal suture line. The gun's central spike is then advanced and the purse-string suture tightened. The spike is then removed and the anvil in the proximal colon snapped into place on the shaft of the gun so that the anastomosis can be completed in the usual fashion.

Double staple technique
This technique avoids the requirement for a distal purse-string suture, the laparoscopic placement of which is technically demanding and time consuming. The rectum is instead transected with a linear stapling device (Fig. 10.13). This markedly reduces contamination from the stump. The construction of the anastomosis thereafter proceeds according to a sequence of events identical to that described above.

Figure 10.11
A laparoscopic distal purse-string suture during a left-sided end-to-end anastomosis.

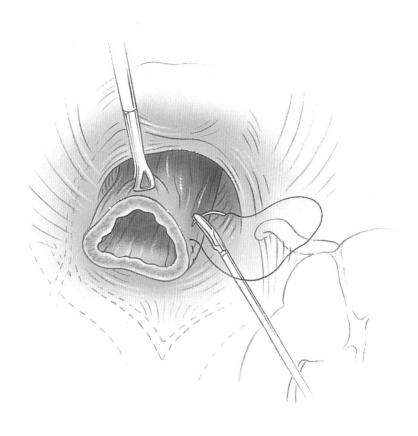

Figure 10.12
An anvil inserted into the proximal bowel during a left-sided end-to-end anastomosis.

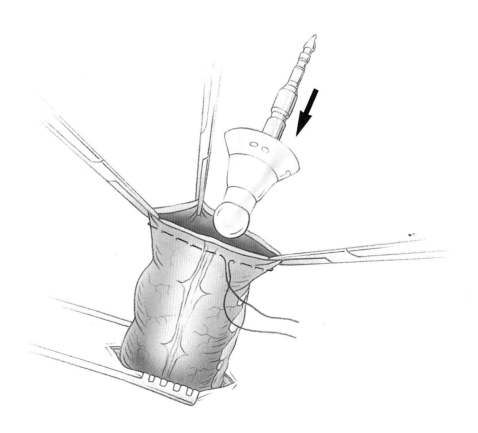

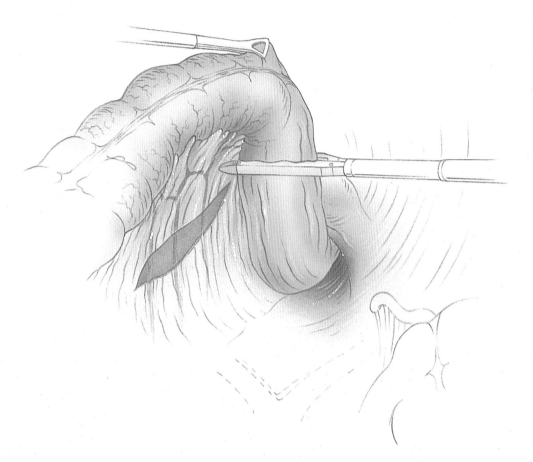

Figure 10.13
Transection of the rectum with a linear stapler.

Triple staple technique

Using this method no purse-string suture is required. Under colonoscopic guidance the anvil is introduced, via the anus, to a position in the sigmoid colon higher than the intended proximal resection margin (Fig. 10.14). Transection of the bowel, proximally and distally, is performed by a linear stapler and the resected specimen is delivered through an enlarged port site. Once pneumoperitoneum had been re-established the shaft of the anvil is guided laparoscopically through an enterotomy in the proximal staple line. The staple gun is then inserted transanally and the anastomosis completed as outlined above. Though no purse string is required the laparoscopic and colonoscopic manipulation of the components of the stapling device still render this method technically demanding and time consuming.

Extracorporeal anastomosis

We remain to be convinced, for reasons outlined earlier in this chapter, of the benefits of those methods of intracorporeal anastomosis currently available. We elect to negotiate the problem of specimen delivery by performing a small abdominal incision in almost all instances. It seems sensible to us to use this access in order to perform an extracorporeal anastomosis, so that this remains standard in our practice. Our procedures are therefore best termed 'laparoscopically assisted'. The technical details of the recognized

Figure 10.14
Colonoscopic guidance of the anvil above the proximal resection margin.

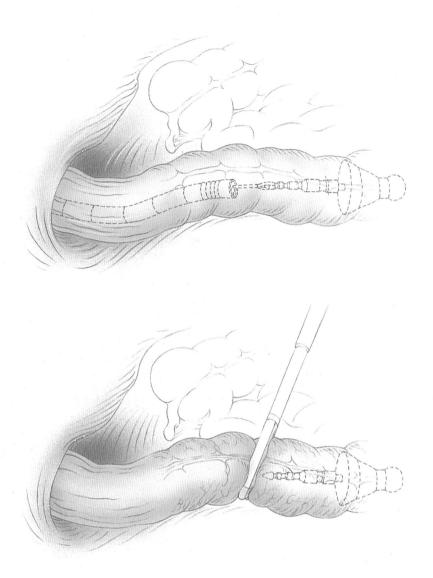

laparoscopically assisted colorectal resections are presented in individual chapters; however, the principal steps will be discussed here.

Firstly, the relevant segment of colon is mobilized laparoscopically thereby avoiding the significant midline incision which is otherwise needed to safely deal with the flexures. Wherever possible, the relevant vascular pedicle is dealt with during the laparoscopic phase of the operation, for example we routinely perform high ligation of the inferior mesenteric artery flush with the aorta (using a linear stapler with a vascular cartridge) (Fig. 10.15) when undertaking an anterior resection. Thereafter bowel resection and anastomosis can be performed through a relatively small low abdominal incision. It is often very difficult to deal with the inferior mesenteric or right colic pedicle through this limited access, so that if it has not proved possible to achieve this laparoscopically the incision will often have to be extended with consequences for cosmesis and wound-associated morbidity. Barring this eventuality, an abdominal incision 5–6 cm in length will usually suffice, and if possible this is centred on one of the port sites. The mobilized bowel is then delivered and transected and an extracorporeal anastomosis completed by a handsewn or stapled technique according to the surgeon's preference. The clear advantage of laparoscopically assisted colectomy

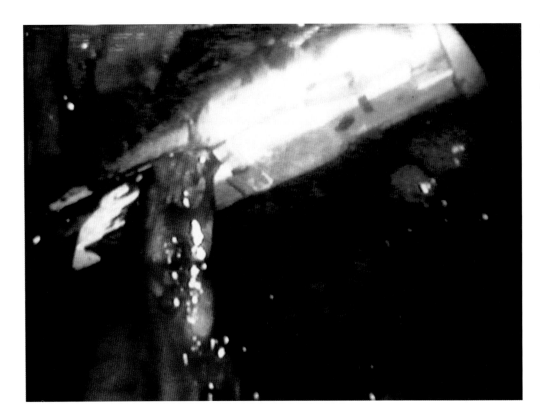

Figure 10.15
Flush ligation of the inferior mesenteric artery with the aorta using a linear stapler.

lies in the facility with which the surgeon can constructed the final anastomosis by whatever technique he or she is most familiar and most comfortable with. We therefore see no reason why laparoscopically assisted colectomy should be associated with any increase in morbidity arising from anastomotic complications.

The authors have thus far successfully completed over 100 laparoscopically assisted segmental colorectal resections, mostly for malignant disease. Anastomotic leaks, diagnosed on clinical grounds, have occurred in four patients, giving a leak rate of less than 4%. All these occurred in patients who had undergone a total mesorectal excision as part of a low anterior resection of the rectum, a procedure described in detail elsewhere in this volume.

Conclusion

The technical difficulties associated with performing an intracorporeal anastomosis, as outlined above, along with the current requirement for an abdominal incision for specimen delivery, lead us to elect to construct extracorporeal anastomoses routinely as part of a laparoscopically assisted approach to colorectal surgery. We currently perform only the reversal of Hartmann's procedures, rectopexy and abdominoperineal excisions of the rectum as true laparoscopic procedures.

There are few data available concerning complications following intracorporeal anastomosis since this is, at this time, not widely practised. However, findings from the largest series done so far are in support of our experience, which suggests that extracorporeal anastomosis can be performed as part of a laparoscopically assisted colorectal procedure, with acceptable morbidity. A number of randomized controlled trials, set up to evaluate all aspects of laparoscopic colorectal surgery, are now under way on both sides of the Atlantic and are expected to confirm this.

It is possible to envisage a number of scenarios by which intracorporeal anastomosis may become more acceptable to a wider number of laparoscopic surgeons. Firstly, accurate histological staging of colorectal cancer requires an intact specimen to be delivered to the pathologist, and at present provides the most important criteria for the selection of patients for adjuvant therapy. If newer, less toxic and more efficacious, adjuvant therapies were to become available it is conceivable that they would be offered to all patients. The delivery of an intact specimen would no longer, therefore, be required rendering intracorporeal anastomosis a potentially more worthwhile pursuit. Secondly, the impending arrival of newer, improved, flexible and articulating laparoscopic instruments, as well as those specifically designed for intracorporeal suturing, may make intracorporeal anastomoses technically less demanding. Under these circumstances the more widespread use of intracorporeal anastomosis may be supported, but this should only be introduced after evaluation by proper clinical trials.

Bibliography

Darzi A, Super P, Guillou PJ, Monson JRT. Laparoscopic sigmoid colectomy: total laparoscopic approach. *Dis Colon Rectum* 1994; **37**: 268–71.

Dean PA, Beart RW, Nelson H, Elftmann TD, Schlinkert RT. Laparoscopic-assisted segmental colectomy: early Mayo Clinic experiences. *Mayo Clin Proc* 1994; **69**: 834–40.

Falk P, Beart R, Wexner S *et al.* Laparoscopic colectomy: a critical appraisal. *Dis Colon Rectum* 1993; **36**: 28–34.

Guillou PJ, Darzi A, Monson JRT. Experience with laparoscopic surgery for malignant disease. *Surg Oncol* 1993; **2**(Suppl. 1): 43–9.

Hoffman G, Baker J, Fitchett C, Vansant J. Laparoscopic-assisted colectomy. Initial experience. *Ann Surg* 1994; **219**: 732–43.

MacFarlane J, Ryall R, Heald R. Mesorectal excision for rectal cancer. *Lancet* 1992; **341**: 457–60.

Monson J, Darzi A, Carey P, Guillou P. Prospective evaluation of laparoscopic-assisted colectomy in an unselected group of patients. *Lancet* 1992; **340**: 831–3.

Phillips E, Franklin M, Carroll B, Fallas M, Ramos R, Rosenthal D. Laparoscopic colectomy. *Ann Surg* 1992; **216**: 703–7.

Roe AM, Harper R, Eltringham WK, Espiner HJ. Intracorporeal laparoscopic resections for colorectal cancer: report of cases of abdominoperineal rectal excision and right hemicolectomy with 2 year follow-up. *J R Soc Med* 1994; **87**: 519–21.

Chapter 11

Physiological changes in laparoscopic surgery

R.J. Delicata, B.I. Rees and P.D. Carey

Introduction

The cardiovascular, respiratory, metabolic and immunological changes that occur as a result of open surgery have been extensively studied and documented and are dealt with at length in standard surgical textbooks. There are, however, four features of laparoscopic surgery which distinguish it from conventional surgery:

1. creation of a pneumoperitoneum using carbon dioxide (CO_2), resulting in:
2. increased intra-abdominal pressure persisting throughout the laparoscopic procedure;
3. absence of a large wound; and
4. a 'microscopical' approach to dissection.

These features produce specific cardiovascular and pulmonary changes and, like their open counterparts, laparoscopic procedures remain events which stimulate a series of hormonal, metabolic and inflammatory changes constituting the stress response. The four cardinal features, however, dictate that the stress response elicited in minimally invasive therapy is different in magnitude from that observed with conventional surgery.

In this chapter we will discuss the physiological changes resulting from laparoscopic surgery. Most of the data available at present relate to laparoscopic cholecystectomy, but the basic physiological changes which occur should apply to other laparoscopic procedures even if these are of an extended nature.

Cardiovascular effects

The intra-abdominal pressure for most laparoscopic procedures is usually kept to a maximum of 15 mmHg. The pressure in the inferior vena cava is normally about 5.5 mmHg [1]; there follows, therefore, a drop in venous return and, since venous return is directly related to the cardiac output, the latter will also fall. Figure 11.1 shows the haemodynamic changes resulting from the establishment of a pneumoperitoneum. Westerbrand et al. [2] showed that the cardiac index falls by about 30% and that the total peripheral resistance index rises by 80%. The systolic blood pressure and the mean arterial pressure also rise. The central venous pressure (CVP) and the pulmonary capillary wedge pressure (PCWP), however, do not fall as expected, but remain largely unchanged because the

Figure 11.1
Changes in cardiovascular parameters following induction of CO_2 pneumoperitoneum. Data are means +/– SD. *p<0.05, **p<0.01, ***p<0.005. (From Ishikazi et al. [4] by kind permission of the publishers.)

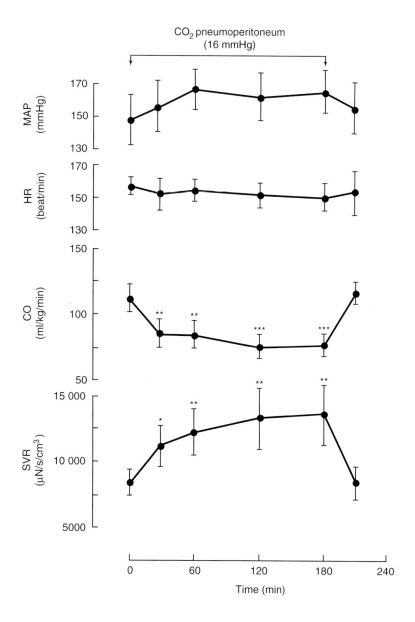

intrathoracic pressure also rises as a consequence of the raised intra-abdominal pressure. The drop in cardiac output is made worse by tilting the patient into a reverse Trendelenburg (head-up) position and ameliorated by tilting the patient to a Trendelenburg position [3]. These changes revert to normal upon deflation. During the procedure the work of the heart is increased overall. This may not be of any great consequence in the fit and healthy patient but may prove hazardous in the elderly and where the myocardium is already damaged.

Alterations in venous bloodflow

Increased intra-abdominal pressure not unexpectedly causes profound changes in flow in the major abdominal veins. Ishikazi *et al.* [4] confirmed this in canine experiments by establishing a pneumoperitoneum with an intra-abdominal pressure of 16 mmHg. These authors demonstrated that inferior vena caval pressure (IVCP) and portal venous pressure (PVP) both rise significantly

(Fig. 11.2) while portal vein flow undergoes significant reduction with the onset of the pneumoperitoneum (Fig. 11.3).

In these circumstances peripheral venous stasis is also enhanced. Following insufflation, Beebe *et al.* [5] demonstrated a rise in femoral venous pressure (10.2 ± 4.1 (mean ± SD) mmHg vs 18.2 ± 5.1 (mean ± SD) mmHg; *P*<0.001) and a decrease in peak blood velocity in the common femoral vein (4.9 ± 8.5 (mean ± SD) cm/s vs 18.5 ± 4.5 (mean ± SD) cm/s; *P*<0.05). A coincidental loss of venous pulsatility (Fig. 11.4) and an increase in the cross-sectional area of the common femoral vein was also shown. All these values returned to normal after deflation of the pneumoperitoneum. Similar findings were reported by other workers [6,7]. Of particular note in these findings is the fact that they were observed in patients undergoing laparoscopic cholecystectomy in the horizontal position; it is reasonable to assume that the values obtained after insufflation would be greater if they were measured with the patient in the reverse Trendelenburg position.

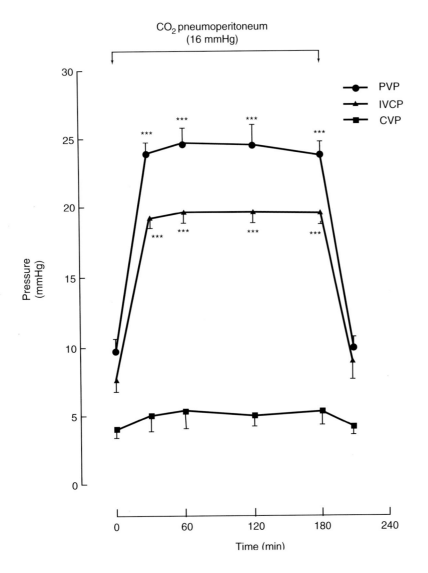

Figure 11.2
*Changes in pulmonary vein pressure, inferior vena caval pressure and central venous pressure after induction of a CO_2 pneumoperitoneum. Data are means +/– SD. ***p<0.005. (From Ishikazi et al. [4] by kind permission of the publishers.)*

Figure 11.3
Changes in splanchnic blood flow following induction of a CO_2 pneumoperitoneum. Data are means +/− SD. *p<0.05, **p<0.01. (From Ishikazi et al. [4] by kind permission of the publishers.)

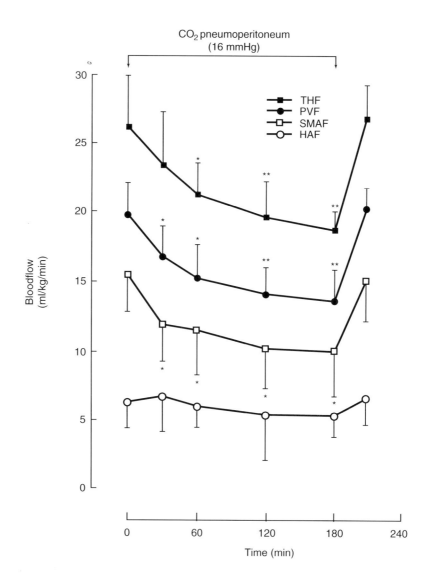

Figure 11.4
Changes in venous pulsatility in the common femoral vein (L) in a patient undergoing laparoscopic cholecystectomy. (a) pre insufflation; (b) post insufflation (By permission of Surgery, Gynecology & Obstetrics, *now known as the* Journal of the American College of Surgeons.)

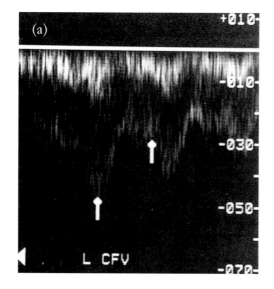
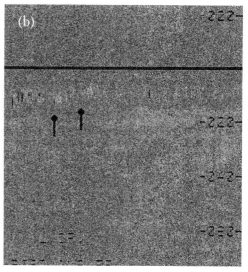

Most early reports demonstrated that laparoscopic procedures take a longer time than their conventional counterparts. Longer procedures predispose to thromboembolic episodes; thus, in the light of the changes in venous pressure described above, does the incidence of deep venous thrombosis rise during laparoscopic surgery? Beebe et al. [5] and Scott et al. [7] were unable to report evidence of deep vein thrombosis at 1 day or 1 week postoperatively. Jorgensen et al. [6], however, reported three thromboembolic episodes in a total of 438 laparoscopic cholecystectomies (one deep vein thrombosis, and one non-fatal and one fatal pulmonary embolism). Kavoussi et al. [8], reporting on a series of 372 patients undergoing laparoscopic pelvic lymph node dissection, describe five patients as developing postoperative deep vein thrombosis. In a confidential inquiry into more than 50 000 gynaecological laparoscopies, both diagnostic and interventional [9], the incidence of thromboembolic complications of laparoscopy was 0.2 per 1000. An important difference, however, is that gynaecological laparoscopies are conducted with the patient in the Trendelenburg position and they have a short procedure duration. Both Peters et al. [10] and Stoker et al. [11] reported no deep vein thrombosis in respective series of 100 and 252 laparoscopic cholecystectomies. However, these same authors report one episode of deep vein thrombosis in a similar number of open cholecystectomies. Furthermore, in a large number of laparoscopic general surgical procedures performed in the authors' hospital (>900 procedures), the incidence of clinically recognized deep vein thrombosis or pulmonary embolism was negligible. Finally, the Southern Surgeons Club reported the largest series so far, with a total number of 1518 laparoscopic cholecystectomies, with no reported deep vein thrombosis [12].

Alterations in arterial bloodflow

Following diminished venous return there must be a resultant change in splanchnic arterial bloodflow. In the canine model mentioned above, Ishikazi et al. [4] also showed that bloodflow in the superior mesenteric artery decreased within 30 min after the onset of the pneumoperitoneum. Similarly hepatic artery bloodflow (HAF) also decreased and total hepatic bloodflow (portal venous flow + HAF) decreased significantly after 1 hour of insufflation. These findings are summarized in Fig. 11.3, and are probably brought about by a combination of the following factors.

1 The action of antidiuretic hormone (ADH), which is released in response to increased intra-abdominal pressure and by occlusion of the portal vein and inferior vena cava [13].

2 The hypercapnia resulting from the use of CO_2 as the insufflating gas. This is due to absorption of the gas into the bloodstream causing an increase in the arterial CO_2 tension.

3 Increase in the caval and portal venous pressures, which it is thought may trigger intrinsic myogenically mediated vasoconstriction.

Blood loss, heat changes and fluid requirements

Cuesta et al. [14], when comparing laparoscopic colon resection and conventional surgery, found that blood loss was significantly less in the laparoscopic group.

These authors speculated that this was due to the more microscopical approach to dissection as in laparoscopic surgery vision of the operating field is magnified and vessels not normally bothered about in open surgery are cauterized. There is therefore less blood in the operating field to prevent light absorption. Similarly, the fluid needs and heat losses were also much reduced in the laparoscopic group. Although insufflation utilizes gases that are at room temperature, the fact that there is no handling or exposure of the bowel to the exterior to a large extent accounts for these observations. However, Jakeways et al. [15], when studying the metabolic and inflammatory changes associated with laparoscopic surgery, showed that body temperature and haematocrit fell in both the laparoscopic and open surgery groups. All the above patients underwent cholecystectomy, which does not require the large incision that is required for a standard colon resection, thus the heat-losing surface is considerably reduced.

Pulmonary changes

Abdominal surgery alters respiratory function in a number of important ways. The vital capacity is reduced to 40% of preoperative values and remains depressed, but less so, for 10–14 days. Likewise, the functional residual capacity (FRC) decreases to about 70% of preoperative levels and gradually returns to normal by days 7–10. The forced expiratory volume in 1 second (FEV_1), peak expiratory flow rate (PEFR) and postoperative oxygen saturation are also reduced. The drop in FRC results in changes in intrapleural pressures that result in narrowing or closing of the smaller airways (<1.0 mm). Ventilation to affected regions is therefore reduced and a ventilation/perfusion ($\dot{V}/\dot{Q}$) inequality results leading to impaired gas exchange and consequently hypoxia. The closure of small airways also leads to collapse of the lung unit subserved by the small airway (atelectasis) [16]. This is the result of a combination of factors: the effects of anaesthetic agents, the presence of an abdominal wound which causes pain and the drugs used to treat this pain. All these factors are also associated with patient immobility. Most authors agree that laparoscopic surgery, by virtue of a smaller wound size, reduces postoperative pain. However, the presence of a pneumoperitoneum with its resultant increase in intra-abdominal pressure has profound effects on respiratory function. Stretching of the peritoneal pain fibres can cause severe pain and the effects of CO_2 insufflation on the acid–base status of the body all serve to produce unique changes in respiratory function [17–19].

Ventilatory changes

Upon induction of a pneumoperitoneum there is a rise in peak airways pressure, end-tidal CO_2 tension ($Pe\mathrm{CO}_2$) and arterial CO_2 tension ($Pa\mathrm{CO}_2$) (Figs 11.5 and 11.6). The consequences of the rise in the latter are discussed under acid–base changes (see below) but in order to maintain a normal $Pa\mathrm{CO}_2$, the minute ventilation ($\dot{V}_E$ must be increased. The respiratory rate (f) also rises and there is a small decrease in the tidal volume ($\dot{V}_t$). The mean vital capacity (VC) decreases significantly. These changes are shown in Fig. 11.7.

Since the pneumoperitoneum causes a rise in intra-abdominal pressure and consequential splinting of the diaphragm, one would expect a degree of basal lung compression to occur. This will give rise to ventilation and perfusion ($\dot{V}/\dot{Q}$) inequalities. The $Pa\mathrm{CO}_2$ to $Pe\mathrm{CO}_2$ difference ($Pa\mathrm{CO}_2 - Pe\mathrm{CO}_2$) depends upon $\dot{V}/Q$

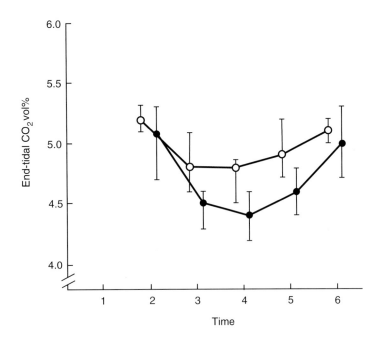

Figure 11.5
Changes in end-tidal CO_2 vol% during halothane anaesthesia (—●—●—) and balanced anaesthesia (—○—○—). (From Johannsen et al. [17] by kind permission of the publishers.)

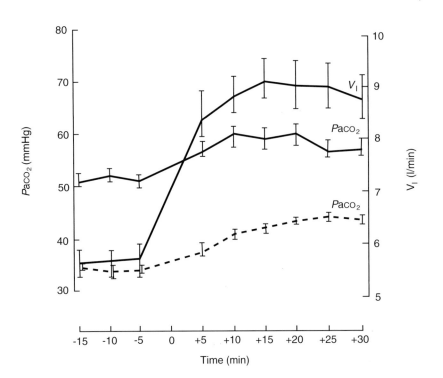

Figure 11.6
*Changes in arterial CO_2 tension (Pa_{CO_2}) and inspired minute volume (V_I) induced by pneumoperitoneum with CO_2 as insufflating gas.
(—|—|—) patients undergoing laparoscopic surgery under anaesthesia with spontaneous ventilation.
(-|--|-) patients undergoing laparoscopic surgery with controlled ventilation.
(Modified from Hodgson et al. [18] by kind permission of the publishers.)*

ratios. Therefore, if $\dot{V}/\dot{Q}$ inequalities result from the pneumoperitoneum, this should show up as a change in $Pa_{CO_2} - Pe_{CO_2}$. McMahon *et al.* [20] did not, however, observe any changes in this parameter.

Laparoscopic surgery is also associated with a perioperative decrease in VC, FEV_1 and PEFR. However, Mealy *et al.* [21] and McMahon *et al.* [22] showed that these changes were significantly less after laparoscopic surgery than after open surgery, and the average postoperative oxygen saturation was also found to be

Figure 11.7
Changes in respiratory rate (f), tidal volume (VT), vital capacity (VC), and minute ventilation (V_E) at various stages during induction of pneumoperitoneum.
Stage I = preoperative control period in the supine position.
Stage II = period after narcotic administration in supine position.
Stage III = period after 20° Trendelenburg tilt.
Stage IV = period after establishment of pneumoperitoneum in Trendelenburg tilt.
Stage V = postoperative control period in the supine position.
(From Brown et al. [19] by kind permission of the publishers.)

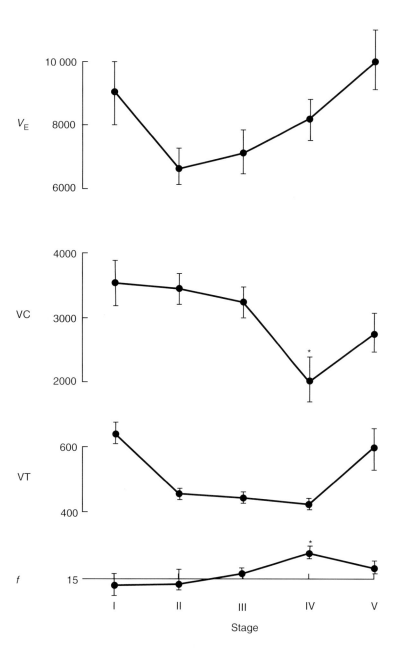

significantly higher in the laparoscopic group. The greater reduction in postoperative pulmonary function in open surgery is likely to produce more small airways collapse leading to increased shunting. The clinical consequence as shown by McMahon *et al.* is a higher incidence of postoperative chest infection following open surgery. It would appear that the increased intra-abdominal pressure leading to increased shunting in laparoscopic surgery has a negligible effect on postoperative pulmonary function.

Pain

The postoperative pulmonary changes in open surgery can be summarized in the following way. An upper abdominal wound produces pain which results in an altered pattern of breathing in order to minimize wound discomfort.

Diaphragmatic breathing is inhibited with synchronous abdominal and lower intercostal muscles undergoing reflex spasm, thus allowing breathing to become shallow and rapid with loss of the ability to sigh. The opiates which are used in pain relief compound the problem by themselves inducing hypoventilation and therefore hypoxaemia.

Most authors are agreed upon the fact that laparoscopic surgery is associated with less postoperative pain than either minilaparotomy or formal open surgery. After laparoscopic cholecystectomy, less analgesia is demanded by patients on patient-controlled analgesic delivery systems and pain severity assessment on linear analogue scales also favours laparoscopic surgery [21,22]. Perhaps the most obvious source of pain in laparoscopic surgery is the inflation of the abdomen with gas, which distends the peritoneum with its rich supply of pain fibres. The abdominal wounds inflicted are much smaller than in conventional surgery and are therefore more easily amenable to infiltration with local anaesthetic agents. Pain is also reduced by the fact that less tissue is disturbed at operation and the need for wound retractors and the assistant's hand to retract bowel away from the operative field are obviated.

Acid–base changes

The cardiovascular and respiratory effects of a pneumoperitoneum are modified further by changes in the acid–base status. CO_2 is currently the gas of choice for the majority of laparoscopic procedures. It is highly soluble in water and therefore diffuses easily across the peritoneal surface into the bloodstream. It is then either eliminated via the lungs or stored. Farhi and Rahn [23] showed that bone is the largest organ of storage of CO_2 followed by skeletal muscle. The longer the duration of the pneumoperitoneum, the greater is the use of the peripheral storage .facilities and consequently the longer is the duration of elevated blood CO_2 level as these storage depots return to normal levels. Under normal circumstances a rise in $PaCO_2$ would induce hyperventilation in an attempt to blow off excess gas with expiration. Nunn and Hill [24] reported that, in patients undergoing laparoscopy under regional anaesthesia, the minute ventilation increased by a mean of 1 l/min in order to keep the $PaCO_2$ within normal limits. When the minute ventilation volume was fixed, the mean $PaCO_2$ rose by 0.6–1.4 kPa.

Wittgen et al. [25] confirmed these findings but went on to report that, in those patients with cardiopulmonary disease, the $PaCO_2$ rose by 2.0 kPa in spite of an increase in minute ventilation of 1.2 l. These data were confirmed in a canine model by Fitzgerald et al. [26] and are naturally of considerable clinical significance in elderly patients and those with chronic obstructive airways disease. Conversion to open procedures owing to difficulty experienced in eliminating CO_2 via the lungs has been reported [27]. Increased $PaCO_2$ results in a fall in blood pH and a respiratory acidosis has been observed both in humans and in animals. It is possible that inability to adequately eliminate CO_2 could be due to shorter respiratory excursions of the diaphragm consequent upon the increased intra-abdominal pressure. Even when helium is used as the insufflating gas in comparative studies with CO_2 a slight rise in $PaCO_2$ does occur [28] and can only be explained by this phenomenon (Table 11.1). However, diffusion of CO_2 into the bloodstream accounts for the greater part of the difference in CO_2 retention observed when CO_2 and helium are compared as insufflating gases.

Table 11.1a
pH changes in insufflation with CO_2 and helium.

	With CO_2	With helium
Pre-insufflation	7.434 ± 0.014	7.428 ± 0.011
Mid-insufflation	7.313 ± 0.015	7.397 ± 0.012
Post-insufflation	7.286 ± 0.018	7.392 ± 0.012

Table 11.1b
$PaCO_2$ changes in insufflation with CO_2 and helium

	With CO_2 (mmHg)	With helium (mmHg)
Pre-insufflation	35.7 ± 1.0	36.7 ± 0.7
Mid-insufflation	46.3 ± 2.2	37.6 ± 1.2
Post-insufflation	50.4 ± 3.2	37.3 ± 1.2

Data from Bongard *et al.* [28] reproduced by kind permission of the publishers.

There are several implications of a prolonged rise in $PaCO_2$. We have already seen above how the cardiac output falls as a direct result of the raised intra-abdominal pressure. Hypercapnia *per se* causes a decrease in the peripheral vascular resistance which will further enhance this fall in cardiac output. Thus a cycle is established which results in a low cardiac output and a further decrease in elimination of $PaCO_2$. The vascular dilatation thus produced gives rise to cerebrovascular effects and subsequent postoperative headaches. This is a known effect of laparoscopic surgery. Further effects of raised $PaCO_2$ were shown by Leighton *et al.* [29] in a porcine model where hypercapnia produced a rise in pulmonary artery pressure. The raised $PaCO_2$ subsequently stimulates the sympathetic nervous system to produce a tachycardia and vasoconstriction. The observed clinical picture is the result of all the above features put together. An added danger of a raised $PaCO_2$ is the tendency to give rise to cardiac arrhythmias [30].

Effects on intestinal motility

Schippers *et al.* [31] studied the effects of gas insufflation of the peritoneal cavity in dogs on small bowel motility. At a formal laparotomy three electrodes were placed on the jejunum at 30 cm intervals. The dogs were allowed to recover and 2 weeks later half of them were subjected to a laparoscopic cholecystectomy whilst the other half had an open cholecystectomy. The period of ileus following the laparoscopic procedure was significantly less (5.5 ± 1 (mean ± SD) h) than that observed following the open procedure (46 ± 5 (mean ± SD) h). Clinical evidence so far supports these observations. The early institution of oral intake after laparoscopic cholecystectomy is now regular practice, as is early discharge from hospital.

Endocrine and metabolic responses

Elective surgery and trauma produce similar physiological responses, which include the release of stress hormones resulting in complex changes in intermediary metabolism (Fig. 11.8), negative nitrogen balance and the

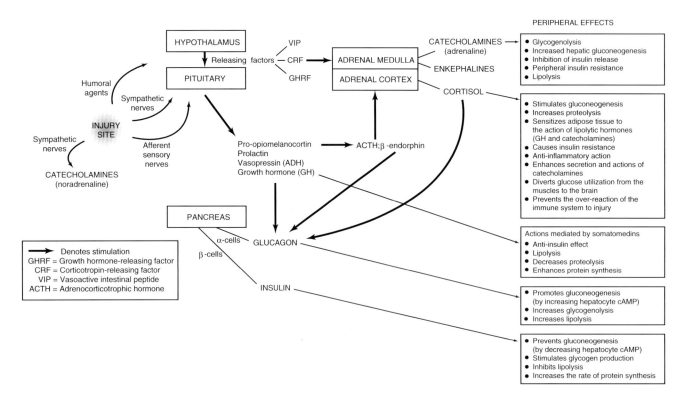

Figure 11.8
*Endocrine and metabolic
response to surgery*

production of a variety of acute phase reactants by the liver. At least some of these changes are mediated by the release of cytokines such as tumour necrosis factor, interleukin (IL)-1 and IL-6. The circulating levels of cortisol, the catecholamines, growth hormone and glucagon all increase in response to stress as outlined in Fig. 11.8. Newsome and Rose [32] showed that the quantitative secretory response of adrenocorticotrophic hormone (ACTH) and cortisol, as well as the length of time over which they are secreted, correlate well with the degree of surgical trauma. Surgery is also known to cause an increase in the glucagon:insulin ratio. Although the level of insulin does increase following surgery it remains inappropriately low for the observed levels of hyperglycaemia after surgery and trauma [33].

Jakeways *et al*. [15], comparing the hormonal and metabolic changes observed after laparoscopic and open cholecystectomy, showed that there was a rise in serum cortisol in both groups but the rise was less in laparoscopic subjects. Mealy *et al*. [21] also showed a rise in both groups, however the opposite was observed and there was a greater rise in the laparoscopic group. Catecholamine breakdown products, namely vanillylmandelic acid (VMA), were also significantly higher in the laparoscopic group than they were in the open group. This excess cortisol response in laparoscopic surgery may represent afferent neural stimuli from the pneumoperitoneum. McMahon *et al*. [34] compared the stress response between laparoscopic, minilaparotomy and open cholecystectomy and showed that cortisol production was less for both minimally invasive groups when compared with open surgery. The changes observed so far with the adrenal hormones have not always shown a consistent pattern, but the rise in blood glucose levels has behaved a little more consistently. The rise in blood glucose levels following laparoscopic surgery is significantly lower compared with open procedures, but no change could be detected in lactate levels following either form of surgery [33].

Immunological changes

Kloosterman *et al.* [35] observed significant increases in granulocyte count and IL-6 levels after open surgery. These changes did not occur following laparoscopic surgery. Lymphocyte numbers did not change in either group, however human leucocyte antigen (HLA-DR) expression on monocytes was significantly reduced in the open group. Monocyte HLA-DR expression is required for presentation of exogenous antigens to T-helper cells, in both the initiation and the effector phases of bacterial immunity. Surface expression of HLA-DR on peripheral blood monocytes has been shown to correlate well with patient outcome after major surgery or trauma, in both the development of and recovery from infection and sepsis. In a similar vein, skin phytohaemagglutinin responsiveness was lost in the open group. This test provides a sensitive indicator of T cell function irrespective of antigen specificity. Neutrophils respond to activation by generating short-lived oxidant forms such as the superoxide anion (O^-) which is unstable and rapidly dismutes to hydrogen peroxide (H_2O_2). H_2O_2 is subsequently converted into hypohalous acids by neutrophil myeloperoxidase in the presence of halide ions. Hypochlorous acid (HOCl) is the most abundant and potent of the neutrophil antimicrobial oxidants. Carey *et al.* [36], examining the effects of laparoscopic surgery on neutrophil HOCl production, compared patients after open and laparoscopic procedures. The type of surgery performed varied from cholecystectomy to major colorectal surgery. There were no significant preoperative or postoperative differences in total or differential white cell counts in either group, but the data suggest that uncomplicated open abdominal surgery caused diminished HOCl production and that no such impairment occurs after laparoscopic surgery. The data so far suggest a lesser degree of suppression of immunological and antibacterial function following minimally invasive therapy. However, this oversimplifies the complex cellular differences which occur and further detailed study is required.

By minimizing the wound size and offering a more microscopical approach to dissection, laparoscopic surgery should in theory reduce the response of the body from both a metabolic and an immunological point of view. Establishing a pneumoperitoneum, however, may stimulate local responses that have stress response characteristics as yet unresearched, which may annul the benefits gained from having a smaller wound. Laparoscopic surgery, therefore, is an exciting field which offers a means of determining the contribution of the wound to the physiological and metabolic responses to surgery.

The future

Several workers have studied the advantages of a helium pneumoperitoneum over a CO_2 pneumoperitoneum [28,37]. The problem arising from the effects of a raised $PaCO_2$ as outlined above are therefore obviated. Helium, however, is very poorly soluble and this poses the higher risk of gas embolism. Various suggestions have been put forward in order to lessen this risk, such as the induction of a pneumoperitoneum with CO_2 and subsequently switching over to helium for maintenance of the pneumoperitoneum. The use of gasless laparoscopy has also been described and may eventually prove to be the way ahead. This will also help in further diminishing heat losses intraoperatively and the likelihood of technical problems such as lens fogging.

The effects of the raised intra-abdominal pressure on venous haemodynamics and postoperative deep vein thrombosis is also currently under study in our and other departments.

The use of intracorporeal anastomotic techniques is theoretically likely to diminish further the magnitude of the immunological responses to laparoscopic surgery. Nothing has so far been reported in the literature about the possible effects of raised intra-abdominal pressure and the consequent changes in splanchnic bloodflow on the intestinal mucosa and hence on bacterial translocation. Clearly more investigative work is required in this field.

References

1   Ganong WF. *Review of Medical Physiology*, 16th edn. Appleton and Lange, 1993.
2   Westerbrand A, Van de Water JM, Amzallag M *et al*. Cardiovascular changes during laparoscopic cholecystectomy. *Surg Gynecol Obstet* 1992; **175**: 535–8.
3   Williams MD, Murr PC. Laparoscopic insufflation of the abdomen depresses cardiopulmonary function. *Surg Endosc* 1993; **7**: 12–16.
4   Ishikazi Y, Bandai Y, Shimomura K, Abe H, Ohtomo Y, Idekuzi Y. Changes in splanchnic blood flow and cardiovascular effects following peritoneal insufflation of carbon dioxide. *Surg Endosc* 1993; **7**: 420–3.
5   Beebe DS, McNevin MP, Crain JM *et al*. Evidence of venous stasis after abdominal insufflation for laparoscopic cholecystectomy. *Surg Gynecol Obstet* 1993; **176**: 443–7.
6   Jorgensen JO, Hanel K, Lalak AK *et al*. Thromboembolic complications of laparoscopic cholecystectmy (letter). *BMJ* 1993; **306**: 518–19.
7   Scott DJA, Paige J, Last C *et al*. Venous haemodynamics during laparoscopic cholecystectomy; a cause for concern (abstract). Association of Surgeon of Great Britain and Ireland Annual Scientific Meeting, Harrogate, 1994. *Br J Surg* (in press).
8   Kavoussi LR, Sosa E, Chandoke P *et al*. Complications of laparoscopic pelvic lymph node dissection. *J Urol* 1993; **149**: 322–5.
9   Chamberlain G, Brown JC. *Gynaecological Laparoscopy*. The report of a working party in a confidential enquiry of gynaecological laparoscopy. Royal College of Obstetricians and Gynaecologists, London, 1978.
10   Peters JH, Ellison EC, Innes JT *et al*. Safety and efficacy of laparoscopic cholecystectomy. A prospective analysis of 100 initial patients. *Ann Surg* 1991; **213**(1): 3–12.
11   Stoker ME, Vose J, O'Mara P, Maini BS. Laparoscopic cholecystectomy — a clinical and financial analysis of 280 operations. *Arch Surg* 1992; **127**: 589–95.
12   Meyers WC. A prospective analysis of 1518 laparoscopic cholecystectomies. The Southern Surgeons Club. *N Engl J Med* 1991; **324**(16): 1073–8.
13   Anderson RJ. Cronin RE, McDonald KM, Schrier RW. Mechanism of portal hypertension-induced alteration in renal haemodynamics, renal water excretion and renin secretion. *J Clin Invest* 1976; **58**: 964–70.
14   Cuesta MA, Meijer S, Borgstein PJ. Physiological responses and advantages of minimally invasive surgery. In: Cuesta MA, Nagy AG (eds) *Minimally Invasive Surgery and Gastrointestinal Cancer*. Churchill Livingstone, London, 1993.
15   Jakeways MSR, Mitchell V, Hashim IA *et al*. Metabolic and inflammatory responses after open or laparoscopic cholecystectomy. *Br J Surg* 1994; **81**: 127–31.
16   Craig DB. Postoperative recovery of pulmonary function. *Anesth Analg* 1981; **60**(1): 46–52.
17   Johannsen G, Andersen M, Juhl B. The effect of general anaesthesia on the haemodynamic events during laparoscopy with CO_2 insufflation. *Acta Anaesthesiol Scand* 1989; **33**: 132–6.
18   Hodgson C, McClelland RMA, Newton JR. Some effects of the peritoneal insufflation of carbon dioxide at laparoscopy. *Anaesthesia* 1970; **25**(3): 382–90.
19   Brown DR, Fishburne JI, Roberson VO, Hulka JF. Ventilatory and blood gas changes during laparoscopy with local anaesthesia. *Am J Obstet Gynecol* 1976; **124**(7): 741–5.
20   McMahon AJ, Baxter JN, Kenny G, O'Dwyer PJ. Ventilatory and blood gas changes during laparoscopic and open cholecystectomy. *Br J Surg* 1993; **80**: 1252–4.
21   Mealy K, Gallagher H, Barry M, Lennon F, Traynor O, Hyland J. Physiological and metabolic responses to open and laparoscopic cholecystectomy. *Br J Surg* 1992; **79**: 1061–4.

22 McMahon AJ, Russel IT, Ramsay G *et al*. Laparoscopic and minilaparotomy cholecystectomy: a randomized trial comparing postoperative pain and pulmonary function. *Surgery* 1994; **115**(5): 533–9.

23 Farhi LE, Rahn H. Gas stores of the body and the unsteady state. *J Appl Physiol* 1955; **7**: 472–80.

24 Nunn JD, Hill DW. Respiratory dead space and arterial to end-tidal carbon dioxide tension difference in anaesthetised man. *J Appl Physiol* 1960; **15**: 383–9.

25 Wittgen CM, Andrus CH, Fitzgerald SD *et al*. Analyses of the haemodynamic and ventilatory effects of laparoscopic cholecystecomy. *Arch Surg* 1991; **126**: 997–1001.

26 Fitzgerald SD, Andrus CH, Baudendistel LJ, Dahms TE, Kaminski DL. Hypercarbia during carbon dioxide pneumoperitoneum. *Am J Surg* 1992; **163**: 186–90.

27 Wolfe BM, Gardiner BN, Leary BF *et al*. Endoscopic cholecystectomy: an analysis of complications. *Arch Surg* 1991; **126**: 1192–8.

28 Bongard FS, Pianim NA, Leighton TA *et al*. Helium insufflation for laparoscopic operations. *Surg Gynecol Obstet* 1993; **177**: 140–6.

29 Leighton TA, Se-Yuan L, Bongard FS. Comparative cardiopulmonary effects of carbon dioxide versus helium pneumoperitoneum. *Surgery* 1993; **113**(5): 527–31.

30 Scott DB, Julian DG. Observations on cardiac arrythmias during laparoscopy. *BMJ* 1972; **1**: 411–13.

31 Schippers E, Ottinger AP, Anurov M *et al*. Intestinale motilitat nach laparoskopischer vs. konventioneller cholezystektomie. Eine tierexperimentelle studie und klinische beobachtung. *Langenbecks Arch Chir* 1993; **337**: 14–18.

32 Newsome HH, Rose JC. The response of adrenocorticotrophic hormone and growth hormone to surgical stress. *J Clin Endocrinol* 1971; **33**: 481–7.

33 Weismann C. The metabolic response to stress: an overview and update. *Anesthesiology* 1990; **73**: 308–27.

34 McMahon AJ, O'Dwyer PJ, Cruikshank AM *et al*. Comparison of metabolic responses to laparoscopic and minilaparotomy cholecystectomy. *Br J Surg* 1993; **80**: 1255–8.

35 Kloosterman T, von Blomberg ME, Borgstein P. Unimpaired immune functions after laparoscopic cholecystectomy. *Surgery* 1994; **115**(4): 424–8.

36 Carey PD, Wakefield CH, Thayeb A *et al*. Effects of minimally invasive surgery on hypochlorous acid production by neutrophils. *Br J Surg* 1994; **81**: 557–60.

37 McMahon AJ, Baxter JN, Murray W, Imrie CW, Kenny G, O'Dwyer PJ. Helium pneumoperitoneum for laparoscopic cholecystectomy: ventilatory and blood gas changes. *Br J Surg* 1994; **81**: 1033–6.

Chapter 12

Liver assessment during laparoscopic colorectal surgery

T.G. John and O.J. Garden

Introduction

The development of video laparoscopic techniques in the treatment of tumours of the large bowel requires the adoption of the same fundamental oncological principles which have emerged during the era of conventional colorectal cancer surgery. The challenge of achieving an adequate tumour resection, with safe restoration of intestinal continuity where appropriate, has been covered in detail elsewhere in the text. However, the laparoscopic surgeon must also overcome the constraints of restricted access in performing a full examination of the abdominal cavity in order to fully stage the tumour, just as one might anticipate during exploratory laparotomy. Intraoperative assessment of the liver is of particular importance in this respect.

Rationale for liver assessment during minimal access colorectal cancer surgery

As many as 50% of patients with a diagnosis of colorectal carcinoma will eventually develop liver metastases. This factor alone has a profound influence on prognosis and is the predominant cause of death within 3 years of resection of the primary tumour [1]. Synchronous liver metastases discovered around the time of the primary operation, either by preoperative radiological investigations or by intraoperative palpation of the liver, have been reported with an incidence of 15–20% [1,2]. However, a further group of patients are known to harbour 'occult' liver metastases which may not be apparent until their metachronous discovery in the postoperative period. Goligher recognized the existence of occult liver metastases and their implication in early postoperative death [3]. Postmortem examinations were performed in 31 patients who had died shortly after colorectal cancer resection and these revealed previously undiscovered liver metastases in five (16%) [3]. Of 1193 patients undergoing apparently curative colorectal cancer resections in the Massachusetts General Hospital during the 1960s, Welch and Donaldson reported the appearance of liver metastases in 71% of 177 patients who represented with recurrent disease [4]. More recently, Finlay and McArdle reported the detection of overt hepatic metastases in six out of 43 patients (14%) undergoing laparotomy for colorectal carcinoma [5]. However, occult hepatic metastases were subsequently discovered by transabdominal ultrasonography, computed tomography (CT) scanning and radioisotope scintigraphy in 11 of the remaining 37 patients (29%) in whom a curative resection had been anticipated [6]. Their long-term follow-up of a larger cohort of patients revealed occult hepatic metastases in 24% [5]. The crude 5-year survival rate of patients with occult tumour dissemination was only 6%, whereas the disease-related 5-year survival rates for patients without evidence for occult metastases were 100, 76 and 59% in those with 'corrected' Dukes' stage A, B and C tumours, respectively (Fig. 12. 1) [5].

Thus, a basic tenet of colorectal cancer surgery holds that accurate tumour staging at the time of the primary resection has profound implications for the continuing management of the patient, and that this should not be restricted solely to an examination of the resection specimen. The early detection of occult liver metastases is important if informed decisions are to be made regarding the appropriateness of additional regional or systemic therapies. Such variables may substantially affect the outcome of clinical trials designed to evaluate both novel surgical procedures and regimens of adjuvant therapy. Prompt detection of localized liver lesions may identify patients suitable for hepatic resection with curative intent. Moreover, if accurate staging could identify patients at low risk from tumour recurrence, then the need for intensive follow-up with its economic implications might be averted.

The most sensitive method for detecting space-occupying lesions within the liver during exploratory laparotomy is the combination of careful bimanual palpation of the organ and intraoperative contact ultrasound scanning. This is the 'gold standard' by which newer techniques should be judged. However, manual palpation of the abdominal organs is precluded during laparoscopic procedures, and laparoscopic instruments convey only limited tactile feedback to the operator. Although the laparoscopic view of the surface of the abdominal viscera is unrivalled in its resolution and detail, there is little perception of the composition and texture of the underlying tissues. The limitations of a laparoscopic inspection may now be addressed with the advent of laparoscopic ultrasonography whereby high resolution intraoperative ultrasound technology has been modified for laparoscopic use. This strategy seems destined to supplant

Figure 12.1
Patient survival rates following 'curative' resection of colorectal carcinomas based upon traditional Dukes' staging (A–C). The survival of patients in whom occult hepatic metastases (OHM) were detected intraoperatively is shown for comparison.

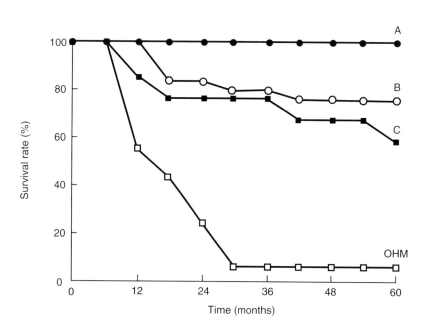

the surgeon's palpating hand as a method of assessing the abdominal organs during laparoscopic procedures, and may well become regarded as an indispensable means of achieving a full staging assessment of the liver during minimal access colorectal cancer operations.

Background

Preoperative hepatic assessment

Preoperative investigations have little value in the detection of colorectal liver metastases in patients for whom an exploratory laparotomy is already inevitable. Prospective comparative studies evaluating the accuracy of liver function tests, serum tumour markers, radioisotope scintigraphy, CT scans (variously enhanced with intravenous water-soluble or lipid contrast, or by arterial portography), transabdominal ultrasonography and/or magnetic resonance imaging (MRI) have shown little benefit over intraoperative assessment in detecting hepatic metastases in advance of exploratory laparotomy [7–11]. Irrespective of whether the findings of these tests were considered alone or in combination, preoperative staging investigations were unable to satisfactorily define the exact number and location of hepatic lesions compared with direct liver palpation, especially when the metastases measured less than 3 cm in diameter. Thus, screening methods for the detection of liver metastases have become redundant in favour of a more informative operative assessment in patients facing an open operation to resect colorectal carcinoma.

Operative assessment of the liver

For many years before the development of cross-sectional radiological scanning techniques, bimanual palpation of the liver during exploratory laparotomy was the only method for the evaluation of the abdomen for hepatic metastases. Two groups of researchers highlighted the apparent remarkable accuracy of detecting such metastases by operative palpation of the liver. Forty years ago, Hogg and Pack evaluated a series of 100 patients who had undergone postmortem examination following death within 30 days of surgery for a variety of primary malignancies [12]. The liver had been regarded as disease free at the time of laparotomy in each case and unsuspected metastatic liver deposits were demonstrated in just 5% of examinations. In a similarly designed study of 116 patients, Gray later reported that the surgeon had failed to define metastatic liver disease in 6% of patients, with a 'false positive' rate of 8% [13]. When patients with only macroscopically obvious lesions were considered, the 'excusable' error rates were just 2 and 3%, respectively.

Intraoperative ultrasound assessment of the liver during hepatic resection

Interest in intraoperative ultrasonography of the liver was stimulated by the availability of high resolution, linear array contact ultrasound probes which were compact, sterilizable, watertight and easily applied, and which provided readily interpretable dynamic B-mode images [14]. Intraoperative ultrasound has also been successfully exploited during operations for benign and malignant pancreatic disease, renal calculi and biliary calculi, and in neurosurgery and vascular surgery. However, it is in the operative assessment of the liver that high resolution contact ultrasonography has had its most dramatic impact over the last 10 years, a period notable for advances in the practice of resectional liver surgery based upon segmental hepatic anatomy. At the same time, the fallibility of exploratory laparotomy in detecting hepatic masses has been recognized [15] along with a general desire to improve the operative detection of 'occult' liver metastases.

The advantage of contact ultrasound over conventional forms of imaging stems from the direct apposition of the ultrasound tranducer with the underlying organ. The smooth moist capsule of the non-diseased liver is an ideal interface for intraoperative ultrasound. The absence of interposed bowel gas and body wall tissues permits the use of high frequency ultrasound probes (≥ 5 MHz), which provide images of exceptional resolution and quality.

Several studies have testified to the sensitivity of intraoperative ultrasound compared with conventional preoperative investigations in detecting established hepatic metastases in patients under consideration for liver resection [16,17]. Intraoperative ultrasound may be used to demonstrate precisely the pattern of intrahepatic disease and so determine the feasibility of the various strategies of anatomical liver resection [18–22]. Targeted needle biopsy of intrahepatic lesions is facilitated, and the advancing plane of the liver resection may be accurately directed so as to maintain adequate margins of tumour clearance thus minimizing the risk of tumour recurrence [23,24]. The value of intraoperative hepatic ultrasound is even more apparent during operations for hepatocellular carcinoma in patients with hepatic cirrhosis where the operator's tactile ability to localize intrahepatic tumour is substantially impaired by the rigid and nodular liver. Thus, small tumours may be distinguished from cirrhotic nodules [25], and intraoperative ultrasound used to devise precise parenchyma-sparing anatomical resections in attempts to diminish operative blood loss and preserve postoperative hepatic function [26–29].

Intraoperative ultrasound detection of occult hepatic metastases

A series of studies has demonstrated that intraoperative ultrasound is the most sensitive available method for the detection of metastatic liver disease at the time of open colorectal cancer operations. When comparisons between tests were made on a 'lesion-by-lesion' basis, sensitivities for intraoperative ultrasound ranged from 90–98%, compared with 41–49% for preoperative ultrasonography, 47% for preoperative CT scanning, and 66–75% for intraoperative inspection and palpation [19,30–32]. Despite careful operative assessment of the liver, intraoperative ultrasound may be the only method sensitive enough to detect impalpable lesions in 14–24% of those patients ultimately documented as having liver metastases (Table 12.1). Impalpable intrahepatic tumours detected by intraoperative ultrasonography alone were 4–18 mm in maximum diameter and situated 1–6 cm below the liver surface in one study [30]. Conversely, those palpable lesions which were undetected by intraoperative ultrasound were superficially located and measured 2–5 mm in diameter. However, the apparent large disparity between intraoperative ultrasound and other methods of detection is diminished when its impact in detecting liver metastases is analysed on a 'patient-by-patient' basis (Table 12.1) [31,33–36]; in some cases the data were reported without the benefit of long-term follow-up.

Reference	No. of patients	Palpation only	Palpation and IOUS	IOUS only (% of all patients with metastases)
Boldrini et al. [33]	86	18/21 (86%)	21/21 (100%)	3/21 (14%)
Charnley et al. [34]	99	18/26 (69%)	24/26 (92%)	6/26 (23%)
Stadler et al. [31]	85	21/27 (78%)	25/27 (93%)	4/27 (15%)
Stewart et al. [35]	100	13/17 (76%)	17/17 (100%)	4/17 (24%)
Stone et al. [36]*	56	4/13 (31%)	7/13 (54%)	3/13 (23%)

* Takes into account 'false negatives' determined by 22.7-month follow-up.

Table 12.1

Sensitivity of operative palpation and intraoperative ultrasound (IOUS) in the detection of patients with liver metastases during laparotomy for colorectal cancer resection.

Machi and colleagues reported the results of a prospective study comparing the accuracy of intraoperative ultrasound with operative inspection and palpation of the liver as well as preoperative ultrasonography and CT scanning in detecting hepatic metastases on a 'lesion-by-lesion' basis in patients undergoing colorectal cancer resections (Table 12.2) [19,30]. Significantly, superior results for intraoperative ultrasound were demonstrated. This study was notable in that patients were followed up for 18–52 months after surgery, whereby the diagnostic accuracies originally obtained were modified in the knowledge that liver metastases had subsequently been discovered in 13 out of 144 patients (9%) thought to have been free of hepatic disease at the time of primary surgery (6.9% of the original 188 patients examined) (Table 12.3). Nevertheless, intraoperative ultrasonography was still shown to have been significantly superior to each of the other methods with respect to its sensitivity, negative predicitive value and overall accuracy in detecting metastases.

Some authors have questioned the incremental benefit and cost-effectiveness of intraoperative ultrasound as a screening procedure in individual patients undergoing exploratory laparotomy at the time of colorectal cancer surgery [36,37]. Stone and colleagues reported that truly 'occult' hepatic metastases were detected solely by intraoperative ultrasound in only 5% of patients screened in this way [36]. However, when a subgroup of patients with T3 and T4 primary tumours only were considered, the incremental benefit for intraoperative ultrasound over all other methods increased to 10%, rising to

	USS (%)	CT (%)	Surgical exploration (%)	IOUS (%)	P value
Sensitivity	41	47	66	93	<0.0001
Specificity	97	94	90	95	–
PPV	90	85	81	92	<0.05
NPV	71	72	80	95	<0.0001
Accuracy	74	75	80	94	<0.0001

NPV, negative predictive value; PPV, positive predictive value.
From Machi et al. [19,30].

Table 12.2

Comparison of the diagnostic accuracy of preoperative ultrasound (USS), CT scanning, intraoperative inspection and palpation, and intraoperative ultrasound (IOUS) in the detection of liver metastases at the time of primary colorectal cancer resection in 189 patients.

Table 12.3

Comparison of the diagnostic accuracy of preoperative ultrasound (USS), CT scanning, intraoperative inspection and palpation, and intraoperative ultrasound (IOUS) in the detection of liver metastases re-evaluated after more than 18 months' follow-up in 189 patients.

	USS (%)	CT (%)	Surgical exploration (%)	IOUS (%)	*P* value
Sensitivity	38	43	60	82	<0.0005
Specificity	97	93	88	92	–
PPV	90	83	80	89	–
NPV	67	68	74	87	<0.005
Accuracy	71	71	76	88	<0.001

NPV, negative predictive value; PPV, positive predictive value.
From Machi *et al.* [30].

12.5% for T3 N0 lesions [36]. It was also evident that repeated palpation of the liver with the benefit of the knowledge of the intraoperative ultrasound findings had led to the discovery of intrahepatic metastases which had not been previously recognized, thus confirming the mutual benefit of operative palpation and intraoperative ultrasonography during open operations.

Diagnostic laparoscopy in the assessment of hepatic malignancy

Laparoscopy was developed as a diagnostic modality long before its exploitation as a means of undertaking therapeutic manoeuvres. Ott, a Russian gynaecologist, has been attributed with performing the first reported laparoscopy in 1901 [38], and Kelling described the feasibility of inspecting the abdominal cavities of dogs using a cystoscope [39]. Jacobeus performed *laparoskopie* in human patients having introduced room air into the peritoneal cavity to create a pneumoperitoneum, and in common with the aforementioned laparoscopic pioneers, he used an early cystoscope and was able to diagnose liver cirrhosis, metastatic liver tumours and tuberculous peritonitis [40]. The technique of diagnostic laparoscopy was subsequently refined with the introduction of the Veress needle [41], the carbon dioxide or oxygen pneumoperitoneum [42] and the forward-viewing laparoscope which was successfully used to evaluate liver disease, ascites, and gastric, colorectal and gynaecological malignancies [43,44]. The development of the Hopkins rod–lens optical system and the fibreoptic bundle finally allowed enhanced light transmission leading to the development of contemporary video laparoscopy systems providing high resolution laparoscopic images for multiple observers.

The utility of laparoscopy in the diagnosis of liver malignancy is beyond doubt. In the absence of adhesions, much of the liver surface is available for laparoscopic inspection, and the high resolution imaging provided by modern optical systems can identify tiny superficial and capsular hepatic lesions measuring less than 1 cm in diameter and which are beyond the threshold of detection of even the highest resolution and optimally enhanced CT or MRI scanning systems (Fig. 12.2). Laparoscopic identification of hepatic malignancy requires that the tumour encroaches upon the liver surface, or that the liver contour be distorted by the intrahepatic lesion. It has been estimated that approximately two-thirds of liver metastases may be detected laparoscopically and are amenable to laparoscopically directed needle biopsy. Bleiberg and co-workers reported that 36% of negative laparoscopies performed in the staging of cancer

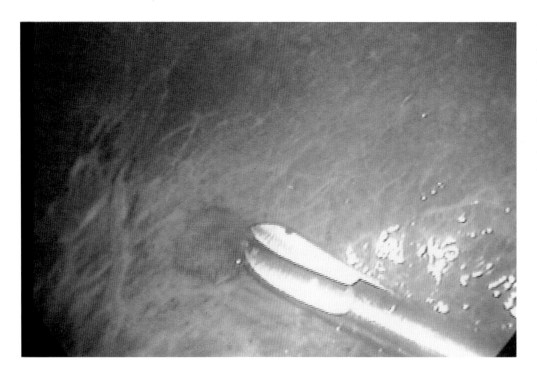

Figure 12.2
A capsular deposit of metastatic adenocarcinoma measuring 5 mm discovered at staging laparoscopy in a patient thought to have resectable pancreatic cancer and undergoing excision biopsy.

patients had failed to demonstrate hepatic involvement subsequently confirmed at autopsy [45]. In a series of 50 consecutive laparoscopic examinations in patients with suspected hepatic malignancy recently performed in Edinburgh, direct visualization of the reference liver tumour was possible in 34 patients (68%) [46].

Staging laparoscopy

Staging laparoscopy is of proven benefit in the detection of the small liver and peritoneal metastases which characterize a variety of primary malignancies, although, perhaps surprisingly, surgeons have generally been resistant to the adoption of this strategy. The laparoscopic discovery of distant metastases may preclude an unnecessary exploratory laparotomy in a significant proportion of patients in whom a curative or palliative operation may no longer be appropriate [47]. Although this philosophy is not applicable to the majority of patients presenting with colorectal malignancy for whom operative intervention will be inevitable, there is strong evidence supporting the rationale for mandatory preoperative laparoscopy in patients with pancreatic and periampullary carcinoma [48–53], gastric and oesophageal carcinoma [54–57], gallbladder carcinoma [58] and ovarian tumours [59]. Its sensitivity in detecting liver metastases has also been reported in the staging of bronchogenic carcinoma [60], carcinoma of the breast [61], malignant melanoma [62] and lymphoma [63,64] in which the laparoscopic findings directly influenced patient management. Paradoxically, there has been little inclination to employ laparoscopy as a preoperative staging tool in the selection of patients with known hepatic malignancy for liver resection. Lightdale employed staging laparoscopy in 16 patients with potentially resectable hepatocellular carcinoma, and discovered factors conferring irresectability in 13 patients (80%) (multifocal tumour, peritoneal dissemination and/or severe cirrhosis) [65]. Similarly, Jeffers and colleagues were able to exclude the possibility of resection in all of their series of

27 patients with hepatocellular carcinoma following laparoscopic assessment [66]. In our own institution, experience with staging laparoscopy in the assessment of 50 patients (colorectal liver metastases in 28 cases) under consideration for curative liver resection revealed previously unsuspected factors contraindicating further operative intervention in 23 patients (46%) [46]. Dissemination of tumour to extrahepatic sites (peritoneal or omental surfaces) was identified in 18 patients and a bilobar liver tumour was defined in 11 patients. All patients had previously been examined by CT scanning (employing a variety of enhancement techniques), and it was clear that the adoption of staging laparoscopy in the preoperative assessment of such patients had made a substantial impact upon their management [46].

Nevertheless, laparoscopic inspection alone is insufficient for the detection of liver tumours in the remaining one-third of patients who present with intrahepatic lesions situated away from the visible organ surface, and in those in whom the liver is partially obscured by adhesions. Nor can the laparoscopist determine their exact relationships with the intrahepatic vascular structures since the liver bears few surface anatomical markings. Documentation of the site, size and number of liver tumours, and their pattern of involvement with respect to the segmental hepatic anatomy is fundamental to the planning of hepatic resectional surgery and to the follow-up of patients who are managed without operation. Laparoscopic ultrasonography presents the means by which these goals may be achieved.

Laparoscopic ultrasonography

Early attempts at laparoscopic B-mode contact ultrasound imaging of the abdominal organs involved the development of prototype laparoscopic probes which incorporated the ultrasound transducer within the telescope shaft. These instruments were called 'echo laparoscopes'. In the early 1980s, several reports from Japanese workers testified to the feasibility of such devices in providing recognizable, high resolution images of intrahepatic lesions during diagnostic laparoscopy, in some cases succeeding where transabdominal ultrasonography had failed [67,68]. Furukawa and colleagues employed a 5–7.5 MHz 360° sectoral scanning probe which was introduced through a separate port from the laparoscope, and reported 'diagnostic value' in 36/42 cases of liver tumour and 8/10 cases of liver cysts [69]. The readily interpretable, high resolution, real time images obtained immediately upon contact of the B-mode transducer with the liver surface was an exciting concept, and more appealing to the laparoscopic surgeon than the unidimensional A-mode images obtained with the embryonic laparoscopic ultrasound devices which had been described during the preceding 20 years [70,71].

Further technological refinements which have stimulated interest in laparoscopic ultrasonography of the liver particularly concern the development of linear array laparoscopic ultrasound probes which appear better suited to examination of the liver than sectoral scanning probes [72]. The potential limitations of the radial scanning systems in examination of the liver was illustrated by Fornari and colleagues who reported their experience with a prototype rigid 180° sector scanning laparosocopic ultrasound probe. Lesions in the posterolateral sector of the liver were undetected, adequate ultrasound penetration of the hepatic parenchyma was not always achieved and orientation of the image with respect to the intrahepatic vasculature was difficult with this transducer configuration [73]. However, the stable and more easily manipulated rectilinear image obtained with linear array laparoscopic ultrasound systems is better suited for cross-sectional hepatic imaging [72], and can even be used to obtain guided needle biopsies of small intrahepatic tumours which are not visible laparoscopically [74,75]. Okita and colleagues described their success in imaging hepatocellular carcinomas while demonstrating tumour invasion of the portal vein [76].

Despite these technical advances, laparoscopic ultrasonography remained an essentially experimental procedure and laparoscopic ultrasound probes were not commercially available until interest re-emerged with the boom in minimal access surgery in the early 1990s.

Laparoscopic ultrasonography in the staging of established liver tumours

Laparoscopic ultrasonography was initially performed at the Royal Infirmary, Edinburgh in the staging of patients with liver tumours. An improvised technique was developed whereby a 16 mm diameter 5 MHz linear array ultrasound probe designed for endorectal ultrasonography was introduced into the abdominal cavity via a custom-built large port assembly [77]. The improved resolution of this system over preoperative CT scanning (unenhanced and iodized oil emulsion-enhanced), transabdominal ultrasonography and hepatic angiography was illustrated by the additional information obtained in seven patients with primary and secondary liver tumours under consideration for liver resection. Laparoscopic inspection firstly identified extrahepatic tumour spread and/or bilobar liver tumours in two patients. Irresectability was further demonstrated in four patients in whom bilobar liver tumour and portal vein invasion were defined [77].

Staging laparoscopic ultrasonography was then utilized to determine tumour resectability in a cohort of patients thought to have potentially resectable liver tumours on the basis of preoperative investigations [46]. Laparoscopic ultrasonography was performed using a commercially available 7.5 MHz linear array probe during staging laparoscopy (Aloka UST-5521-7.5 probe with an Aloka SSD-500 monitor, KeyMed Ltd, Southend-on-Sea, UK). Additional staging information was obtained in this way in 18 out of 43 patients examined (42%) (bilobar or multifocal liver tumour, hilar lymphadenopathy and main portal or hepatic venous invasion). In seven patients, laparoscopic ultrasonography was the only investigation to demonstrate tumour irresectability and so averted unnecessary laparotomies [46]. When compared with historical control patients in whom no attempt at laparoscopic staging had been made, a significant increase in tumour resectability was observed for those evaluated laparoscopically (58 vs 93%) [46].

Laparoscopic ultrasonography as a method of screening for liver metastases during minimal access colorectal cancer operations

In view of the insensitivity of preoperative scanning investigations in accurately assessing the liver of patients undergoing large bowel surgery, and given that the surgeon's ability to manually palpate the liver is denied during laparoscopic procedures, laparoscopic intraoperative ultrasonography is a logical and inevitable development. However, experience with this novel technique is still relatively restricted. So far there have been no published studies evaluating its role in screening for liver metastases during primary laparoscopic cancer resections. Nevertheless, laparoscopic ultrasonography has been shown to be useful in detecting metastases which were otherwise imperceptible [46,78], and these observations seem certain to be reproduced in the context of the detection of occult liver metastases during minimal access colorectal cancer operations.

Technique of laparoscopic ultrasonography

General considerations

A variety of commercially available laparoscopic ultrasound systems are now available and refinements in design are continually being implemented. All probes are introduced into the abdominal cavity through a separate cannula under direct vision of the camera. Although laparoscopic sector scanning probes may have a role in the examination of the extrahepatic biliary tree and pancreas, a linear array transducer configuration is undoubtedly preferred for examination of the liver parenchyma. The system employed in Edinburgh comprises a 9 mm diameter rigid probe incorporating a 4 cm long 7.5 MHz multi-element linear array transducer at its tip (Aloka SSD-5521-7.5) (Fig. 12.3). Following sterilization in glutaraldehyde, the probe is connected to a portable multipurpose ultrasound machine and monitor (SSD-500) which are positioned alongside the operating table. A higher specification system also used offers facilities for Doppler spectral analysis, colour Doppler flow imaging and quantitative flow measurement (Aloka SSD-680), although the laparoscopic ultrasound probe

Figure 12.3
Linear array laparoscopic ultrasound probe in position on the right hemiliver via a 10 mm umbilical port.

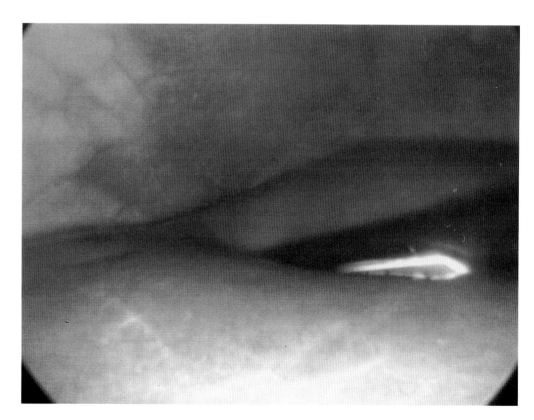

dimensions are similar. Few adjustments to the control settings are required during the procedure (image direction, magnification and gain (or 'brightness')), and these may easily be performed by the operating theatre nursing staff. It is convenient to view both laparoscopic and ultrasound images simultaneously on the theatre monitors, and this may be achieved using the 'picture-in-picture video mixing' facility of an audiovisual mixing desk (Panasonic Digital AV mixer WJ-AVE5, KeyMed Ltd).

The only absolute requirement for port site positioning is that which permits comfortable positioning of the ultrasound probe upon the diaphragmatic surface of the liver (Fig. 12.4). Our experience with over 300 laparoscopic ultrasound examinations indicates that a 10–11 mm port sited at the umbilicus is nearly always adequate for a complete examination of the liver, although a more superiorly placed portal may be required in a very large or obese patient. An additional 10–11 mm port in the right side of the abdomen is useful in order to vary the scanning plane, but this is not essential. Thus, the access to the peritoneal cavity employed by laparoscopic colorectal surgeons would not preclude adequate examination of the liver by laparoscopic ultrasound.

Figure 12.4

Schematic diagram illustrating the orientation of the sonograms obtained using a linear array laparoscopic ultrasound probe via an umbilical port. (A) Oblique scan through the right hemiliver demonstrating the bifurcation of the right portal vein into its anterior (ARPV) and posterior (PRPV) divisions. The right hepatic vein (RHV) is seen passing in the plane between the anterior (segments V and VIII) and posterior (segments VI and VII) sectors of the right hemiliver.
(B) Parasagittal scan angled slightly to the left through hepatic segment V, the middle hepatic vein (MHV), hepatic segment IV and the caudate lobe (segment I) which separates the hilar structures from the inferior vena cava (IVC). The right hepatic artery (RHA) is depicted passing anterior to the main portal vein (PV).
(C) Oblique scan through the left hepatic lobe demonstrating the branches of the left portal vein (LPV) to segments II and III, which are separated from the caudate lobe (I) by the interlobar fissure, and the left hepatic vein (LHV). The hepatic parenchyma acts as an acoustic window through which the compressed stomach (St), the body of the pancreas (P) and para-aortic region may be identified. Ao, aorta; CA, coeliac axis; SMA, superior mesenteric artery; SV, splenic vein.

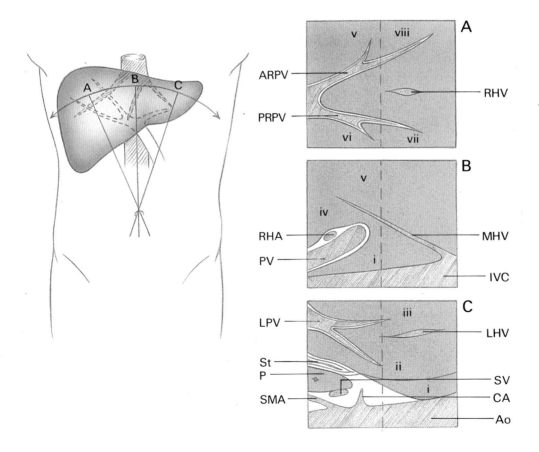

Laparoscopic assessment of the liver

As with any laparoscopic procedure a systematic examination of the peritoneal cavity takes precedence. Thus, the presence of ascites, or tumour dissemination to the serosal surfaces or mesenteric lymph nodes should be sought. The contours and surface texture of the liver are important indicators of the presence of liver disease, especially metastatic tumour. Occasionally, a hepatic mass lesion may compress the portal vein causing splanchnic venous congestion, or a differential in perfusion of one or other hemiliver when portal vein branches are compressed (although this is more commonly observed with portal venous involvement of hepatocellular carcinoma). A 30° telescope is required to obtain the most complete view of the diaphragmatic surface of the right hemiliver. The left hepatic lobe should be lifted to allow inspection of its undersurface and of the lesser omentum, through which the caudate lobe of the liver is visible in most individuals (Fig. 12.5). Scrutiny of this region may be facilitated with the patient in the reverse Trendelenburg position, and following decompression of the stomach and displacement of the bowel loops. The porta hepatis should be examined for malignant lymphadenopathy which might preclude any prospect of liver resection with 'curative intent' in patients discovered to have metastases.

Liver metastases affecting the liver surface usually appear as white umbilicated lesions with fine surface vascular markings (Fig. 12.6). An intraparenchymal tumour should be suspected when a bulge is apparent with a distortion of contour suggesting an underlying mass effect. Palpation of the area with a blunt instrument (a laparoscopic ultrasound probe is ideal) may confirm the presence of a space-occupying lesion.

Figure 12.5
Laparoscopic view of the caudate lobe through the lesser omentum.

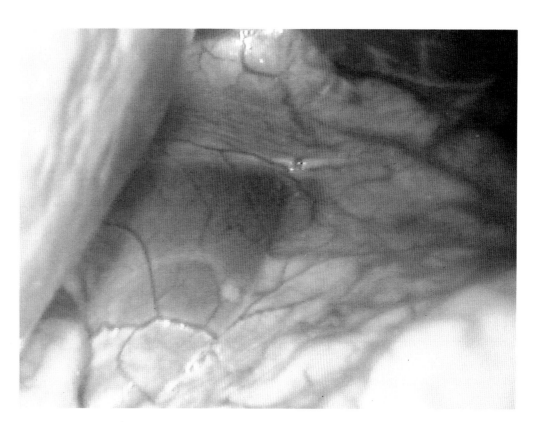

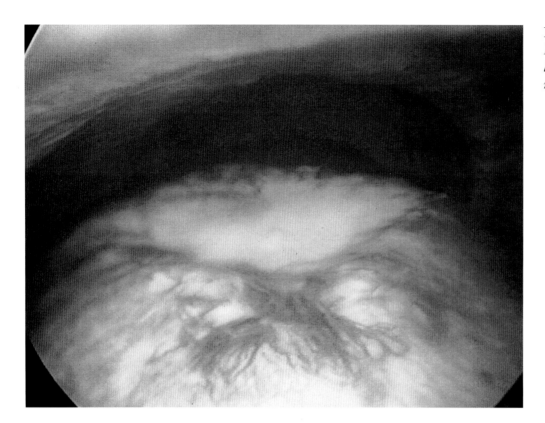

Figure 12.6
Laparoscopic appearance of a large umbilicated liver metastasis.

Laparoscopic ultrasonography — anatomical survey

Screening of the hepatic parenchyma by laparoscopic ultrasonography should be a systematic survey based upon the recognized anatomical landmarks of the liver. This system allows accurate and reproducible documentation of the sites of abnormalities and avoids unnecessary repetitive scanning. An understanding of the segmental hepatic anatomy as described by Couinaud [79] and popularized by Bismuth [80] is fundamental to this process (Fig. 12.7). The segmental ultrasound anatomy may be defined from the interrelationship of the three hepatic veins (right, middle and left) and the portal vein branches. The hepatic veins converge towards their confluence with the inferior vena cava and appear as sinusoidal structures, possessing no fascial wall. Conversely, the portal veins ramify from the porta hepatis and carry a hyperechoic (bright) fascial investment derived from Glisson's capsule of the liver. The flow of blood may be directly visualized within these venous stuctures, whereas the intrahepatic branches of the hepatic artery and bile ducts are not normally visualized.

Orientation
Laparoscopic ultrasound scans of the liver performed with the probe manipulated from a lower abdominal port site are orientated in a narrow range of oblique and parasagittal planes (see Fig. 12.4). Consistent orientation of the 'image direction' is important to avoid confusion and we prefer to orientate the rectilinear sonogram with the superior (cephalad) direction corresponding to the tip of the probe situated to the right of the image (see Fig. 12.4). Movements of the probe should be slow and smooth, and should consist of advancement/withdrawal, rotation (clockwise/anticlockwise) and left and right sweeps.

Figure 12.7
Couinaud's segmental hepatic anatomy.

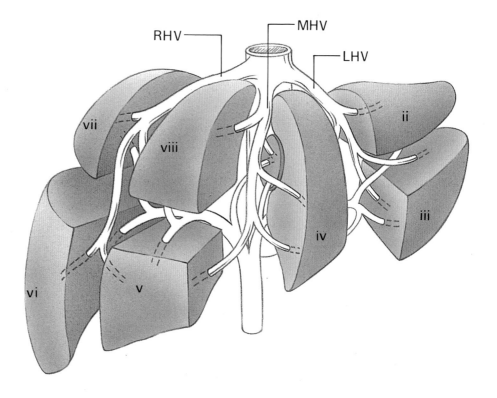

The functional midline separating the right and left hemilivers (the principal fissure) has no surface markings, but passes from the gallbladder fossa to the left edge of the inferior vena cava posteriorly. The middle hepatic vein runs in this plane and is easily identified in longitudinal section with the probe positioned upon the dome of the right liver in line with the gallbladder bed. Clockwise rotation of the probe reveals the parenchyma of the adjacent segments of the right liver (segments V and VIII), whereas anticlockwise rotation allows examination of the quadrate lobe (segment IV). The middle hepatic vein may be identified terminating at the vena cava by advancing the probe through the port, and the vena cava may be traced back behind the liver to the level of the porta hepatis by withdrawal of the probe until it is seen separated from the main portal vein and other hilar structures by the interposed caudate lobe (segment I) (Figs 12.4B and 12.8).

Examination of the right hemiliver
The segmental organization of the right hemiliver may appear complicated at first, but a rudimentary understanding of the segmental anatomy and the application of a systematic approach to scanning rapidly clarifies the terminology. The main portal vein is easily identified bifurcating into right and left branches high in the porta hepatis. The right portal vein itself immediately bifurcates into the anterior and posterior divisions which supply the paramedian sector (segments V (inferiorly) and VIII (superiorly)) and posterolateral sectors (segments VI (inferiorly) and VII (superiorly)) (see Figs 12.4A and 12.7). The paramedian and posterolateral sectors comprise the right hemiliver and are separated by an imaginary plane which bisects the right portal venous bifurcation and is marked by the passage of the right hepatic vein. Once the right hepatic vein has been identified, the anterior and posterior branches of the right portal

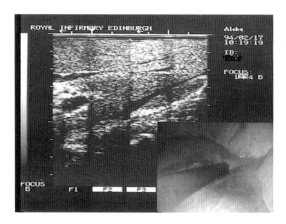

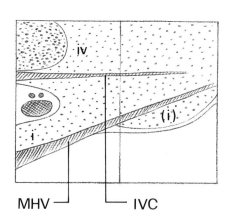

Figure 12.8
A sagittal laparoscopic sonogram through hepatic segment IV demonstrating the middle hepatic vein (MHV), right portal vein, caudate lobe (I) and inferior vena cava (IVC). Note how these venous structures have been compressed by down pressure from the probe.

vein can be seen passing on either side (supplying segments V and VIII, and VI and VII, respectively), and the three-dimensonal organization of the right liver becomes apparent. Segment VI is situated laterally and is seen lying in front of the right kidney (which possesses similar echo texture to the liver), while segment V constitutes the anterior free edge of the liver and is separated by the gallbladder bed from segment IV (quadrate lobe). Segment VIII occupies the angle formed by the converging right and middle hepatic veins posteriorly (Fig. 12.9). Hepatic segment VII is the most posterolaterally situated area of the right liver and its examination may require the insertion of the probe along the right lateral subphrenic space.

Examination of the left hemiliver
The ultrasonographic topography of the left hemiliver is simple. The ligamentum teres insertion and falciform ligament divide the left hemiliver between segment IV and the 'left lobe', which is composed of segments II and III. Having identified the middle hepatic vein in the midline, a slight movement or rotation of the probe to the left demonstrates hepatic segment IV and the hilar structures which pass beneath it (see Fig. 12.4B). The ultrasound probe should then be replaced upon the left hepatic lobe across the falciform ligament (see Fig. 12.4C). Segment III lies anteriorly and is separated from segment II (which lies posterosuperiorly) by the left hepatic vein in its posterior reaches (from where it

Figure 12.9
A parasagittal/oblique laparoscopic sonogram towards the right demonstrating a 2 cm metastasis (Met) wedged between the converging middle hepatic vein (MHV) and right hepatic vein (RHV) within hepatic segment VIII. The anterior branch of the right portal vein (ARPV) is identified anterior to the plane of the right hepatic vein supplying segments V and VIII (note its hyperechoic fascial investment; compare with the

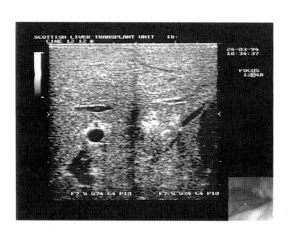

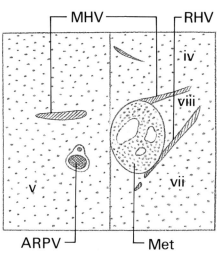

forms a common venous trunk with the middle hepatic vein to join the vena cava). The intrahepatic continuation of the hepatic insertion of the lesser omentum appears as a clearly visible bright line (interlobar fissure) separating segment II from segment I below (caudate lobe). The liver parenchyma of the left hepatic lobe may be used as an 'acoustic window' through which the aorta may be recognized by its pulsatility, and the coeliac axis, superior mesenteric trunks and para-aortic region may be examined for lymphadenopathy. A complete examination of the liver following this procedure may be satisfactorily completed within 10 min.

Laparoscopic ultrasonography — evaluation of abnormal lesions

The normal hepatic parenchyma appears homogeneous with a medium to fine echo texture similar to that of the renal parenchyma. However, the liver texture may appear coarse and hyperechoic when affected by fatty infiltration (e.g. following alcoholic hepatitis or cirrhosis). Slow, smooth movements of the probe according to the above description ensures that the entire liver is scanned, and the real-time images obtained should be perused for the presence of focal lesions. The intrahepatic venous channels which criss-cross the liver are recognizable by their tubular form and are also readily distinguished from a focal tumour by visible blood flow within the vessel lumen (Fig. 12.10).

Laparoscopic ultrasound appearance of metastases
Colorectal liver metastases may affect any part of the liver and are unusual amongst other types of secondary carcinoma in that they may be truly solitary (and therefore resectable). When multiple, the metastases are usually of a similar size. Liver metastases of colorectal origin most commonly appear hypoechoic (dark) relative to the surrounding parenchyma, and typically neither cast 'acoustic shadows' (compare with gallstones) nor produce posterior 'acoustic enhancement' (compare with cysts) (see Fig. 12.10). The classic sonographic appearance of a colorectal liver metastasis is the 'target' or 'bull's-eye' lesion (Fig. 12.11), where the tumour is surrounded by an 'anechoic halo' thought to be due to peritumoral parenchymal compression by the enlarging lesion [81]. However, metastases may appear hyperechoic (brighter) compared with the surrounding tissue (Fig. 12.12), in which case they are more easily identified. Haemangiomas are also

Figure 12.10
An oblique laparoscopic sonogram across the midline of the liver demonstrating a 5 × 8 mm hypoechoic metastasis (Met a) adjacent to a portal venous radicle supplying segment IV (LPV IV), and a 2 cm hypoechoic metastasis (Met b) adjacent to the middle hepatic vein (MHV) in segment IV. Tubular vessels are readily distinguished from focal tumours on laparoscopic ultrasonography by gentle rotation of the probe.

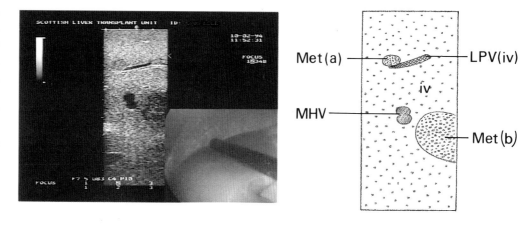

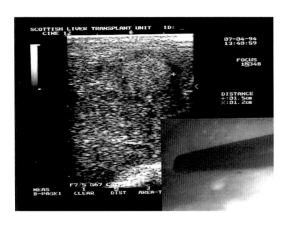
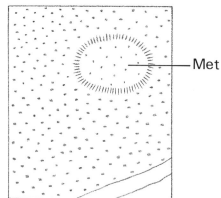

Figure 12.11
*A 'target' or 'bull's-eye'
metastasis (Met)
characterized sonographically
by an anechoic halo. The
metastasis itself appears
isoechoic with the
surrounding hepatic
parenchyma. The ultrasonic
calipers indicate the
dimensions of the lesion as
12 × 15 mm.*

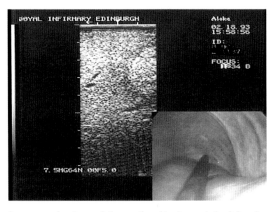
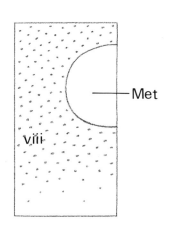

Figure 12.12
*A hyperechoic liver metastasis
(Met).*

hyperechoic, although distinguishable by the posterior acoustic enhancement
associated with these lesions. Larger metastases may become calcified, thereby
casting dense posterior acoustic shadows, or undergo necrosis with cavitation
thus demonstrating an anechoic cystic component (Fig. 12.13). In advanced cases,
extensive confluent metastatic tumour may cause a patchy heterogeneous
appearance throughout the liver in which it is difficult to orientate the
laparoscopic sonograms due to the absence of recognizable normal liver.

Difficulty may occasionally be experienced in imaging the 4–5 mm of tissue
immediately beneath the transducer ('near field'), although pathological changes
in this location are almost always readily visualized laparoscopically. The
instillation of 1 l of crystalloid solution into the peritoneal cavity allows scanning
to be performed with minimal contact between the transducer and liver and
abolishes this problem (Fig. 12.14). This manoeuvre is also useful when
examining the uneven surface of a liver with extensive metastatic disease or
cirrhosis. Measurement of the tumour dimensions may be achieved at a glance by
comparison with the 1 cm gradations along the *y* axis of the rectilinear image.
Alternatively, the 'electronic calipers' installed in the ultrasound machine may be
used to achieve more precise measurements (see Fig. 12.11).

Guided biopsy
It may be desirable to obtain histological proof of the nature of newly discovered
focal liver lesions, and this may be achieved by laparoscopic or laparoscopic
ultrasound-guided needle biopsy. Nevertheless, it is debatable whether this

Figure 12.13
Necrosis and cavitation of a colorectal liver metastasis (Met). Note the anechoic fluid-filled cavities within the tumour which appear as a bulge upon the surface of hepatic segment V (inset).

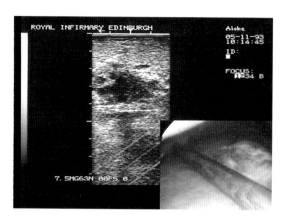
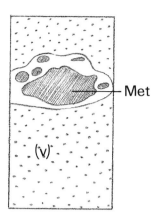

Figure 12.14
Crystalloid solution (NaCl) has been introduced into the peritoneal cavity allowing laparoscopic ultrasonography to demonstrate the subhepatic space behind hepatic segment V with minimal surface contact.

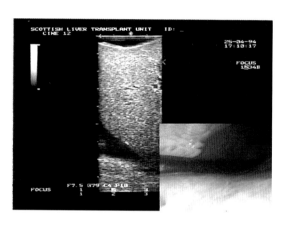
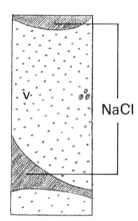

manoeuvre is always justified, particularly when the typical sonographic appearances are those of a metastasis, when the findings are corroborated by other imaging modalities and when the lesion is considered potentially resectable. The well-recognized and probably under-reported phenomenon of needle track seeding of liver tumours should be avoided by not performing unnecessary biopsies in patients being considered for curative resection [82], especially considering the current concern regarding the risk of port site seeding following laparoscopic operations for malignancy [83]. Needle biopsy may be performed by a 'freehand' technique or by utilizing a targeted biopsy system integral to the laparoscopic ultrasound probe. The latter option is preferable for smaller and deeper seated lesions where precision is important. However, such devices, which incorporate a forward-viewing curvilinear extension to the side-viewing linear array transducer along with an integrated biopsy 'gun', are still at the developmental stage (Tetrad Corporation, Englewood, CO, USA). Nevertheless, their further refinement and widespread adoption seems inevitable.

Laparoscopic ultrasound-guided biopsy using a freehand technique requires a degree of skill and three-dimensional spatial awareness. It is necessary to align the needle puncture of the abdominal wall and liver surface with the intrahepatic lesion localized within the ultrasound beam, and the probe position upon the liver surface is used as a reference point. The hyperechoic and highly reflective needle tip may be identified in its passage towards the lesion, and this may be enhanced by lightly abrading the tip of the needle beforehand (Fig. 12.15). Both fine needle aspiration cytology and core-cutting needle biopsy may be achieved in this way.

Future prospects

Laparoscopic ultrasound-guided interstitial laser hyperthermia and cryotherapy

Hepatic cryotherapy is a technique which has shown early promise in the local ablation of inoperable metastatic liver tumours. Early work performed at open surgery confirmed the utility of intraoperative ultrasonography as a means of both accurately guiding the placement of the cryotherapy probes and monitoring the progress of the resultant spherical iceball [84,85]. Similarly, ultrasonography has been shown to be the optimal method for monitoring the ablation of liver tumours using interstitial laser hyperthermia [86,87]. Both these techniques will be performed laparoscopically in the future, and laparoscopic ultrasonography will inevitably play an important role in the success of these novel therapeutic approaches.

Colour flow Doppler

Several laparoscopic ultrasound systems now include a colour flow Doppler capability which is of enormous advantage in the rapid identification and differentiation of ductular and vascular structures (e.g. in the porta hepatis, Fig. 12.16, and in assessment of the peripancreatic vasculature when staging pancreatic tumours), and which has been reported to be useful in localizing the ureter during open exploration of the abdomen [88]. Although its advantages in the assessment of the liver are less well defined, there has been increasing interest in the use of colour flow Doppler ultrasonography in the characterization of liver tumours by virtue of the increased internal vascularity of some lesions [89]. Although colour flow imaging may not be specific enough to distinguish between primary and secondary liver tumours [90], there is some evidence that the detection of colorectal liver metastases may be facilitated by the use of colour flow Doppler ultrasound, especially when the images are enhanced following the administration of intravenous galactose microparticles [91].

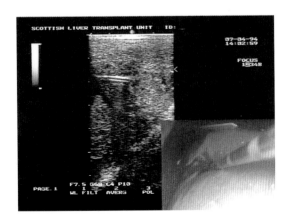 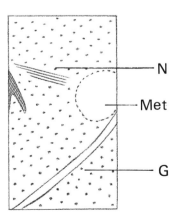

Figure 12.15
Laparoscopic ultrasound-guided needle biopsy of a hyperechoic metastasis (Met) situated posteriorly within the liver. Note the hyperechoic fascial border produced by Glisson's capsule (G). The needle track (N) shows up as hyperechoic 'tramlines'.

Figure 12.16
Colour flow Doppler laparoscopic ultrasonography confirming bloodflow (blue) within a patent portal vein (PV) in a patient with cirrhosis (insert). IVC, inferior vena cava.

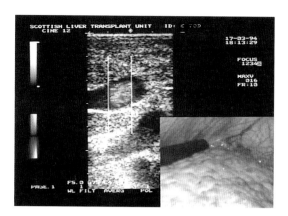
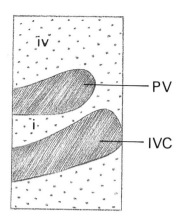

Quantitative Doppler flow assessment of hepatic vascular inflow

A potentially exciting set of observations has recently been made by Leen and co-workers who have used transabdominal duplex sonography to predict the presence of both occult and overt liver metastases with extraordinary accuracy [92]. By exploiting the principle that liver metastases cause subtle microcirculatory changes with an increase in the hepatic arterial : portal venous bloodflow ratio, they measured these parameters in a range of patients and derived a Doppler perfusion index (DPI) for each. They reported a significant separation in DPI values between control subjects and patients with overt liver metastases and also observed elevated DPI values in those patients who, after follow-up, were discovered to harbour occult liver metastases [92]. However, it remains to be seen whether these findings will be widely reproducible. It may be that laparoscopic Doppler ultrasonography will provide an accurate means of assesssment of the haemodynamic changes in the hepatic bloodflow on account of its markedly improved resolution compared with transabdominal ultrasonography. This may diminish the error rate inherent in Doppler flow measurement techniques when undertaken by the transabdominal route.

Conclusion

The rationale for screening the liver for metastases during large bowel cancer surgery is well established. Despite the obvious limitations of access inherent in therapeutic laparoscopy, minimal access colorectal cancer operations provide an excellent opportunity for detailed assessment of the liver by means of laparoscopy and laparoscopic ultrasonography. This technique is theoretically ideal for fully staging the intra-abdominal disease. Early experience has demonstrated its feasibility, sensitivity and ease of implementation in detecting liver tumours, and further prospective studies are required to define its precise role in the management of a variety of conditions [47]. As laparoscopic ultrasonography continues to evolve in concert with further technological refinements, its role within the armamentarium of the laparoscopic surgeon should be assured.

References

1 Bengtsson G, Carlsson G, Hafström L, Jonsson P-E. Natural history of patients with untreated liver metastases from colorectal cancer. *Am J Surg* 1981; **141**: 586–9.
2 Oxley EM, Ellis H. Prognosis of carcinoma of the large bowel in the presence of liver metastases. *Br J Surg* 1969; **56**: 149–52.
3 Goligher JC. The operability of carcinoma of the rectum. *BMJ* 1941; **2**: 393–7.
4 Welch JP, Donaldson GA. Detection and treatment of recurrent cancer of the colon and rectum. *Am J Surg* 1978; **135**: 505–11.
5 Finlay IG, McArdle CS. Occult hepatic metastases in colorectal carcinoma. *Br J Surg* 1986; **73**: 732–5.
6 Finlay IG, Meek DR, Gray HW, Duncan JG, McArdle CS. Incidence and detection of occult hepatic metastases in colorectal carcinoma. *BMJ* 1982; **284**: 803–9.
7 de Brauuw LM, van de Velde CJH, Pauwels EKJ *et al.* Prospective comparative study of ultrasound, CT scan, scintigraphy and laboratory tests to detect hepatic metastases. *J Nucl Biol Med* 1991; **35**: 131–4.
8 Kemeny MM, Ganteaume L, Goldberg DA, Hogan JM. Preoperative staging with computerized axial tomography and biochemical laboratory tests in patients with hepatic metastases. *Ann Surg* 1986; **203**: 169–72.
9 Schreve RH, Terpesta OT, Ausema L, Lameris JS, van Seijen AJ, Jeekel J. Detection of liver metastases. A prospective study comparing liver enzymes, scintigraphy, ultrasonography and computed tomography. *Br J Surg* 1984; **71**: 947–9.
10 Smith T, Kemeny M, Sugarbaker P *et al.* A prospective study of hepatic imaging in the detection of metastatic disease. *Ann Surg* 1982; **195**: 486–91.
11 Ward B, Miller D, Frank J *et al.* Prospective evaluation of hepatic imaging studies in the detection of colorectal metastases: correlation with surgical findings. *Surgery* 1989; **105**: 180–7.
12 Hogg L, Pack GT. Diagnostic accuracy of hepatic metastases at laparotomy. *A M A Arch Surg* 1956; **72**: 251–2.
13 Gray BN. Surgeon accuracy in the diagnosis of liver metastases at laparotomy. *Aust N Z J Surg* 1980; **50**: 524–6.
14 Garden OJ. Operative ultrasonography. *Hosp Update* 1992; **18**: 470–9.
15 Harbin WP, Wittenberg J, Ferrucci JT, Mueller PR, Ottinger LW. Fallibility of exploratory laparotomy in detection of hepatic and retroperitoneal masses. *Am J Roentgenol* 1980; **135**: 115–21.
16 Clarke MP, Kane RA, Steele G Jr *et al.* Prospective comparison of preoperative imaging and intraoperative ultrasonography in the detection of liver tumours. *Surgery* 1989; **106**: 849–55.
17 Parker GA, Lawrence W, Horsley SJ *et al.* Intraoperative ultrasound of the liver affects operative decision making. *Ann Surg* 1989; **209**: 569–77.
18 Rifkin MD, Rosato FE, Branch HM *et al.* Intraoperative ultrasound of the liver. An important adjunctive tool for decision making in the operating room. *Ann Surg* 1987; 466–72.
19 Machi J, Sigel B, Zaren HA, Kurohiji T, Yamashita Y. Operative ultrasonography during hepatobiliary and pancreatic surgery. *World J Surg* 1993; **17**: 640–6.
20 Soyer P, Elias D, Zeitoun G, Roche A, Levesque M. Surgical treatment of hepatic metastases: impact of intraoperative sonography. *Am J Roentgenol* 1993; **160**: 511–14.
21 Traynor O, Castaing D, Bismuth H. Peroperative ultrasonography in the surgery of hepatic tumours. *Br J Surg* 1988; **75**: 197–202.
22 Gozzetti G, Mazziotti A, Bolondi L *et al.* Intraoperative ultrasonography in surgery for liver tumours. *Surgery* 1986; **99**: 523–9.
23 Izumi R, Shimizu K, Kiriyama M *et al.* Hepatic resection guided by needles inserted under ultrasonographic guidance. *Surgery* 1993; **114**: 497–501.
24 Lau WY, Leung KL, Lee TW, Li AKC. Ultrasonography during liver resection for hepatocellular carcinoma. *Br J Surg* 1993; **80**: 493–4.
25 Sheu J-C, Lee C-S, Sung J-L, Chen D-S, Yang P-M, Lin T-Y. Intraoperative hepatic ultrasonography — an indispensable procedure in resection of small hepatocellular carcinomas. *Surgery* 1985; **97**: 97–103.
26 Castaing D, Garden OJ, Bismuth H. Segmental liver resection using ultrasound-guided selective portal venous occlusion. *Ann Surg* 1989; **210**: 20–3.
27 Bismuth H, Castaing D, Garden OJ. The use of operative ultrasound in surgery of primary liver tumours. *World J Surg* 1987; **11**: 610–14.
28 Makuuchi M, Hasegwa H, Yamazaki S, Takayasu K, Moriyama N. The use of operative ultrasound as an aid to liver resection in patients with hepatocellular carcinoma. *World J Surg* 1987; **11**: 615–21.
29 Makuuchi M, Hasegwa H, Yamazaki S. Ultrasonically guided subsegmentectomy. *Surg Gynecol Obstet* 1985; **161**: 346–50.
30 Machi J, Isomoto H, Kurohiji T *et al.* Accuracy of intraoperative ultrasound in diagnosing liver metastasis from colorectal cancer: evaluation with postoperative follow-up results. *World J Surg* 1991; **15**: 551–7.

31 Stadler J, Hölscher AH, Adolf J. Intraoperative ultrasonographic detection of occult liver metastases in colorectal cancer. *Surg Endosc* 1991; **5**: 36–40.
32 Olsen AK. Intraoperative ultrasonography and the detection of liver metastases in patients with colorectal cancer. *Br J Surg* 1990; **77**: 998–9.
33 Boldrini G, de Gaetano AM, Giovannini I, Castagneto M, Colagrande C, Castiglioni G. The systematic use of operative ultrasound for detection of liver metastases during colorectal surgery. *World J Surg* 1987; **11**: 622–7.
34 Charnley RM, Morris DL, Dennison AR, Amar SS, Hardcastle JD. Detection of colorectal liver metastases using intraoperative ultrasonography. *Br J Surg* 1991; **78**: 45–8.
35 Stewart PJ, Chu JM, Kos SC, Chapuis PH, Bokey EL. Intra-operative ultrasound for the detection of hepatic metastases from colorectal cancer. *Aust N Z J Surg* 1993; **63**: 530–4.
36 Stone MD, Kane R, Bothe A, Jessup JM, Cady B, Steele GD. Intraoperative ultrasound imaging of the liver at the time of colorectal cancer resection. *Arch Surg* 1994; **129**: 431–6.
37 Gozzetti G. Operative ultrasonography during hepatobiliary and pancreatic surgery (invited commentary). *World J Surg* 1991; **17**: 645–6.
38 Gunning JE. The history of laparosocopy. *J Reprod Med* 1974; **12**: 223–31.
39 Kelling G. Zur colioskopie (On coelioscopy). *Arch Klin Chir* 1923; **126**: 226–9.
40 Jacobeus HC. Kurze ubersicht uber meine erfahrungen mit der laparoskopie (Brief overview of my experience with laparoscopy). *Munch Med Wochenschr* 1911; **58**: 2017–19.
41 Veress J. Neues instrument zur ausführung von brust oder bauchpunktionen (New instrument for performing chest or abdominal puncture). *Dtsch Med Wochenschr* 1938; **64**: 1480–1.
42 Fervers C. Die laparoskopie mit dem zystoscope (Laparoscopy with the cystoscope). *Med Klin* 1933; **29**: 1042–5.
43 Ruddock JC. Peritoneoscopy. *Surg Gynecol Obstet* 1937; **65**: 523–39, 623–39.
44 Benedict EB. Peritoneoscopy. *N Engl J Med* 1938; **218**: 713–14.
45 Bleiberg H, Rozencweig M, Mathieu M, Beyens N, Gompel C, Gerard A. The use of peritoneoscopy in the detection of liver metastases. *Cancer* 1978; **41**: 863–7.
46 John TG, Greig JD, Crosbie JL, Miles WFA, Garden OJ. Superior staging of liver tumours with laparoscopy and laparoscopic ultrasound. *Ann Surg* 1994; **220**: 711–19.
47 John TG, Garden OJ. Laparoscopic ultrasound: extending the scope of diagnostic laparoscopy. *Br J Surg* 1994; **81**: 5–6.
48 John TG, Greig JD, Carter DC, Garden OJ. Carcinoma of the pancreatic head and periampullary region: tumor staging with laparoscopy and laparoscopic ultrasonography. *Ann Surg* 1995; **221**: 156–64.
49 Cuschieri A. Laparoscopy for pancreatic cancer: does it benefit the patient? *Eur J Surg Oncol* 1988; **14**: 41–4.
50 Cuschieri A, Hall AW, Clark J. Value of laparoscopy in the diagnosis and management of pancreatic carcinoma. *Gut* 1978; **19**: 672–7.
51 Warshaw AL, Gu ZY, Wittenberg J, Waltman AC. Preoperative staging and assessment of resectability of pancreatic cancer. *Arch Surg* 1990; **125**: 230–3.
52 Warshaw AL, Tepper JE, Shipley WU. Laparoscopy in the staging and planning of therapy for pancreatic cancer. *Am J Surg* 1986; **151**: 76–80.
53 Murugiah M, Paterson-Brown S, Windsor JA, Miles WFA, Garden OJ. Early experience of laparoscopic ultrasonography in the management of pancreatic carcinoma. *Surg Endosc* 1993; **7**: 177–81.
54 Possik RA, Franco EL, Pires DR, Wohnrath DR, Ferreira EB. Sensitivity, specificity, and predictive value of laparoscopy for the staging of gastric cancer and for the detection of liver metastases. *Cancer* 1986; **58**: 1–6.
55 Shandall A, Johnson C. Laparoscopy or scanning in oesophageal and gastric carcinoma. *Br J Surg* 1985; **72**: 449–51.
56 Watt I, Stewart I, Anderson D, Bell G, Anderson JR. Laparoscopy, ultrasound and computed tomography in cancer of the oesophagus and gastric cardia: a prospective comparison for detecting intra-abdominal metastases. *Br J Surg* 1989; **76**: 1036–9.
57 Gross E, Bancewicz J, Ingram G. Assessment of gastric carcinoma by laparoscopy. *BMJ* 1984; **288**: 1577.
58 Dagnini G, Marin G, Patella M, Zotti S. Laparoscopy in the diagnosis of primary carcinoma of the gallbladder. A study of 98 cases. *Gastrointest Endosc* 1984; **30**: 289–91.
59 Rosenhoff SH, Young RC, Anderson TC *et al.* Peritoneoscopy: a valuable staging tool in ovarian carcinoma. *Ann Intern Med* 1975; **83**: 37–41.
60 Margolis R, Hansen H, Muggia F, Kanhouwa S. Diagnosis of liver metastases in bronchogenic carcinoma. A comparative study of liver scans, function tests, and peritoneoscopy with liver biopsy in 111 patients. *Cancer* 1974; **34**: 1825–9.
61 Van der Spuy S, Levin W, Smit BJ, Graham T, McQuaide JR. Peritoneoscopy in the management of breast cancer. *S Afr Med J* 1978; **54**: 402–3.
62 Bleiberg H, La Meir E, Lejeune F. Laparoscopy in the diagnosis of liver metastases in 80 cases of malignant melanoma. *Endoscopy* 1980; **12**: 215–18.

63 Huberman M, Bunn P, Matthews M *et al.* Hepatic involvement in the cutaneous T-cell lymphomas. Results of percutaneous biopsy and peritoneoscopy. *Cancer* 1980; **45**: 1683–8.
64 Bagley C, Thomas L, Johnson R, Chretien P, DeVita V. Diagnosis of liver involvement by lymphoma: results in 96 consecutive peritoneoscopies. *Cancer* 1973; **31**: 840–7.
65 Lightdale CJ. Laparoscopy and biopsy in malignant liver disease. *Cancer* 1982; **50**: 2672–5.
66 Jeffers L, Spieglman G, Reddy R *et al.* Laparoscopically directed fine needle aspiration for the diagnosis of hepatocellular carcinoma: a safe and accurate technique. *Gastrointest Endosc* 1988; **34**: 235–7.
67 Aramaki N, Yoshida K, Yamashiro Y, Namihisa T. Ultrasonic laparoscopy (abstract). *Scand J Gastroenterol* 1982; **78** (Suppl. 17): 185.
68 Ota Y, Sato Y, Takatsui K *et al.* New ultrasonic laparoscope. Improvement in diagnosis of intraabdominal disease (abstract). *Scand J Gastroenterol* 1982; **78** (Suppl. 17): 194.
69 Furukawa Y, Sakamoto F, Kanazawa H *et al.* A new method of B-mode ultrasonography under laparoscopic guidance (abstract). *Scand J Gastroenterol* 1982; **78** (Suppl. 17): 186.
70 Look D, Henning H, Yano N. Direkte ultraschallechographie der gallenblasse unter laparoskopischer sicht (Direct ultrasonography of the gallbladder under laparoscopic vision). In: Lindner H (ed.) *Fortschritte der gastro-enterologischen Endoskopie*, Vol. VI. Witzstrock, Baden-Baden, 1975.
71 Hayashi S, Wagai T, Miyazawar R *et al.* Ultrasonic diagnosis of breast tumor and cholelithiasis. *West J Surg Obstet Gynecol* 1962; **70**: 34.
72 John TG, Garden OJ. Clinical experience with sector scan and linear array ultrasound probes in laparoscopic surgery. *Endosc Surg Allied Technol* 1994; **2**: 134–42.
73 Fornari F, Civardi G, Cavanna L *et al.* Laparoscopic ultrasonography in the study of liver diseases: preliminary results. *Surg Endosc* 1989; **3**: 33–7.
74 Fukuda M, Mima S, Tanabe T, Suzuki Y, Hirata K, Terada S. Endoscopic sonography of the liver — diagnostic application of the echolaparoscope to localize intrahepatic lesions. *Scand J Gastroenterol* 1984; **19** (Suppl. 102): 24–8.
75 Bönhof JA, Linhart P, Bettendorf U, Holper H. Liver biopsy guided by laparoscopic sonography. A case report demonstrating a new technique. *Endoscopy* 1984; **16**: 237–9.
76 Okita K, Kodama T, Oda M, Takemoto T. Laparoscopic ultrasonography. Diagnosis of liver and pancreatic cancer. *Scand J Gastroenterol* 1984; **19** (Suppl. 94): 91–100.
77 Miles WFA, Paterson-Brown S, Garden OJ. Laparoscopic contact hepatic ultrasonography. *Br J Surg* 1992; **79**: 419–20.
78 Cuesta MA, Meijer S, Borgstein PJ, Sibinga Mulder L, Sikkenk AC. Laparoscopic ultrasonography for hepatobiliary and pancreatic malignancy. *Br J Surg* 1993; **80**: 1571–4.
79 Couinaud C. *Le Foie Etudes Anatomiques et Chirurgicales* (Anatomical and Surgical Studies on the Liver). Masson, Paris, 1957.
80 Bismuth H. Surgical anatomy and anatomical surgery of the liver. *World J Surg* 1982; **6**: 3–9.
81 Marchal GJ, Pylyser K, Tshibwaba-Tumba EA *et al.* Anechoic halo in solid liver tumors: sonographic, microangiographic, and histologic correlation. *Radiology* 1985; **156**: 479–83.
82 John TG, Garden OJ. Needle track seeding of primary and secondary liver carcinoma after percutaneous liver biopsy. *HPB Surg* 1993; **6**: 199–204.
83 Nduka CC, Monson JRT, Menzies-Gow N, Darzi A. Abdominal wall metastasis following laparoscopy. *Br J Surg* 1994; **81**: 648–52.
84 Onik G, Kane R, Steele G *et al.* Monitoring hepatic cryosurgery with sonography. *Am J Roentgenol* 1986; **147**: 665–9.
85 Ravikumar TS, Kane R, Cady B *et al.* Hepatic cryosurgery with intraoperative ultrasound monitoring for metastatic colon carcinoma. *Arch Surg* 1987; **122**: 403–9.
86 Masters A, Steger AC, Lees WR, Walmsley KM, Bown SG. Interstitial laser hyperthermia: a new approach for treating liver metastases. *Br J Cancer* 1992; **66**: 518–22.
87 Steger AC, Lees WR, Shorvon P, Walmsley K, Brown SG. Multiple-fibre low-power interstitial laser hyperthermia: studies in the normal liver. *Br J Surg* 1992; **79**: 139–45.
88 Smith LE, Wherry D, Marohn M. Use of ultrasound to identify the ureter. *Surg Endosc* 1993; **8**: 467.
89 Tanaka K, Kitamura T, Fujita M *et al.* Colour Doppler flow imaging of liver tumors. *Am J Roentgenol* 1990; **154**: 509–14.
90 Nino-Murcia M, Ralls PW, Jeffrey RB, Johnson M. Color flow doppler characterization of focal hepatic lesions. *Am J Roentgenol* 1992; **159**: 1195–7.
91 Leen E, Angerson WJ, Warren HW *et al.* Improved sensitivity of colour Doppler flow imaging of colorectal hepatic metastases using galactose microparticles: a preliminary report. *Br J Surg* 1994; **81**: 252–4.
92 Leen E, Goldberg JA, Robertson J *et al.* Early detection of occult colorectal hepatic metastases using duplex colour Doppler sonography. *Br J Surg* 1993; **80**: 1249–51.

Chapter 13

Laparoscopic colorectal surgery: the US experience

S.M. Cohen and S.D. Wexner

Introduction

The rapid emergence of the use of the laparoscope in diseases of the biliary system has stimulated surgeons around the world to attempt larger and more complex procedures. To date, laparoscopic nephrectomy, appendicectomy, fundoplication, adrenalectomy, splenectomy and pneumonectomy have all been either attempted or successfully performed. The use of the laparoscope in the field of colorectal surgery is still in its infancy with respect to the ease, efficacy and safety of colonic mobilization, resection and anastomosis. It was initially thought that the benefits of laparoscopic colorectal surgery would be the same as those in other forms of surgery: faster postoperative recovery, smaller incisions and a decreased length of hospitalization. However, many recent reports claim no difference when compared with standard open operations [1–4].

In order to achieve these goals, several precepts are of paramount importance. Firstly, never forsake the fundamental tenets of surgery in the interests of using inadequate technology. The different manufacturing companies are continuing to develop a spectrum of instruments which enable safe application of basic surgical principles. Secondly, accept only those manoeuvres during a laparoscopic procedure which would be acceptable during an open procedure. This statement applies to handling of the bowel, manipulation of the tumour, fashioning of the anastomosis, management of the mesenteric defect and all the other steps in the procedure. If a given technique violates the accepted principles, an alternative technique should be applied. If an alternative technique is not available or not suitable, the laparoscopic phase should be terminated. Thirdly, never consider conversion to a laparotomy a failure, but rather good surgical judgement. Willingness to increase morbidity and mortality rates is unacceptable. Fourthly, never favour a triumph of technology over sound common sense. A case in point is the laparoscopic right colectomy with intracorporeal anastomosis. As a small incision is necessary for the removal of the specimen, an extracorporeal anastomosis can save much time and money and may result in less contamination compared with an intracorporeal anastomosis. Surgeons have described as 'successful' intracorporeal right hemicolectomies utilizing two cameras, two surgeons, up to 14 ports and up to 11 applications of an endoscopic stapler, and requiring double the time and triple the cost needed for a 'standard' right hemicolectomy. In addition to these disadvantages, an incision is still required to remove the specimen [5].

However, laparoscopic colorectal surgery is notably different from all the other procedures being performed at the moment. In point of fact, all of the other attempted procedures have several common denominators. Firstly, they are performed in a relatively fixed intra-abdominal location. From a strictly practical point of view this is fundamental, as there is virtually no need for intraoperative repositioning of instruments, ports, monitors and personnel. The pathology is always in the anticipated position. Secondly, they include either no vascular division (herniorrhaphy or fundoplication) or limited vascular division (cholecystectomy or appendicectomy). Thus vascular control can be rapidly and inexpensively undertaken. Conversely, the colonic mesentery includes numerous large vessels. Thus vascular control requires considerably more time and quite often considerably more cost than in the other procedures. Thirdly, in none of these procedures is an anastomosis fashioned. The dissection, mobilization and mere harvesting of an organ or suturing a defect requires certain skills and instrumentation. However, the more advanced skills and equipment necessary for a tension-free, well-vascularized anastomosis are markedly different. Moreover, although the failure of sutures or staples after laparoscopic hernia or fundoplication may or may not result in recurrence, this complication may be asymptomatic. Conversely, the failure of a bowel anastomosis is a potentially lethal complication associated with significant increases in morbidity, length of hospitalization, cost and survival. Fourthly, the other procedures require either the removal of a small organ or no retrieval at all. Removal of a properly resected segment of colon with its attached mesentery requires either an incision or an extremely large port. Lastly, none of the other currently performed laparoscopic procedures are undertaken to cure a malignancy. This feature again can lead to a marked difference in clinical sequelae between an asymptomatic hernia recurrence and a pelvic recurrence from a rectal carcinoma. Moreover, if such recurrences are asymptomatic, and appropriate prospective randomized trials are not utilized, true laparoscopic rates will be erroneously low in the absence of diligent routine long-term postoperative assessment.

To date, there have been no prospective randomized trials published to demonstrate the superiority or even the equivalence of laparoscopic colectomy. These data will only become available if qualified surgeons learn, develop and apply these new techniques in a responsible and scientific manner. Currently, the steep part of the learning curve is still being ascended. As our skills develop in conjunction with the development of improved instrumentation, results too will hopefully improve and equivalent skills will be compared. It is inappropriate to compare the results of a standard colectomy in the hands of a skilled specialist with the results from a laparoscopic novice.

Results

Recently there have been several studies to document the potential advantages of laparoscopic and laparoscopically assisted colon and rectal surgery. Phillips *et al.* [6] reported 51 laparoscopic colectomies performed by several surgeons at two different institutions in two states. Seven cases (14%) were converted to laparoscopically assisted cases and four (8%) were converted to open procedures. Indications included cancer, diverticulitis, endometriosis, regional enteritis, villous adenoma and polyps. One concern was that the circular stapled anastomosis was incomplete in five instances (18%). Most series of open surgery report incomplete 'doughnuts' in only 2–3% [7]. Thus in the rush to 'prove' the benefits of the completely laparoscopic coloproctostomy the authors have instead beautifully illustrated a compromise in surgical technique to facilitate a technology. Operative time averaged 2.3 h and one patient required blood transfusion. Clear liquids were administered until the third postoperative day. No patient required parenteral narcotics after the second postoperative day. Discharge from the hospital ranged from 1 to 30 days (4.6 ± 4.1 (mean + SD) days). Four patients had postoperative complications (8%), and one patient died from pneumonia. Patients who were working were able to return to work 1 week after the operation.

They concluded that laparoscopic colectomies can be performed safely, but that a surgeon's awareness of his or her limitations and capabilities will be the difference between reckless and safe surgery. One concern is obviously the six to ninefold increase in the incidence of incomplete anastomosis. Although Phillips and co-workers recognized and treated this problem, such technical imperfections are fodder for postoperative disaster in the hands of the laparoscopic neophyte. It is also important to note that eight of 51 patients (16%) underwent colotomy and wedge resection for polyps. This procedure has been shown to increase the rate of local recurrence [8] compared with standard resection. A colotomy is thus not the preferred procedure for neoplasias in the United States. As such it does not form a basis of fair comparison between a laparoscopic colotomy and standard colectomy. Lastly, such a dramatic departure from standard practice represents another departure from accepted surgical practice to facilitate an otherwise difficult technology. Nonetheless, such a compromise may account for shorter hospitalization.

Corbitt [9] was able to complete 15 of 18 attempted laparoscopically assisted colectomies (LACs). In three patients the colonic lesion could not be laparoscopically identified and conversion was performed. Indications for colon resection were adenocarcinoma in 15 patients (five left-sided and 10 right-sided), two large adenomas in the ascending colon and one perforated diverticulum of the sigmoid colon. Five patients had undergone prior abdominal surgery. All intestinal anastomoses were performed extracorporeally using a stapling instrument. No operative complications or mortality were reported. The length of the operative procedure ranged from 45 to 90 min (mean 68 min). Some patients were able to begin oral intake as soon as the first postoperative day, whereas others had no oral intake for 72 h. Nonetheless, the average length of hospitalization was still 4 days (range: 3–6 days). The authors stated there was a 'marked reduction' in postoperative pain and discomfort as reported by the patients, but this was not quantified.

Jacobs and co-workers [10] performed laparoscopically assisted colon resections on 20 patients. Indications for surgery were large villous adenomas or adenocarcinoma in 12 patients, diverticular disease in five, a sigmoid endometrioma in one, caecal volvulus in one, and inflammatory bowel disease in one. The mean length of operative procedures was 170 min (range: 95–255 min) for sigmoid colectomies and 155 min (range: 110–260 min) for right colectomies. There were no reported intraoperative complications, clear liquids were tolerated in 18 of the 20 patients on the first postoperative day and 14 patients were discharged on day 4. Three patients developed a postoperative complication: haemorrhage requiring transfusion, oedema of a rectosigmoid anastomosis requiring a decompressing rectal tube and a mechanical small bowel obstruction requiring a second operation. The authors concluded that, although this procedure is considered in evolution, it 'will become as accepted as laparoscopic cholecystectomy'.

Quattlebaum *et al.* [11] reported on 40 laparoscopically assisted colon resections. Indications included cancer, diverticulitis and a variety of other benign conditions. Procedures were generally completed in 30–90 min. There was no reported intraoperative mortality or morbidity. Gastrointestinal function, defined as intake of solid food with flatus or bowel movements, returned on average 2.5 days after surgery. The average hospital stay for patients with benign colonic lesions was 4.2 days (range: 3–12 days) and was 4.6 days (range: 2–6 days) for those patients with malignant conditions. Postoperative complications occurred in six patients, the most severe being a transient late anastomotic obstruction which resolved spontaneously and a persistent abdominal wall haemorrhage at a trocar insertion site. They also reported one patient with a Dukes' C splenic flexure carcinoma who developed a local recurrence at 1 year. They concluded that this approach is a cost-effective alternative in the therapy of most colon lesions. However, no cost data were included in the study. Moreover, the oncological merit of their approach must be questioned in light of a local recurrence after resection of a *colonic* (not rectal) neoplasm. Ultimately one must question which data represent the better result for the patient — rapid discharge from the hospital or rapid recurrence of carcinoma. Again, one must be honest and detailed during the informed consent procedure.

Scoggin *et al.* [12] also reported shorter hospitalization and less patient discomfort. Twenty patients underwent laparoscopically assisted large and small bowel surgery. Indications for surgery included polyps in 10 patients, carcinoma in two, arteriovenous malformations in two, endoscopic perforation in one and inflammatory bowel disease in five. Operative time ranged from 40 to 280 min (mean: 178 min). Vessel ligation was performed intracorporeally, and all anastomoses were handsewn extracorporeally. There was no reported intraoperative morbidity or mortality. Average time for the return of bowel function (as marked by the patient reporting flatus) was 1.9 days and oral feeding 2.3 days. However, the median postoperative hospital stay was 5 days. No mortalities were noted, and morbidity was 20% including a urinary tract infection, urinary retention, a postoperative blood transfusion and a small bowel obstruction that required laparotomy for an internal hernia.

All of the above studies were performed on unselected groups of patients without comparison to standard open operations. Peters and Bartels [13] reviewed their experience with 28 attempted laparoscopic and LACs and compared them with 33 with similiar open colectomies (OCs) at the same institution by the same surgeon. The two groups were similar with respect to age, weight and the types of procedures performed. Twenty-four were successfully completed. Conversion was due to intraoperative bleeding, invasive carcinoma or an ileosigmoid fistula. The operative times for the LAC group were significantly longer than for the OC group. However, patients also regained bowel function significantly earlier (2.7 vs 4.0 days), tolerated a regular diet earlier (2.3 vs 4.6 days) and their length of stay was markedly diminished (4.8 vs 8.2 days). Postoperative complications were noted in three (13%) patients including a wound infection, urinary retention and a urinary tract infection. Many surgeons claim a subjective decrease in blood loss after laparoscopic compared with standard colectomies [14]. Peters and Bartels [13], however, measured both preoperative and 24 h postoperative haemoglobin levels as an indirect indicator of operative blood loss. They demonstrated no statistically significant difference between the two groups although there was a trend towards a greater fall in the laparoscopic group (more intraoperative blood loss using the laparoscope).

Similarly, Senagore *et al.* [14] assessed 140 colonic resections which included 102 OC cases and 38 LAC cases. There were no significant differences with respect to surgical indications, age or perioperative morbidity. However, the LAC group required significantly more operative time compared with the OC group. Only one conversion was performed secondary to uncontrolled bleeding and one enterotomy was created by a laparoscopic instrument which was successfully repaired laparoscopically. Bowel function returned quicker (3.0 vs 4.9 days) and hospital stay was significantly shorter in the LAC group (6.0 vs 9.0 days). The authors demonstrated that the cost for patients who received laparoscopic colon resections was less than that for patients who underwent a standard laparotomy (US $2300; *P*=NS). These savings came not only from a reduction in hospital stay but also from fewer pharmaceutical agents, intramuscular injections and intravenous infusions. They felt that, the modest increase in operating room cost (approximately US $1000) was offset by reductions in postoperative care. Furthermore, Vayer *et al.* [15] examined the cost-effectiveness of LACs versus open resection. They revealed that, despite the higher cost of operating room time and equipment, the total cost of LACs was not statistically different from that of open resection. Again, they claimed that the cost savings were due to a shortened hospital stay.

Not all laparoscopic colectomy trials have been so favourable in terms of patient benefit. Schmitt *et al.* prospectively compared the time to oral intake and to subsequent discharge from the hospital after LAC and OC procedures [2]. Forty-eight patients were prospectively evaluated and 45 age-, sex- and procedure-matched OC controls were randomly selected and reviewed for comparison. Diagnoses were matched wherever possible. Oral intake was begun on postoperative day 0–7 (mean: day 3.4) after LAC and on postoperative day 0–8 (mean: day 4) for OC patients. The patients were discharged from the hospital on postoperative day 5–16 (mean: day 8.2) for the LAC group and on postoperative day 5–18 (mean: day 8.1) for the OC group. The authors concluded that LACs did not appear to confer any advantage over OCs in the time to oral intake or the length of hospitalization. Similarly, this same group stratified their patients and individually assessed patients undergoing laparoscopically assisted ileal pouch anal anastomosis (LAC) and prospectively compared them to age-, sex- and diagnosis-matched controls (OC) [16]. There were 22 and 20 patients each in the LAC and OC group, respectively. Ileus resolved on the fourth postoperative day in both groups: LAC mean 4.1 days (range: 0–5 days) and OC mean 4.3 days (range: 2–7 days). Hospital discharge was on the eighth postoperative day in both groups: LAC mean 8.4 days (range: 6–13 days) and OC mean 8.9 days (range: 7–18 days). Again, they demonstrated that neither the length of time for ileus resolution nor the length of hospitalization was reduced in the LAC group.

Milsom *et al.* [17] reported their initial experience with laparoscopically assisted ileocolectomy in patients with Crohn's disease of the terminal ileum. Nine patients underwent operation; there was no reported morbidity or mortality. The median time of operation was 170 min (range: 150–210 min). All patients did well in the postoperative period and the median time interval to the first bowel movement was 5 days (range: 4–6 days). The median postoperative hospital stay was 7 days (range: 5–12 days). Although laparoscopically assisted surgery is feasible in Crohn's disease, the authors noted no apparent differences from what is seen following conventional surgery with respect to resumption of bowel function or length of hospital stay.

Similarly, Larach and co-workers [3] recently described their early experience with LAC. Eighteen patients underwent laparoscopic procedures for benign and malignant colorectal pathology. In three of these cases resections were not carried out secondary to abdominal wall bleeding, tumour infiltrating the abdominal wall or diagnostic intervention alone. Seven patients (39%) had nine complications directly related to the laparoscopic procedure: two enterotomies, a partial ureteral obstruction and resection of the wrong bowel segment. The mean length of operative procedures was 3 h 32 min (range: 1 h–8 h 35 min). There was one postoperative death. The mean length of hospital stay was 7.2 days (range: 4–14 days). They concluded that LAC will take more time to be assimilated into the armamentarium of surgeons than did laparoscopic cholecystectomy because of the greater technical difficulties. Furthermore, they stated that as instrumentation improves and the technique evolves both the surgical results and operative time will likewise improve and they predict 'wide acceptance' in the near future.

Some of the 'benefits' of laparoscopic colectomy may diminish by altering the management of standard laparotomy patients. Binderow and co-workers performed a prospective randomized study to evaluate whether or not early postoperative feeding can be solely claimed as a unique benefit to laparoscopic surgery [18]. Sixty-four consecutive patients over a 3-month period underwent standard laparotomy with either a colonic or an ileal resection. In all cases the nasogastric tube was removed immediately after the operation Group I consisted of 32 patients (age range: 15–81 years, mean: 52 years) who received a regular diet on the first postoperative morning. Group II consisted of 32 patients (age range: 15–87 years, mean: 52 years) who were fed in a traditional manner: regular food was permitted after resolution of ileus as defined by resumption of bowel movements in the absence of abdominal distension, nausea or vomiting. The rate of nasogastric tube re-insertion for distension with vomiting was 19% (six patients) in group I and 12% (four patients) in group II (*P*=NS). In the 26 patients from group I who did not require nasogastric tube reinsertion, there was shorter hospitalization (6.7 vs 8.0 days, respectively). Thus, the laparoscopic surgeons' claim of shorter hospitalization and earlier tolerated oral intake may not be unique to laparoscopy.

Another potential problem that has recently been recognized is one of local wound recurrence of tumour cells in port sites of patients undergoing laparoscopic or laparoscopically assisted colectomies for cancer. The Paul–Mikulicz operation, popularized in the early part of this century, involves performing resections on loops of large bowel by an extracorporeal technique [19]. Although initially popular because of a reduction in operative mortality, this procedure lost its appeal due to the high incidence of local recurrence, with recurrence of the wound being the most common.

Alexander and co-workers, in a letter to the editor of the *Lancet*, reported a 67-year-old female who, 3 months after a curative laparoscopically assisted right hemicolectomy for a Dukes' C adenocarcinoma, presented with a wound recurrence of her tumour [20]. There have also been numerous other early port site recurrences after curative resection [21–23]. The real concern is not only wound recurrences in patients with Dukes' C disease, but also that some of these patients had Dukes' B lesions. O'Rourke and co-workers described an 82-year-old woman who 10 weeks' postoperatively presented with two port site recurrences. Her initial lesion was moderately well differentiated with no lymph node involvement (Dukes' B) [24].

Furthermore, not all port site recurrences have occurred in the port of retrieval of the specimen. Fusco and co-workers reported a trocar site abdominal wall recurrence 10 months after a laparoscopically assisted right hemicolectomy [25]. At colonoscopy, the patient was felt to have an early cancer. The final pathology reveal a T3N1M0 lesion, with four of 11 resected lymph nodes positive for metastatic carcinoma. They concluded that the questions surrounding the efficacy of laparoscopic colectomy in the eradication of colorectal carcinoma support the need for prospectively randomized trials. Similarly, Walsh and co-workers described a 92-year-old man who underwent an uncomplicated right hemicolectomy for a Dukes' C lesion [26]. Pathological examination of the specimen revealed a moderate to poorly differentiated adenocarcinoma with six of seven mesenteric nodes containing tumour. He presented 6 months later with a biopsy-proven port site recurrence. Interestingly, only later did tumour masses develop at the site of the 5 cm incision through which the specimen was retrieved. Moreover, this problem does not seem to be limited to laparoscopic colectomy. There have been several reports of port site recurrences in relation to gallbladder, pancreatic, gastric and ovarian carcinoma [27–30].

There still remain many unanswered questions in the management of diseases of the colon and rectum. Firstly, current resident training programmes are teaching laparoscopy; however, a 1-day course does not constitute adequate knowledge to safely perform all types of resections. Secondly, the number of laparoscopic colon and rectal resections necessary to surpass the learning curve has not yet been established. Thirdly, the 'significant cost savings' analysis never includes the cost of the expensive instruments including the cameras, video, insufflator, monitors, recorders, printers and cables. Nor does cost analysis ever include the expensive extra operating room time needed during the setup and takedown of the myriad of equipment necessary to perform 'cost-effective minimally invasive surgery'. Fourthly, the cost-effectiveness of both reusable and disposable instruments must be assessed.

Lastly, it is important that science prevails and adequate prospective randomized trials are performed in order to answer the question of acceptability of the technology for the cure of cancer.

Conclusion

Laparoscopy is a good tool that should be a part of every surgeon's armamentarium. There is no question that laparoscopic cholecystectomy has changed abdominal surgery forever. However, we must approach laparoscopic colon and rectal surgery with cautious enthusiasm in order to live up to the most important part of the Hippocratic oath: *Primum non nocere* — First, do no harm.

It is of paramount importance that the surgeon tells the patient honestly whether, if he of she required the same operation for the same pathology, it would be undertaken with a laparoscope. Informal polls at major national and international meetings to date, including over 5000 surgeons, have revealed that the majority of surgeons are happy to advocate the laparoscope for both benign and malignant disease. However, only 30 and 1% would themselves undergo a laparoscopic operation for benign and malignant disease, respectively. We must not in our enthusiasm create a dual standard of acceptability – one for our patients and a different one for us.

References

1   Monson JRT, Darzi A, Carey PD, Guillou PJ. Prospective evaluation of laparoscopic-assisted colectomy in an unselected group of patients. *Lancet* 1992; **340**: 831–3.

2   Schmitt SL, Cohen SM, Wexner SD *et al*. Does laparoscopic-assisted ileal pouch anal anastomosis reduce the length of hospitalization? *Int J Colorect Dis* 1994; **9**: 134–7.

3   Larach SW, Salomen MC, Williamson PR, Goldstein E. Laparoscopic assisted colectomy: experience during the learning curve. *Colo-proctology* 1993; **1**: 38–41.

4   Tate JJT, Kwok S, Dawson JW *et al*. Prospective comparison of laparoscopic and conventional anterior resection. *Br J Surg* 1993; **80**: 1396–8.

5   Wexner SD, Johansen OB. Laparoscopic bowel resection: advantages and limitations. *Ann Med* 1992; **24**: 105–10.

6   Phillips FH, Franklin M, Carroll BJ *et al*. Laparoscopic colectomy. *Ann Surg* 1992; **216**(6): 703–7.

7   Lazorthes F, Chiotassol P. Stapled colorectal anastomosis: operative integrity of the anastomosis and risk of postoperative leakage. *Int J Colorect Dis* 1986; **1**: 96–8.

8   Morson BC, Whiteway JE, Jones EA *et al*. Histopathology and prognosis of malignant colorectal polyps treated by endoscopic polypectomy. *Gut* 1984; **25**: 437–44.

9   Corbit JD. Preliminary experience with laparoscopic-guided colectomy. *Surg Laparosc Endosc* 1992; **2**(1): 79–81.

10 Jacobs M, Verdeja JC, Goldstein MS. Minimally invasive colon resection (laparoscopic colectomy). *Surg Laparosc Endosc* 1991; **1**(3): 144–50.

11 Quattlebaum JK, Flanders HD, Usher CH. Laparoscopic assisted colectomy. *Surg Laparosc Endosc* 1993; **3**(2): 81–7.

12 Scoggin SD, Frazee RC, Snyder SK *et al*. Laparoscopic-assisted bowel surgery. *Dis Colon Rectum* 1993; **36**: 747–50.

13 Peters WR, Bartels TL. Minimally invasive colectomy: are the potential benefits realized? *Dis Colon Rectum* 1993; **36**: 751–6.

14 Senagore AJ, Luchtefeld MA, Macheigan JM, Mazier WP. Open colectomy versus laparoscopic colectomy: are there differences? *Am Surg* 1993; **59**(8): 549–54.

15 Vayer AJ, Larach SW, Williamson PR *et al*. Cost effectiveness of laparoscopic colectomy. *Dis Colon Rectum* 1993; **36**: P34.

16 Cohen SM, Schmitt SL, Wexner SD *et al*. Does laparoscopy confer an advantage over standard colectomy? *Surg Endosc* 1993; **7**(3): 265.

17 Milsom JW, Lavery IC, Böhm B, Fazio VW. Laparoscopic-assisted ileocolectomy in Crohn's disease. *Surg Laparosc Endosc* 1993; **3**(2): 77–80.

18 Binderow SR, Cohen SM, Wexner SD *et al*. Must early postoperative oral intake be limited to laparoscopy? *Dis Colon Rectum* 1993; **36**(4): P33.

19 von Mikulicz J. Small contributions to the surgery of the intestinal tract. *Boston Med Surg J* 1903; **148**: 608–11.

20 Alexander RJT, Jaques BC, Mitchell KG. Laparoscopically assisted colectomy and wound recurrence (letter). *Lancet* 1993; **341**: 249–50.

21 Goh P. Laparoscopic colon resection — the Singapore experience. Presented at the Tripartite Colorectal Meeting, 1993, Sydney, Australia.

22 Stitz R. Presented at the Tripartite Colorectal Meeting, 1993, Sydney, Australia.

23 Franklin M. *Laparoscopic Colectomy*. International Symposium on Advances in Laparoscopic Colectomy 1993, Indianapolis, Indiana, USA.

24 O'Rourke N, Price PM, Kelly S, Sikora K. Tumour inoculation during laparoscopy (letter). *Lancet* 1993; **342**: 368.

25 Fusco MA, Paluzzi MW. Abdominal wall recurrence after laparoscopic-assisted colectomy for adenocarcinoma of the colon. *Dis Colon Rectum* 1993; **36**: 858–61.

26 Walsh DCA, Waitchow DA, Wilson TG. Subcutaneous metastases after laparoscopic resection of malignancy. *Aust N Z J Surg* 1993; **63**: 563–5.

27 Siriwardena A, Samarji WN. Cutaneous tumour seeding from a previously undiagnosed pancreative carcinoma after laparoscopic cholecystectomy. *Ann R Coll Surg Engl* 1993; **75**: 199–200.

28 Fong Y, Brennan MF, Turnbull A *et al*. Gallbladder cancer discovered during laparoscopic surgery. *Arch Surg* 1993; **128**: 1054–6.

29 Cava A, Román J, Quintela AG *et al*. Subcutaneous metastasis following laparoscopy in gastric adenocarcinoma. *Eur J Surg Oncol* 1990; **16**: 63–7.

30 Gleeson NC, Nicosia SV, Mark JE *et al*. Abdominal wall metastases from ovarian cancer after laparoscopy. *Am J Obstet Gynecol* 1993; **169**: 522–3.

Chapter 14

The Laparoscopic Bowel Surgery Registry: preliminary results

R.W. Beart Jr

Introduction

The introduction of laparoscopic cholecystectomy in 1988 was associated with the enormous task of training and credentialing American surgeons in a new operative approach which was unprecedented in the history of surgery. While a number of centres published excellent experiences with the technique in terms of safety and efficacy, concerns regarding a higher morbidity, pariticularly with respect to biliary injuries, became apparent. The rapid proliferation of other laparoscopic procedures and a concern for the prevention of the untoward sequelae associated with the 'learning curve' prompted the establishment of the Laparoscopic Bowel Surgery Registry by the American Society of Colon and Rectal Surgeons and the American College of Surgeons. The aim of this project was to identify potential pitfalls in the application of laparoscopy to colorectal surgery early in its development. The complete results of this experience have been submitted to the journal *Diseases of the Colon and Rectum* for publication. This chapter summarizes the initial experience as subsequently submitted to this journal.

A registry was initially approved by the American Society of Colon and Rectal Surgeons. In an effort to promote broad compliance, the American College of Surgery Commission on Cancer consented to house and analyse the data accumulated. This organization is accustomed to managing large amounts of data accumulated through the Commission on Cancer Patient Care Evaluation Studies [1]. SAGES endorsed the registry and has promoted it since its inception. The registry was promoted through presentations at meetings and advertisements in national peer-reviewed surgical journals. Registry data forms were available through the American College of Surgery, SAGES and the American Society of Colon and Rectal Surgeons. Forms were entered in the CDC database EP15 which also performed the data analysis. Statistical calculations were not considered appropriate for this type of voluntary registry.

Two hundred and fifty-two or 45% of the 565 patients within the registry underwent a laparoscopic procedure whilst having a diagnosis of cancer. Inflammatory disease was the indication in 106 patients (19%) and polyps in 117 patients (21%). Eighty-three patients (15%) had 'other' indications. The precise diagnosis was not provided in six patients (1%).

The predominant site of pathology was the right colon in 197 patients (35%), the sigmoid colon in 173 (31%), the rectum in 91 (16%), the left colon in 22 (4%), the transverse colon in nine (2%) and the small bowel in 17 patients (3%). Disease in various other segmental combinations were reported in 56 patients (8%).

Resection was the single most commonly performed procedure undertaken in 520 patients (92%). Twenty-four patients underwent a bypass procedure (4%) and polypectomy was performed in seven cases (1%). The operative procedure was not reported in 13 patients (3%).

Completion of the intended procedure was possible in 425 instances (75%). Three hundred and forty-four extracorporeal anastomoses (61%) and 90 intracorporeal anastomoses (16%) were performed. One hundred and thirty cases initiated laparoscopically were converted to open laparotomy, or 23% of the total group. The most common reason stated for conversion to open surgery was unclear anatomy in 47 cases (40%) followed by bleeding in seven (6%) and perforation in three instances (3%). In 61 patients (50%), there was some other reason for conversion unrelated to anatomy, bleeding or perforation. The authors assume most of these consisted of either adhesions and/or sheer frustration.

Thirty cases (6%) were associated with strictly intraoperative laparoscopic complications consisting of bleeding in 10, perforations in seven and contamination in one patient. 'Other' unspecified intraoperative problems occurred in 12 patients.

The registry form queried surgeons specifically whether a violation in the principles of cancer surgery occurred. Four hundred and ninety-nine of responders (97%) answered no. Twelve answered yes. In these 12 cases the primary indication for the procedure was cancer in only three cases and polyps in one. Therefore, the overall subjective incidence of non-observance of the technical and anatomical considerations of cancer surgery was four of 499 cases (0.8%). In 53 cases, this consideration was not applicable and no affirmative response was given.

Postoperative complications occurred in 98 patients or an overall rate of 18%. Seventeen of these were laparoscopically related or 17% of the group with postoperative morbidity. When complication rates are examined between patients whose anastomoses were performed either intra- or extracorporeally, the incidences were 17 and 18%, respectively. The occurrence of laparoscopically related postoperative complications is also identical for both types of anastomoses (4%). The registry did not allow for the identification of the type of postoperative complication. Many contributors did identify specific complications but these could not be analysed because of incomplete data.

While comparisons between these patients whose procedures were completed laparoscopically and those requiring conversion to open surgery are problematic since the two groups are not strictly comparable, it is, however, worth highlighting the difference between the two groups in terms of length of postoperative hospital stay. Patients whose bowel surgery was performed and completed laparoscopically were discharged on average 5.5 days postoperatively (median: 5 days, range: 0–51 days). Those converted to open surgery went home 7.8 days postoperatively on average (median: 7 days, range: 0–45 days). There were no significant differences in hospital stay in patients having intracorporeal versus extracorporeal anastomoses performed.

Studies of this type are necessarily limited in the conclusions which can be drawn [2]. Contributed cases are by definition selected. Because of strong professional encouragement, we feel these cases reflect national experience.

This database underscores a number of important findings in the preliminary experience with laparoscopic bowel surgery. Clearly the laparascopic approach to malignancy is suspect in the estimation of many surgeons [3–7]. However, 45% of patients in the present series were operated upon for cancer. While data are lacking with respect to the average length of the margins of resection and yield of lymph nodes, at least each surgeon's subjective report of the maintenance of standards for cancer surgery suggests that the laparoscopic approach does conform to each surgeon's perception of these principles. Further study and long-term follow-up is clearly necessary before any valid conclusions can be drawn about the efficacy of laparoscopic bowel resection for malignancy.

Another important finding is the relative success of laparoscopic bowel procedures in terms of the relatively low incidence of conversion to open procedures [8–10]. One-fourth of patients had their laparoscopic procedure abandoned in favour of open laparotomy. Given the technically demanding nature of laparoscopic bowel resections, this conversion rate is not only entirely acceptable, but suggests a greater margin for improvement as surgeons advance on the learning curve. The predominance of extracorporeal anastomotic techniques over the intracorporeal by a margin of 4:1 is less surprising. These techniques did not differ in terms of complication rates or postoperative hospital stays. Given the relative greater degree of difficulty in intracorporeal techniques and the concomitant necessity for a small incision of some type for the extraction of specimens from the abdominal cavity, extracorporeal anastomosis seems to be the more logical method at this time.

The incidence of intraoperative complications was 6%. Preliminary fears concerning massive contamination, bleeding and vascular and ureteral injuries is not identified. Intraoperative bleeding, perforation or contamination occurred with overall rates of 1.7, 1.5 and 0.2%, respectively. The overall incidence of postoperative complications was 18% which is similar to other reported series using open techniques. The incidence of postoperative complications which were directly laparoscopically related was 3.4%.

Finally, the data presented here are consistent with other reports about foreshortened hospital stays in patients undergoing laparoscopic bowel surgery. On average patients whose operations were completed laparoscopically were discharged 2 days earlier than those having the procedure converted to an open operation. While this comparison is obviously unfair in many respects, it does evoke a number of provocative questions. Are patients discharged earlier when operated upon laparoscopically because they do so much better than patients undergoing laparotomy, or do surgeons change their postoperative management depending upon whether a patient has endoscopic or open surgery? Is there less paralytic ileus following laparoscopic surgery on the intestine and what are the factors responsible for this phenomenon? Moreover, can the experience with laparoscopic bowel surgery actually change our postoperative management of patients operated on via laparotomy in terms of when patients are given liquids, regular diets and ultimately discharged?

Laparoscopic colectomy and other minimally invasive procedures of the small and large intestine are safe. Its application for the treatment of malignancy seems reasonable *vis-à-vis* the observation of the principles of cancer surgery, but further study is necessary. There is no evident advantage of intracorporeal anastomosis in preference to those performed extracorporeally. Given the greater technical ease of the latter, an argument can be made that extracorporeal techniques are the method of choice at the present time. Patients operated upon laparoscopically appear to have shorter hospital stays, but the factors associated with this finding deserve greater scrutiny.

References

1   Lawrence W Jr, Donegan WL, Natarajan N, Mettlin C, Beart R, Winchester D. Adult soft tissue sarcomas. A pattern of care survey of the American College of Surgeons. *Ann Surg* 1987; **205**: 349–59.

2   Beart RW Jr. Laparoscopic colectomy: status of the art. *Dis Colon Rectum* 1994; **37** (Suppl.): S47–S49.

3   Braithwaite BD, Ritchie AWS, Earnshaw JJ. Laparoscopic surgery for colorectal cancer. *Br J Surg* 1994; **81**: 313.

4   Cirocco WC, Schwartzman A, Golub RW. Abdominal wall recurrence after laparoscopic colectomy for colon cancer. *Surgery* 1994; **116**: 842–6.

5   Decanini C, Milsom JW, Böhm B, Fazio VW. Laparoscopic oncologic abdominoperineal resection. *Dis Colon Rectum* 1994; **37**: 552-8.

6   Monson J, Darzi A, Carey P, Guillou P. Prospective evaluation of laparoscopic-assisted colectomy in an unselected group of patients. *Lancet* 1992; **340**: 831–3.

7   Ramos JM, Gupta S, Anthone GJ, Ortega AE, Simons AJ, Beart RW. Laparoscopy and colon cancer: is the port site at risk? A preliminary report. *Arch Surg* 1994; **129**: 897–9.

8   Franklin ME Jr, Ramos R, Rosenthal D, Schuessler W. Laparoscopic colonic procedures. *World J Surg* 1993; **17**: 51–6.

9   Jacobs M, Verdeja JC, Goldstein HS. Minimally invasive colon resection (laparoscopic colectomy). *Surg Laparosc Endosc* 1991; **1**: 144–50.

10 Redwine DB, Sharpe DR. Laparoscopic segmental resection of the sigmoid colon for endometriosis. *J Laparoendosc Surg* 1991; **1**: 217–20.

Chapter 15

Laparoscopic colorectal surgery: the experience in the Far East

P.D. Carey, S.P.Y. Kwok, R.J. Delicata and A.K.C. Li

Introduction

Following the huge success of laparoscopic cholecystectomy and its rapid acceptance as the procedure of choice for removal of the diseased gallbladder, it was only a matter of time before laparoscopic techniques were applied to other areas such as colorectal surgery. From a purely technical point of view, laparoscopic mobilization of the healthy colon or rectum is not a difficult concept to grasp and accept as reasonable surgical practice. However, mobilizing the malignant colon, guaranteeing clear resection margins, performing adequate vascular and, therefore, nodal clearance and developing techniques for both intraperitoneal and intraluminal cytocidal washout are all subjects of concern and debate and have proved to be too much of an anathema to traditional colorectal surgeons. Understandably, these questions raised doubts about the viability of laparoscopic colorectal surgery. While these techniques are in their infancy, such questions remain and need to be addressed and satisfactorily answered by proponents of laparoscopic resection. For these reasons, our observations during the development of laparoscopic colectomy in the Chinese University of Hong Kong (at the Prince of Wales Hospital (PWH), Shatin, New Territories) are particularly pertinent as there is little in the way of benign colorectal disease and up to 200 malignant cases present to a single surgical unit in one calendar year. The purpose of this chapter is to discuss these observations.

The 'setup' in Hong Kong

Surgical specialization in Hong Kong is developing in tandem with similar developments in the United Kingdom and elsewhere. A significant proportion of the six million population are treated in the private sector. Thus many general surgeons treat colorectal cancer; however, until mid-1993, none of these surgeons had any experience of, or indeed interest in, laparoscopic colorectal resection. The 40% of the population who are treated at the university hospitals by and large are cared for by surgeons who have a special interest in colorectal disease. In the PWH, which has a catchment area of 1.5 million people, between 170 and 200 new colorectal cancers present per year. Almost all of these are seen and treated by a single surgical team. This unit is also the hepatobiliary unit and unlike other units worldwide, where colorectal surgeons do not have access to laparoscopic biliary work, the team of surgeons at PWH all had considerable experience in laparoscopic techniques prior to embarking on this new venture.

The first attempted laparoscopically assisted colectomy (LAC) was performed in April 1992. At the outset, strict criteria were laid down within the unit concerning the selection of cases. Procedures in the first 30 patients were performed in those with proven metastatic disease who were deemed medically fit for prolonged anaesthesia and pneumoperitoneum. Informed consent was obtained in all patients. Thus, despite the large case load presenting to the unit, the number of laparoscopic colectomy procedures was initially restricted. The details and results of these cases, over the subsequent 2 years, are presented in this chapter. Furthermore, various other colorectal procedures were performed in the unit, and included routine procedures such as appendicectomy and rectopexy. This experience is also discussed.

The distal first technique

One major significant development locally was the accomplishment of the excision of the left side of the colon using a 'distal first' technique. This procedure was developed in the laparoscopic sphere because of the importance of obtaining optimum access to the vessels at the root of the left colonic mesentery and the need to attain as high a tie on these vessels as possible. The authors had noted that when the rectosigmoid junction had been transected at the pelvic brim, traction on the proximal 'tumour-bearing' colon facilitated access to the vessels at the root of the sigmoid mesentery and it was apparent that easier access could be obtained to the inferior mesenteric artery (IMA) (Fig. 15.1).

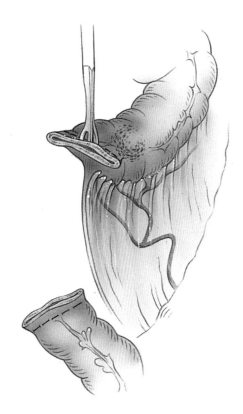

Figure 15.1
Traction on the proximal part of the large bowel after division some 5 cm below the tumour causes the mesentery to be stretched, thus facilitating dissection and division of the mesenteric vessels.

Figure 15.2 shows the proposed resection margins for a tumour situated in the sigmoid or lower descending colon. Debate still exists about the extent of left colon resection for tumours situated in the sigmoid colon, namely a sigmoid colectomy as opposed to a formal left hemicolectomy. What is not in doubt is the fact that if a high tie is performed on the IMA, then the laparoscopist, in the same way as in the equivalent open procedure, must adequately mobilize the splenic flexure and distal transverse colon in order to be able to perform a tension-free anastomosis in the upper pelvis. Frequently, excision of the sigmoid colon requires division of the lienocolic attachments and full mobilization of the descending colon to the level of the splenic flexure.

The procedure commences along the lines which have come to be seen as standard for laparoscopically assisted colorectal excision. Figure 15.3 shows the standard placement of ports. We routinely use an infra-umbilical port 10 mm in size for initial camera positioning and two 10 or 12 mm ports spaced along the right flank as indicated in the figure. By inserting a 10 mm diameter Babcock-type forceps in the lower one of the right flank ports and a further atraumatic grasping forceps in the other port, one can perform the initial assessment of the peritoneal cavity and the tumour. The former examination includes in every case the pelvic cavity, the rectum, the liver and the total intra-abdominal colon. By a combination of palpation using atraumatic grasping forceps and direct vision, a search for synchronous lesions is carried out.

After confirmation of the site of the lesion in the sigmoid or descending colon, dissection is commenced along the left lateral peritoneal fold (Fig. 15.4) and where possible a no-touch technique is employed. The patient is positioned in a moderate Trendelenburg position and rotated to the right side, towards the operator. This enables, firstly, the loops of small intestine to be drawn out of the pelvis and retracted to a stable position in the upper right abdomen and, secondly, it facilitates traction on the colon to the right side thus putting the plane of lateral dissection under a greater degree of stretch (Fig. 15.4). With each

Figure 15.2

The extent of laparoscopic bowel resection for tumours of the sigmoid colon is shown between the horizontal lines. Laparoscopic mobilization is carried as high as the splenic flexure.

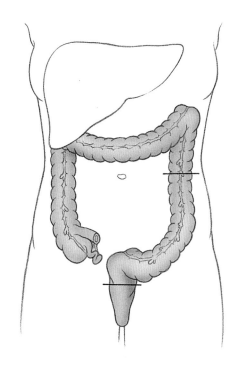

(a)

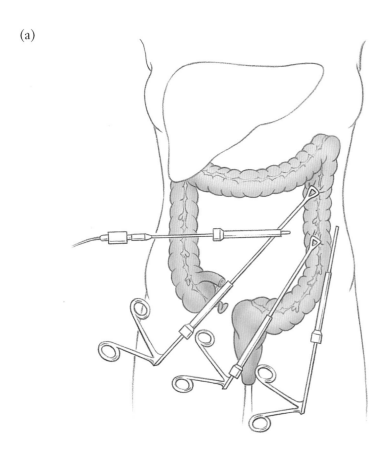

(b)

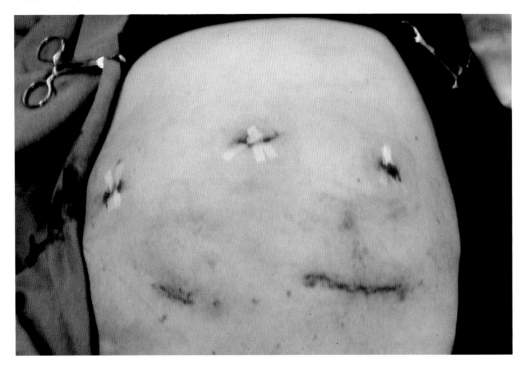

Figure 15.3
(a) A schematic representation of the port sites with the instruments in position. (b) The abdominal wall of a patient at the end of a laparoscopically assisted sigmoid colectomy. The left iliac fossa incision is the site through which the specimen was delivered.

Figure 15.4
Traction of the large bowel to the right using atraumatic tissue-grasping forceps facilitates dissection along the line of peritoneal dissection.

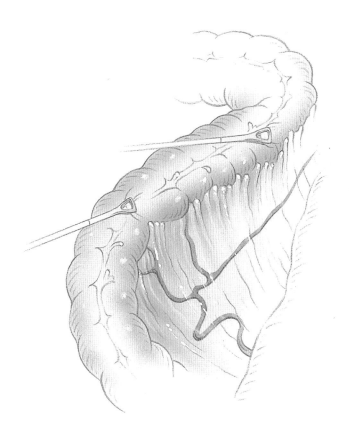

excursion of the dissecting scissors the colon is mobilized further and further to the right side, thus opening up the left lateral aspect of the sigmoid and descending colonic mesentery. This dissection can be carried out from the pelvic brim to the level of the splenic flexure. It is during this initial mobilization that extra port sites may be introduced, particularly to facilitate the dissection around the splenic flexure. The camera position is frequently varied, particularly to the right-hand ports to enable instruments to be placed in the infra-umbilical port.

On a number of occasions the initial dissection was commenced at the splenic flexure where it was felt that the mobilization would be easily achieved and usually when the flexure was low lying. Once the whole extent of the large bowel from pelvic brim to the splenic flexure is mobilized, a thorough search for the ureter is performed and this was successful in more than 90% of cases. A mesenteric window is created and the bowel is then divided at a point 5 cm or more distal to the tumour using an Endo-GIA (Autosuture, Ascot, UK). This is inserted via the 12 mm port in the right iliac fossa. By lifting the distal end of the colon bearing the tumour, traction can then be exerted on the mesentery in order to facilitate adequate mesenteric and therefore nodal clearance (see Fig. 15.1). This division of the mesentery is carried out by a combination of scissor dissection and diathermy. In order to ensure secure clipping of the large vessels (the IMA just distal to the origin of the upper left colic branch), these are first skeletonized using an ultrasonic dissector or diathermy scissors (Fig. 15.5). Polydioxanone (PDS) clips (Ethicon Ltd, Edinburgh, UK) are then applied as shown in Fig. 15.6.

Once the larger vessels are ligated and divided, the leaf of mesentery leading up to the splenic flexure at the proposed level of the proximal division of the

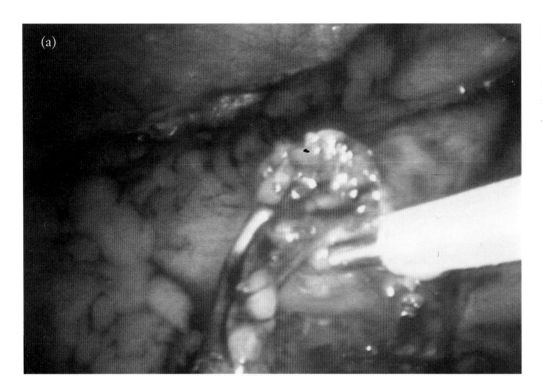

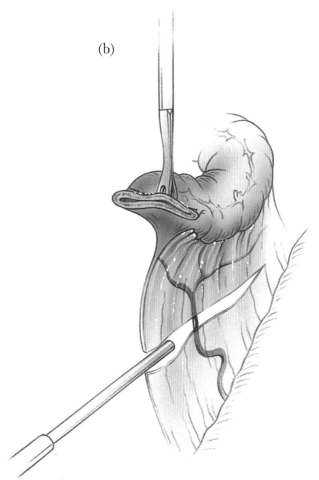

Figure 15.5
(a) The ultrasonic dissector in use during skeletonization of the mesenteric vessels; (b) a line drawing representing the same.

Figure 15.6
The mesenteric vessels are very clearly seen after skeletonization with the ultrasonic dissector. The figure shows PDS clips being applied on these skeletonized vessels.

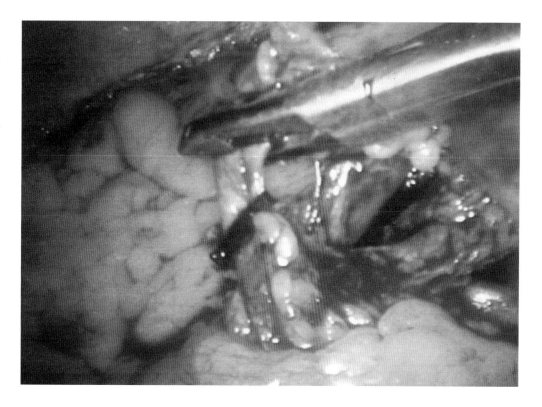

bowel is divided again using a combination of scissor dissection and diathermy. A 5–10 cm incision is then made in the left iliac fossa (see Fig. 15.3); this is developed in order to gain access into the peritoneal cavity. The closed sigmoid and descending colon are then brought out through this incision (Fig. 15.7). Various wound protectors or sheaths can be employed at this stage to protect against tumour implantation. The proximal colon is then divided at the proposed level. The anvil of an end-to-end anastomosis (EEA) stapling gun is inserted into the lumen of the proximal colon for anastomosis and a purse-string suture is applied. The proximal colon and anvil component of the EEA gun are then replaced inside the abdomen and the left iliac fossa wound closed. The pneumoperitoneum is re-established. In the meantime a perineal operator inserts the EEA gun through the anal canal and under guidance from the intraperitoneal views seen on screen via the laparoscope camera, the spike of the EEA gun is opened. Any organ coming in the way of the spike inside the abdomen is gently lifted away by a grasping forceps. The laparoscopist then guides the anvil of the EEA gun downwards towards the spike of the gun (Fig. 15.8). Once again any organ or tissue coming in the way is gently retracted away. The colorectal anastomosis is thus completed under direct vision. Figure 15.9 shows the specimen of colon obtained in this way. This was an example of a Dukes' B tumour and resected specimen contained a minimum of 24 lymph nodes, all of which were examined.

Patient selection

During the period between April 1992 and July 1994, a total of 91 patients underwent a LAC. Five operations were for benign colorectal conditions

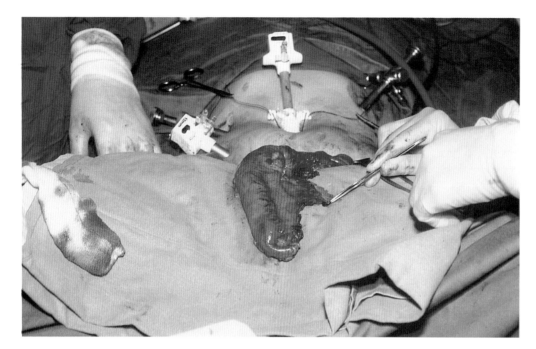

Figure 15.7
The sigmoid colon is delivered via the left iliac fossa wound. Resection of the tumour is carried out outside the abdomen and the anvil of the end-to-end anastomosis stapler is introduced into the end of the residual loop of bowel and secured by a purse-string suture. This loop is then replaced inside the abdominal cavity.

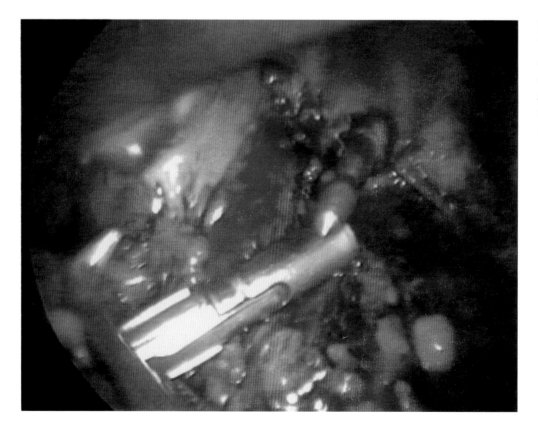

Figure 15.8
The spike of the end-to-end anastomosis stapler has emerged from the rectal stump and is being connected to the shaft of the anvil (bottom left).

Figure 15.9
A specimen of sigmoid colon obtained by laparoscopically assisted sigmoid colectomy (see text).

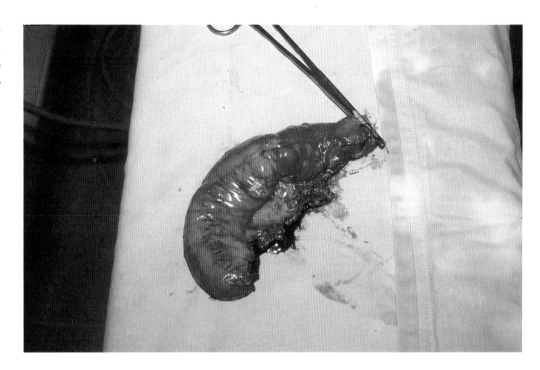

(Table 15.1) and 86 were for colorectal cancer. In 17 of the cancer patients, initial laparoscopy revealed advanced disease and laparoscopic dissection was therefore not attempted. The total number of LACs for cancer was therefore 69 (Table 15.2). In the initial phase of the series, only patients aged over 65 and those with distant metastases were selected for LAC (*n*=30). With the experience accrued from phase 1 patients and following analyses of the early reasons for conversions (see below), patients in the latter phase were of all ages. However, bulky tumours, locally advanced disease and very low anterior resections were not attempted (*n*=39).

Table 15.1
Benign colorectal conditions treated laparoscopically.

Condition	No. of operations
Sigmoid volvulus	1
Rectal prolapse	1
Polyps	3

Table 15.2
The types and numbers of procedures performed and the number of procedures that were eventually converted.

Operation	Total number	Completed	Converted
Abdominoperineal resection	13	11	2
Anterior resection	19	14	5
Sigmoid colectomy	23	22	1
Left hemicolectomy	3	2	1
Transverse colectomy	2	1	1
Right hemicolectomy	9	7	2

Preoperative investigations

Colonoscopy was performed routinely in all patients as was ultrasound scan of the liver. However, the use and role of computed tomography (CT) and double contrast barium enema (DCBE) in the preoperative evaluation of the tumour are discussed later.

Results

There were 35 male and 34 female patients with an age range of 32–87 years (68.3 ± 11.5 (mean ± SD) years). The period of follow-up ranged between 3 and 23 months with a median of 10 months. The overall mean duration of these procedures was 189.6 ± 43.0 (mean ± SD) min. Completed operations lasted 190.2 (± 44.0) min and those operations which necessitated conversion lasted 186.8 (± 41.0) min. The blood loss ranged between 100 and 3000 ml with a median loss of 200 ml.

Dukes' staging and treatment intent

Fifty-five operations were deemed to be curative resections and the other 14 palliative. The staging of these tumours is shown in Table 15.3.

Postoperative progress

Resumption of a normal diet occurred within 4 days on average (range: 1–15 days); the average analgesic requirements (assessed by patient demand using patient-controlled analgesia) was two demands per 24 h with a range of 0–39 demands; the average hospital stay was 6 days with a range of 2–33 days.

The complications which were encountered are listed in Table 15.4.

Dukes' stage	Distribution (%)
A	8
B	40
C	33
D	19

Table 15.3
Distribution of tumours by Dukes' staging.

Complications	No. of patients
Wound infection	4
Small bowel perforation	1
Ureteric injury*	1
Retention of urine	2
Deep vein thrombosis	1

* This occurred during open surgery after conversion.

Table 15.4
Complications encountered in the laparoscopically assisted colectomies performed.

Early recurrence

There were three instances of recurrence; one patient presented with lung metastases and one with ovarian secondaries; both had seemingly curative resections. The single incidence of port site recurrence was in a patient who had a non-curative resection.

Mortality

There were five deaths in total; one following a cerebrovascular accident, one following aspiration pneumonia and three from disseminated disease. The latter were all patients in whom the resection was deemed from the start to be palliative.

Conversion analysis (early assessment)

Following the first year's experience it became clear that there was a high rate of conversion from laparoscopic to open colorectal resection. Though there is an obvious learning curve for all such new adventures it was felt that conversion was unacceptably high since, as stated above, the three surgeons involved had individually accumulated significant laparoscopic expertise and all had formal training in colorectal surgery. Therefore it was felt that the high conversion rate (see the figures below) was probably due to inappropriate case selection. Thus, at the end of the first year the data were analysed with reference to preoperative assessment and subsequent reasons for conversion to open surgery. The importance of analysing converted cases cannot be stressed enough. Laparoscopic surgery for colon cancer, especially if attention is paid to established rules of oncological clearance, requires prolonged operation time and exposes patients to enhanced cardiovascular side effects. Identification of factors which contraindicate laparoscopic dissection may eliminate or minimize inappropriate case selection. Thus appropriate preoperative assessment could reduce costs and facilitate the development of this type of surgery.

The aim was to determine factors influencing conversion to open surgery. The patients analysed were the initial consecutive series of patients (n=33). All were elderly or had proven metastatic colorectal disease (liver or lung). Fifteen male and 18 female patients underwent colorectal surgery in the period April 1992 to March 1993. Patients had a mean age of 72.4 ($\pm$ 9.4 SD) years and 30 had malignant disease while the remaining three were operated on for benign disease.

Table 15.5 gives the details of the types of resections performed and the number of conversions in this group. Three of these patients were, at initial laparoscopy, deemed to be inoperable by the laparoscopic route. Of the remaining 30, the majority had left-sided colon resections which were either sigmoid colectomy or anterior resection. Rectal tumours were all in the upper rectum and involved anastomosis in the upper pelvis. There were no low colorectal anastomoses performed in this initial series. The mean operative time was 230 min (range: 130–340 min). Five of the sigmoid colectomies had full intracorporeal mobilization and transanal stapled anastomosis, with the tumours being removed via a 5 cm incision in the left iliac fossa. Table 15.5 also lists the converted cases, which included five of the anterior resections.

For this analysis any case which required an abdominal wound (any size) for the purpose of colonic or rectal mobilization prior to division of the vascular

Resections	No. attempted	No. converted	Diagnostic laparoscopy
Right hemicolectomy	4	2	–
Sigmoid colectomy	11	2	1
Anterior resection	10	4	2
Abdominoperineal resection	2	1	–
Benign polypectomy	2	1	–
Benign rectopexy	1		
Total	30	10 (30%)	3

Table 15.5
The types and number of resections performed together with the type and number of procedures that required conversion.

pedicle was defined as a conversion to open surgery (excluding the diagnostic laparoscopy cases). In total, 10 of 30 (33%) cases required conversion to formal open procedures. The stated reasons for converting are listed in Table 15.6. One sigmoid colectomy which required conversion was complicated by a large bulky tumour obliterating the sigmoid mesentery. This tumour was prolapsing into the pelvis and was adherent to the bladder roof. Four of the anterior resections were converted due to tumour fixity as assessed by the mobility of the tumour and trial dissection in the upper pelvis. In one instance a further difficulty was cited and that was an inability of the operating surgeon to satisfactorily retract the small intestine out of the operating field. Similarly, the conversion of the one abdominoperineal resection cited was due to difficulty with small bowel retraction which obscured the operative field. One patient having a large polyp removed from her transverse colon was converted due to an inability of combined on-table colonoscopy and laparoscopy to localize her lesion. At a previous colonoscopy her polyp was identified in the transverse colon (80 cm) and felt to be too large for routine endoscopic polypectomy; the polyp was not marked at that time with indian ink or stains which might have facilitated its subsequent localization. A further difficulty cited for one of the anterior resections was the obese nature of the patient (a female weighing 110 kg) who not surprisingly had a thick, fatty sigmoid mesentery which was difficult to dissect and locate the vascular pedicle with safety. The final reason cited was a technical problem relating to the availability of satisfactory equipment for the assisted dissection of an ascending colon cancer.

Stated reason for conversion	No. of occurrences
Tumour fixity:	
Adjacent organs	4
Pelvic side wall/retroperitoneum	2
Tumour not localized	1
Mesenteric tumour spread	1
Small bowel obscuring operative field	2
Obesity (mesenteric bulk)	1
Technical	1

Table 15.6
Reasons necessitating conversion in 10 patients from the first group of 33 patients.

Following this retrospective review it was felt that all the reasons cited for conversions, bar the small bowel retraction problems, could have been predicted by extensive preoperative assessment. Indeed more aggressive reverse Trendelenburg positioning of the patient, strongly resisted by the anaesthetists at the time, would have ensured that small intestinal retraction from the pelvic dissection field was optimal. Extensive reverse Trendelenburg positioning, though of some cardiovascular concern in the more elderly patients, is the norm now for laparoscopic rectopexy procedures. Thus it was felt that only the technical conversion was of absolute necessity in this group of patients.

A further analysis was now performed which looked at the preoperative assessment of these patients. All 30 patients (100%), as is routine in the unit, had attempted full colonoscopy and biopsy of suspected lesions. Colonoscopy, of course, has the advantage that lesions can be seen and biopsied to determine their nature. In addition, a search for synchronous cancers and polyps can be undertaken and snare removal performed if appropriate. However, colorectal endoscopy is inaccurate at localizing lesions to those parts of the colon between the extremes of the fixed rectum and the ileocaecal area. It has, however, been suggested that indelible dyes can be used for subsequent localization of these lesions.

The alternative is on-table colonoscopy. Use of colonoscope in the theatre is attended by a number of problems. These include the availability of state-of-the-art equipment, which in the present day must be considered to be the widely available videoendoscope systems. This, however, would require the frequent transfer of such equipment between the endoscopy suite and theatre or the purchase of a duplicate system for the operating department. The obvious follow-on is that in the former instance, scheduling is of paramount importance, to make sure that equipment is available at the right time, whereas in the latter a considerable cost is incurred.

However, even if endoscopy equipment of sufficient standard is available other constraints come into play. Many colorectal surgeons are not expert endoscopists. The use of an insufflating instrument in the colonic lumen by an inexperienced technician, without the guiding hand of an able assistant inside the peritoneal cavity, is fraught with many hazards. Air insufflation is a necessary requirement for the proper viewing of the colonic lumen and rarely, if ever, is adequate desufflation completed following the examination. Thus the laparoscopist is faced with a blown, distended colon when viewed through the laparoscope. The risks of perforating this thinned, attenuated colonic wall with a grasping instrument and the possible inability to view the area to be resected compound an already difficult procedure. The two options to circumvent such difficulties are the use of good DCBE preoperatively or, as already stated above, the use of marking dyes at preoperative colonoscopy. The colonoscopy option, however, requires that the colorectal surgeon performs his or her own endoscopy.

Anatomical variations may be a cause of considerable confusion and delay during laparoscopic mobilization and are not likely to be identified on colonoscopic examination. A barium enema was performed in only 17% of the completed cases and 4% of the converted cases in this reported series. None of these examinations contributed to the recognition of factors adversely influencing resection rates. Twenty-seven of the 30 patients (90%) had an ultrasound examination looking for liver metastases, however a very low proportion (two out of 30 patients (7%)) had an examination of the tumour by this method. Thus the usefulness of tumour assessment by real-time ultrasound examination cannot be commented upon. Similarly, the use of CT in tumour assessment could not be evaluated because again only two of 30 patients had the tumour mass evaluated by this technique. In each instance neither of the patients evaluated were in the converted group.

Computed tomography and ultrasound scanning in preoperative assessment

Following the above retrospective analysis a prospective series of 22 consecutive patients having laparoscopic colorectal resections for carcinoma were assessed. This analysis was designed to yield information regarding the usefulness of CT scanning and real-time ultrasound. All patients had laparoscopy and an attempted laparoscopic resection and the findings were recorded and analysed with respect to the preoperative assessment. Above all, patients had colonoscopy and a biopsy confirming malignancy. Patients were aged 32–87 years (four patients were less than 60) and the group contained 11 males and 11 females. Of this group 12 (54%) had successfully completed procedures while six (27%) were converted. Three patients had laparoscopy only and were immediately converted, while the remaining patient underwent a planned open procedure. Nine sigmoid colectomies were performed, three upper rectal and three descending colon lesions were resected while the rest were made up of lesions in the splenic flexure (one), transverse colon (one), hepatic flexure (one) and ascending colon (one). In total, seven intracorporeal anastomoses were performed in this group. In all 22 patients real-time ultrasonography and CT scanning were performed and in four selected patients attempted assessment of upper rectal tumours with transrectal ultrasound was performed. The CT technique involved the use of standard oral and intravenous contrast with rectal air insufflation. All 22 lesions were identified on CT while only 15 of the 22 were seen on transabdominal ultrasound. Each investigation was performed by a separate radiologist blinded to the results of the other. Each radiologist, with the results of the above retrospective analysis in mind, independently predicted the resectability of each tumour stating the relevant reasons. Surgery was then undertaken in all patients and all tumours were found to be resectable. All patients except one, who had a large mass extensively invading the left flank, had at least laparoscopy performed.

Following the surgical procedure, the surgeon and two radiologists analysed each case and retrospectively reassessed the preoperative investigations. The following conclusions were drawn. Ultrasound, when the tumour was well visualized, appeared to give the most useful information and CT did not further contribute to the evaluation. If the tumour was not seen on ultrasound it was tempting to assume that the lesion was small and thus amenable to laparoscopic resection. However CT is recommended. Despite optimal preoperative investigation there will be cases where laparoscopic resection is not feasible due to adhesions, mesenteric obesity or mesenteric invasion (which obscures vessels) and tethering adhesions, all of which could not be fully evaluated. Ultrasound, though it proved to be the more valuable technique, failed to visualize a certain percentage of tumours due to their small size and intraluminal gas. There was also a problem in distinguishing the plane between tumours and the dome of the bladder. However, the ability to assess the movement of tumours relative to adjacent structures and the transrectal option which, like its transabdominal counterpart, is quick, easy, cheap and involves no contrast and no radiation seems the most satisfactory option at present. (Detailed results of this study are currently being prepared for publication elsewhere.)

Experience with other colorectal conditions

Considerable experience has been gained in the technique of laparoscopic appendicectomy and the results of a prospective trial comparing laparoscopic and conventional appendicectomy involving a total of 155 patients have been reported elsewhere [1]. A modified technique of laparoscopic appendicectomy is also being used at the PWH. This 'two-handed' technique [2] differs from Semm's technique in that the camera is held by an assistant rather than by the surgeon's right hand. In this way, the procedure mimics the procedure of laparoscopic cholecystecomy with which most surgeons are more familiar.

A further contribution to laparoscopic surgery from the PWH has been the Hong Kong tissue retriever [3]. This is a modified sigmoidoscope used for the retrieval of inflamed or bulky tissue and it has successfully been used in the retrieval of an inflamed appendix and resected colon during polypectomy. It consists of a metal guide rod, a tissue retrieval unit, a screw-tapered obturator and a reducing cannula. Following excision of the inflamed organ, the metal guide rod is introduced under direct vision via a suitably placed pre-existing 10 mm port. The existing skin incision is extended and the assembled retrieval unit with the obturator in position is inserted. The guide rod and the obturator are then removed and the reducing cannula is inserted into the retrieval unit. A 10 mm grasping instrument is then introduced and the tissue to be removed is grasped by the forceps. The tissue is then withdrawn into the barrel of the reducing instrument and this is then removed. Because of the presence of the outer cannula, the inflamed tissue does not come into contact with skin or subcutaneous tissue; furthermore, because of the presence of a spring-loaded metal valve in the (outer) barrel of the tissue retriever unit, the pneumoperitoneum is maintained. Work is progressing on a modification of this device for the retrieval of the malignant colon.

A technique of laparoscopic rectopexy has also been developed in the unit [4]. This makes use of four port sites: a 10 mm infra-umbilical port for the video laparoscope; two 12 mm ports in the right iliac fossa; and a further 12 mm port in the left iliac fossa. The rectum is retracted upwards using an atraumatic grasping forceps introduced via the left iliac fossa port and mobilized down to the level of the levators ani in much the same way as described above for LAC. The lateral ligaments of the rectum are divided. An 8 × 8 cm polypropylene mesh is then introduced via one of the 12 mm ports in the right iliac fossa and stapled in position.

The future

Controversy will always exist between laparoscopic surgeons and conventional surgeons regarding the radicality of laparoscopic surgery in colorectal cancer. The only way to solve this controversy is to perform prospective randomized trials comparing both procedures. The extent of nodal clearance in the above series of patients was not specifically studied but each laparoscopic procedure consistently yielded more than 20 lymph nodes with each specimen. Falk *et al.* [5] reported on 66 patients who underwent laparoscopic colorectal procedures comparable to the ones that we have presented; the lymph node harvest in the specimens thus obtained was comparable with that obtained by traditional means. Careful preoperative patient selection as well as operative experience should decrease the incidence of conversion.

Several reports have so far appeared in the literature regarding the use of a biofragmentable anastomotic ring (BAR) [6,7]. Employment of this method of anastomosis, especially after right hemicolectomy and transverse colectomy, should minimize further the size of the incision required to retrieve the resected colon and for subsequent anastomosis.

Acknowledgements

The authors would like to thank Mrs Janice Sharp, Department of Medical Illustration, University of Wales College of Medicine, for the illustrations that appear in this chapter.

References

1   Tate JJT, Chung SCS, Dawson J *et al.* Conventional versus laparoscopic surgery for acute appendicitis. *Br J Surg* 1993; **80**: 761–4.
2   Tate JJT, Chung SCS, Li AKC. Laparoscopic appendicectomy: a two-handed technique. *Br J Surg* 1993; **80**: 764.
3   Carey PD, Lau WY, Kwok SPY, Li AKC. Laparoscopic removal of inflamed or bulky tissue: preservation of the pneumoperitoneum. *Aust N Z J Surg* 1994; **64**: 434–6.
4   Kwok SPY, Carey PD, Lau WY, Li AKC. Laparoscopic rectopexy. *Dis Colon Rectum* 1994; **37**: 947–8.
5   Falk PM, Beart RW Jr, Wexner SD *et al.* Laparoscopic colectomy: a critical appraisal. *Dis Colon Rectum* 1993; **36**: 28–34.
6   Polglase AL, Skinner SA, Johnson WR. Laparoscopic assisted right hemicolectomy with Valtrac BAR (biofragmentable anastomotic ring) ileotransverse anastomosis. *Aust N Z J Surg* 1993; **63**: 481–4.
7   Sackier JM, Slutzki S, Wood C, Negri M, Moor EV, Halevi A. Laparoscopic endocorporeal mobilization followed by extracorporeal sutureless anastomosis for the treatment of carcinoma of the left colon. *Dis Colon Rectum* 1993; **36**: 610–12.

Chapter 16

Laparoscopic surgery for benign colorectal disorders

P. Reissman and S.D. Wexner

Introduction

Laparoscopic surgery for colorectal disorders has rapidly gained increased popularity among general and colorectal surgeons [1–9]. Unlike malignant disorders, laparoscopic surgery for benign colorectal disorders is free of scrutiny concerning some crucial yet unresolved issues such as long-term survival, local and distant recurrences, port site recurrences and the adequacy of the oncological principles of the surgical procedure [4–6]. This chapter will outline the various laparoscopic colorectal procedures which have been successfully performed for a wide range of benign colorectal disorders (Table 16.1).

General considerations

These general principles apply to all laparoscopic colorectal procedures: all patients who undergo elective or urgent operations will have a standard mechanical bowel preparation with oral antibiotics and perioperative intravenous broad-spectrum antibiotics. After induction of general anaesthesia, a nasogastric or orogastric tube and a bladder catheter are inserted. The patient is placed in the modified lithotomy position with the legs flattened to avoid interference with the laparoscopic instruments. This position has several advantages:

1 It provides the option of intraoperative colonoscopy in case the pathology is unidentifiable by the laparoscope [10].
2 The colonoscope may also be used for retraction of the hepatic or splenic flexures and thereby facilitates the dissection of these segments [11].
3. Rigid or flexible proctoscopy may be required to confirm that the margins of resection are adequate and free of inflammation, diverticular disease or other pathology. Similarly, the rigid proctoscope may be used to provide rectal retraction during pelvic dissection.
4 This position will enable the transanal introduction of a circular stapler when an end-to-end, stapled ileorectal or colorectal anastomosis is performed.
5 If required, another assistant or the camera holder may stand between the legs.

Pneumoperitoneum is usually established by using a Veress needle introduced trans-, supra- or infra-umbilically. In patients in whom previous surgery has been performed, an open Hasson technique is used [12]. Alternatively, the Veress needle is introduced in a 'virgin' area away from previous surgical scars, including

Procedure	Indications
Segmental colonic resection (right, transverse, left, sigmoid, anterior)	Polyps or other benign tumours such as lipomas or leiomyomas Diverticular disease Volvulus Endometriosis Sigmoidocele
Hartmann procedure	Diverticular disease Colo/rectovesical fistula Ischaemic colitis Volvulus Following segmental resection in unprepared colon or poor condition patients
Hartmann reversal procedure	All patients after the Hartmann procedure
Total abdominal colectomy (with end ileostomy, ileorectal anastomosis or restorative proctocolectomy and ileo-anal reservoir)	Mucosal ulcerative colitis Crohn's colitis Familial adenomatous polyposis Colonic inertia
Abdominoperineal resection	Intractable Crohn's proctitis Irradiation proctitis
Management of rectal prolapse Laparoscopic rectopexy ± resection Laparoscopically assisted perineal rectosigmoidectomy	Full-thickness complete rectal prolapse
Ileocolic and small bowel resection	Crohn's disease Benign tumours Symptomatic Meckel's diverticulum
Ileostomy/colostomy (loop, end)	Acute sphincter injury Faecal incontinence Rectovaginal fistula Colo/rectovesical fistula Severe perineal Crohn's disease Necrotizing fasciitis Irradiation proctitis
Appendicectomy (emergency or elective)	Acute appendicitis Familial Mediterranean fever After peri-appendicular abscess
Adhesiolysis	Chronic recurrent intestinal obstruction Acute intestinal obstruction in selected cases

Table 16.1
Laparoscopic procedures in the management of benign colorectal diseases.

laparoscopic scars. In cases in which cosmesis is a major consideration, preoperative port selection can be undertaken by the enterostomal therapist [13]. Another consideration in patients after previous pelvic surgery is the insertion of ureteric stents. Either ordinary or illuminated stents may expedite the identification of the ureters during a laparoscopic procedure in the presence of multiple adhesions and distorted anatomy.

Initially, all cannulae are 10–12 mm to enable flexibility of instruments and camera relocation as dictated by the anatomical findings. The number of ports used may vary between three and five, according to the procedure performed. Three ports are commonly used for a stoma creation and four or five for a resection. As the procedure progresses, some cannulae are replaced with a larger size (18 or 33 mm) using a Seldinger technique with a 10 mm exchange rod (Ethicon Endosurgery Inc., Cincinatti, OH, USA). This manoeuvre enables the use of linear and circular stapler devices and facilitates the specimen retrieval. Frequent relocation of personnel and instruments may be required during the procedure, as colorectal operations often involve several anatomical regions. Frequent alterations in the patient's position, such as steep Trendelenburg, anti-Trendelenburg and tilt to the sides, may improve exposure of the surgical field.

The more commonly used instruments include a 0 or 30° laparoscope, atraumatic Babcock clamps, Denis bowel clamps, 10 mm diameter scissors, Kelly, right-angle and modified Alis clamps, short (35 mm) and long (60 mm) linear stapler devices, circular 29–33 mm stapler devices, 10–12, 18 and 33 mm cannulae, bowel retractors, endoloops, endoclips and a hernia stapler. The latter instrument can be employed for either closure of the mesenteric defect or marking of the planned resection margins.

The importance of the exact localization of a benign colonic lesion before segmental resection cannot be overemphasized as the loss of tactile sensation is one of the major disadvantages of laparoscopic colorectal procedures. Accurate localization can be achieved by either preoperative colonoscopic injection of various compounds such as indian ink, methylene blue, indocyanine green or indigo carmine, or intraoperative colonoscopy with extraluminal marking using clips or hernia staples applied adjacent to the lesion.

In general, for rectal and left-sided colonic resection such as anterior resection, sigmoidectomy or left hemicolectomy, a completely laparoscopic procedure may be performed with an intracorporeal, double stapled, end-to-end anastomosis using a circular stapler. Alternatively, for right-sided or small bowel resections such as right hemicolectomy, ileocolic resection or small bowel resection, a laparoscopically assisted procedure is performed with an extracorporeal anastomosis.

Fascia closure at all port sites is another important principle to follow. An increasing number of port site hernias have been reported with occurrences between several hours to 1 month after surgery [14,15]. The fascial opening of all ports equal to or greater than 10 mm in diameter should be closed under direct vision or by using one of the several specially designed instruments.

Finally, in the postoperative management, the same criteria as those for open colorectal procedures should be followed. In our experience, in elective laparoscopic as well as in open colorectal procedures, the nasogastric or orogastric tube may be removed immediately after surgery and a clear liquid diet may be started the following day. The majority of patients tolerate a regular diet within 48 h [16,17].

Segmental resections of the colon

Indications for these procedures in the management of benign colorectal disease include colonoscopically unresectable polyps, benign lesions such as lipomas or leiomyomas, Crohn's disease of the terminal ileum, diverticular disease, volvulus, sigmoidocele or rectal prolapse [1–10,18,19].

Right hemicolectomy and ileocolectomy

For right-sided resection, four 10–12 mm ports are used in the following locations: umbilical, left para-umbilical, left lower and right para-umbilical areas (Fig. 16.1). If necessary, another right lower quadrant or suprapubic port may be placed. After complete mobilization of the terminal ileum and right colon past the hepatic flexure and identification of the right ureter, a 3–5 cm midline transumbilical incision is made for exteriorization of the segment to be resected. After complete mobilization, if laparoscopically performed, the right colon is easily exteriorized through a midline incision rather than a right paramedian or a right transverse incision. The midline incision is closer to the mesenteric root and may also be easily extended if further exposure is needed. The lesion's location may be reconfirmed by palpation and the involved segment is resected using the standard surgical technique for mesenteric vessel division and bowel transsection. After the anastomosis is fashioned and the mesenteric defect is closed, the bowel is placed back into the abdominal cavity, the incision closed and the abdomen re-insufflated for a final inspection.

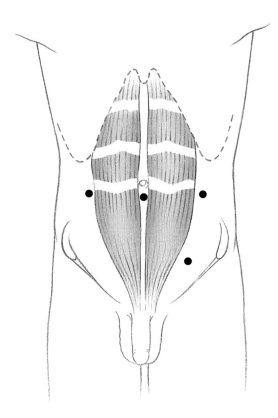

Figure 16.1
Port site placement for laparoscopic right colectomy or ileocolic resection.

Left colectomy, sigmoidectomy and anterior resection

For left-sided and anterior resections, we also use four 10–12 mm ports: umbilical, right para-umbilical, right lower quadrant and left paraumbilical ports (Fig. 16.2). An additional left lower quadrant or suprapubic port may be placed, as needed. The patient is positioned in a steep Trendelenburg position with tilt to the right to facilitate the retraction of the small bowel out of the pelvis and away from the surgical field. The involved segment is mobilized and intracorporeal division of the mesenteric vessels is performed after the left ureter has been identified. Although high ligation of the mesenteric vessels is not required, it may help to facilitate the dissection and expedite the procedure as one or two main vessels may be divided close to the mesenteric root as opposed to multiple vessels close to the colonic wall. Vessel division may be carried out by either large endoclips or vascular stapler devices. Frequent assessment of the required extent of resection should be practised to ensure adequate, disease-free margins and a tension-free anastomosis. Marking of the planned distal and proximal margins of resection by endoclips or hernia staples is extremely helpful. In diverticular disease of the sigmoid, special care should be taken to completely resect the sigmoid colon from the level of the sacral promontory at the rectosigmoid junction to the sigmoid descending junction proximally, to avoid potential recurrent diverticulitis.

Distal transection of the bowel is the next step. The right lower quadrant 10–12 mm port is exchanged for an 18 mm port as previously described. A 60 mm linear stapler device is then introduced via the 18 mm port (Fig. 16.3). Before firing, the tips of the instrument are carefully inspected to exclude any trapped tissue. A 'trial run' of approximation of the intended proximal resection margin to

Figure 16.2

Port site placement for laparoscopic left colectomy, sigmoidectomy and anterior resection.

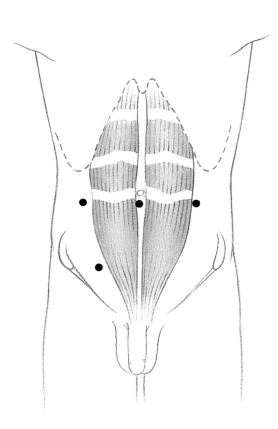

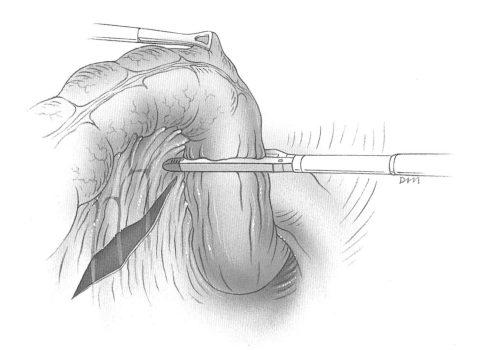

Figure 16.3
The distal colon or rectum is divided by a 60 mm laparoscopic linear stapler device.

the distal rectal stump should be undertaken. The area for proximal resection can be marked with clips or hernia staples either on the appendices epiploicae or on the antimesenteric margin. The reason for this manoeuvre is that it is difficult to gauge the length and absence of tension once the descending colon has been extracorporealized. Thus, the splenic flexure can be mobilized, if necessary. After the transection, the left paraumbilical port is replaced with a 33 mm port (Ethicon Endosurgery Inc.) through which the proximal colon is gently delivered. The port is then removed, the pneumoperitoneum evacuated and the involved segment is resected. A 29 or 33 mm anvil is placed in the proximal end of the colon and secured with a purse-string suture (Fig. 16.4). The proximal colon containing the anvil is placed back in the abdominal cavity and the 33mm port is replaced. Pneumoperitoneum is re-established, the anvil is grasped by a modified Alis clamp (Ethicon Endosurgery Inc.) and guided down towards the pelvis to reach the rectal stump. If needed, additional mobilization is obtained by incising the lateral peritoneal attachments at the splenic flexure or mesentery. A circular stapler is now introduced transanally and advanced to the rectal stump staple line with laparoscopic guidance. The trocar of the circular stapler is advanced to pierce through or close to the staple line (Fig. 16.5). The anvil and shaft are connected and the two ends of the bowel are now approximated. At this point, the laparoscope is positioned in the right lower or left lower port to confirm that no excess tissue is trapped and that the descending colon and rectum are appropriately aligned. After firing, the 'doughnuts' are inspected for completeness and the anastomosis is tested for air tightness by transanal air insufflation while the pelvis is filled with saline and the descending colon is gently occluded proximal to the anastomosis. The procedure is concluded after final inspection of the pelvis and abdominal cavity is performed, the patient is returned to the normal supine position and the irrigation fluid is aspirated. Pelvic drainage is not routinely performed unless a formal pelvic dissection has been undertaken.

Figure 16.4
The anvil of the circular stapler is placed in the proximal colon (a) and secured with a purse-string suture (b).

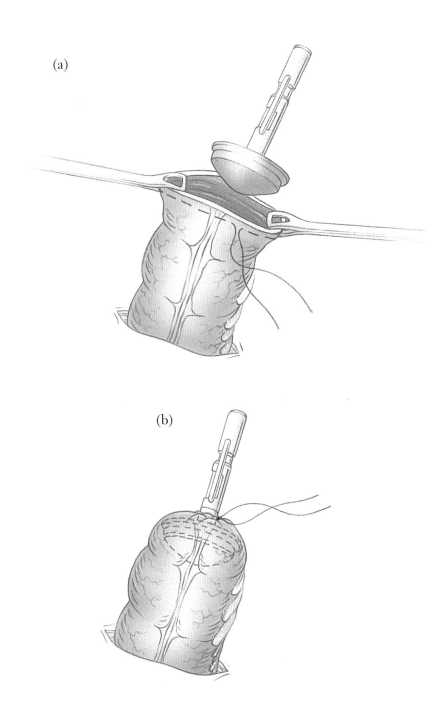

(a)

(b)

Hartmann and Hartmann reversal procedures

Today, the term Hartmann procedure is widely used to include numerous procedures which result in the creation of a variable length of a closed stump of the rectum or colon and an end colostomy or ileostomy. The procedure is performed in cases of high-risk primary anastomosis when faecal diversion is preferred. The indications for a Hartmann procedure in benign disorders include intra-abdominal sepsis, acute diverticulitis, complications of diverticular disease such as a fistula or perforation, toxic colitis, ischaemic colitis, perforation due to a foreign body or trauma, volvulus, following resection in a patient with

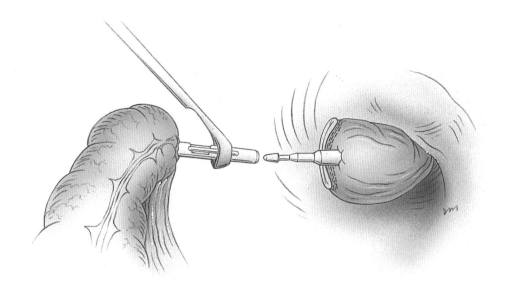

Figure 16.5
Intracorporeal double stapled, end-to-end colorectal anastomosis after a left-sided colonic resection, anterior resection or reversal of a Hartmann procedure. The anvil is guided to the shaft of the circular stapler which has pierced the rectal stump through or close to the previous staple line.

poor general condition or in any event of unprepared bowel. In other conditions such as inflammatory bowel disease, colitis or extensive ischaemic colitis, a total abdominal colectomy with closure of the rectum and creation of an end ileostomy may be performed. The Hartmann procedure may also be used for temporary or permanent faecal diversion in many anorectal disorders including faecal incontinence, sphincter injury, perianal sepsis such as Crohn's disease or necrotizing fasciitis, rectovaginal fistulae and irradiation proctitis.

Since the Hartmann procedure is most frequently performed as an emergency procedure in patients with peritoneal sepsis due to perforation, necrosis, obstruction or severe colitis, laparoscopy may have a limited role. Conversely, reversal of the Hartmann procedure may have a wide application. The reversal is generally an elective procedure in a well-prepared patient. Although all of these patients have an additional incision besides the stoma and may have significant adhesions, laparoscopy performed by an experienced and skillful team is a practical option with several potential advantages [20–23].

The technical principles of a laparoscopic Hartmann procedure are similar to those of a left-sided colonic resection. The main difference is that, instead of an anastomosis, after the proximal colon is exteriorized and the involved segment is resected, an end colostomy is matured (Fig. 16.6). In elective cases, the colostomy site is marked by an enterostomal nurse prior to surgery. The marked site may be used for one of the ports, which is later replaced by the 33 mm port (Ethicon Endosurgery Inc.) for specimen and proximal colon delivery. Alternatively, a formal stoma incision is performed without the use of the 33 mm port. In either case, the fascial opening should be sufficient for safe delivery of the proximal colon and creation of the colostomy.

In laparoscopic reversal of the Hartmann procedure, preparation for surgery, positioning of the patient and the operating room setup are identical to those of the Hartmann procedure or left-sided resection. Intraoperative ureteric stent insertion is extremely helpful. Initially, the stoma is dissected free of the abdominal wall using an ordinary surgical technique. Complete mobilization of the stoma and lysis of adhesions in the proximity of the fascial opening should be carried out. Subsequently, the edges of the previous colostomy are trimmed and

Figure 16.6
Closed port sites and the matured colostomy after a laparoscopic Hartmann procedure or abdominoperineal resection.

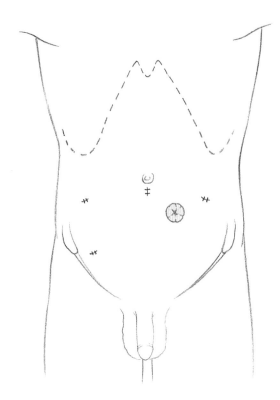

the anvil of a 29 or 33 mm circular stapler device is introduced (see Fig. 16.4). If the vascular supply to the stoma is compromised during the dissection, a limited resection may be required. Similarly, in cases of diverticulitis care must be taken to ensure that the proximal end of the anastomosis will consist of healthy normal bowel. The proximal colon containing the anvil is now placed back into the abdominal cavity. Retraction through the stomal site allows for enterolysis of much of the midline incision. After such enterolysis, several fascial sutures are placed but not tied, and the 33 mm cannula is introduced through the incision. One or two of the fascial sutures may now be tied to prevent carbon dioxide (CO_2) leakage during insufflation of the abdominal cavity. Under direct vision, a 10–12 mm cannula is inserted and the laparoscope is introduced through this 10–12 mm cannula. Any additional adhesions should be carefully lysed. Additional ports are placed after sufficient visualization has been achieved. After adequate exposure is achieved by lysis of adhesions and retraction of the small bowel out of the pelvis, attention is paid to both the proximal colon and the rectal stump. The proximal colon is carefully inspected for sufficient mobility and viability. If needed, additional mobilization can be achieved by incising the lateral peritoneal attachment or mobilizing the splenic flexure or transverse colon. The rectal stump must be clearly identified and dissected free of adhesions. The rectal stump dissection may be facilitated by rigid proctoscopy. Additionally, if one or two long, non-absorbable sutures are placed at the edge of the rectal stump during the initial Hartmann procedure, identification is facilitated during the reversal procedure.

After both the rectal stump and the proximal colon have been adequately mobilized, the anvil is grasped with the modified Alis clamp (Ethicon Endosurgery Inc.) which is introduced through the right upper port. The circular stapler device is now introduced transanally and laparoscopically guided to reach the end of the rectal stump at the staple line. A double stapled end-to-end anastomosis is created similar to that in a sigmoid or anterior resection (see Fig. 16.5), and subsequently tested with transanal air insufflation. It is crucial to anastomose the proximal descending colon to the rectum and not to the sigmoid colon. This is especially true in cases of diverticulitis as the incidence of recurrent diverticulitis inceases multifold if a colosigmoidostomy is achieved. Thus, any residual sigmoid must be resected as detailed earlier in this chapter.

Total abdominal colectomy

Laparoscopic total abdominal colectomy is an uncommonly performed procedure due to its length, complexity and cost. Due to the large specimen, or the need to create an ileo-anal reservoir, total abdominal colectomy is usually a laparoscopically assisted procedure. Indications include mucosal ulcerative colitis, Crohn's colitis, familial adenomatous polyposis and colonic inertia [24–27]. These disorders are commonly found in younger patients and therefore the improved cosmesis achieved by a laparoscopically assisted procedure as opposed to an open procedure may play a significant role.

The patient's preparation, position and operating room setup are similar to those already detailed for other laparoscopic colorectal procedures. Initially, five 10–12 mm ports are placed, as shown in Fig. 16.7. The incision for specimen delivery and/or creation of the ileo-anal reservoir and the future stoma site, if planned, should be all considered when planning port placement. Most frequently, a Pfannenstiel incision or a lower midline incision is performed for that purpose. Complete mobilization of the entire abdominal colon is the first step. Since total abdominal colectomy actually combines right, transverse, left

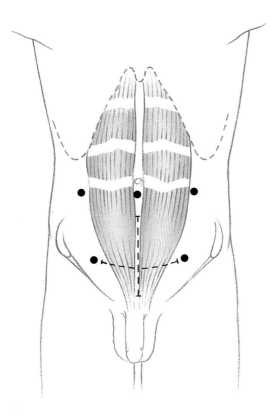

Figure 16.7
Port site placement for total abdominal colectomy. The future stoma in the premarked site and the incision for specimen delivery and/or creation of an ileo-anal reservoir should all be considered before placing the ports. The dashed lines show the optional incisions.

and sigmoid mobilization, frequent relocation of the surgeon, assistants and monitors are required. As for other laparoscopic colonic procedures, principles such as complete inspection of the peritoneal cavity and the pelvis, traction and countertraction, and bilateral ureteric identification are practised. According to the underlying pathology, the extent of mobilization is from the terminal ileum through the right transverse, left and sigmoid colon to the level of the rectosigmoid junction, or, in cases of proctectomy, mobilization of the entire rectum may also be laparoscopically performed. Alternatively, rectal mobilization may be performed during the open phase of the procedure. After adequate mobilization has been achieved, a true Pfannenstiel or an infra-umbilical midline incision is performed and the complete abdominal colon is exteriorized (Fig. 16.8). If a Pfannenstiel incision is chosen, it should incorporate the two lowest right and left port sites. The division of the mesenteric vessels, mesentery and transection of the terminal ileum may be performed either intra- or extracorporeally. According to the planned procedure, the following may be performed.

1 Completion of the rectal dissection and resection with creation of an ileo-anal reservoir and an ileo-anal anastomosis.
2 An end-to-end double stapled ileorectal anastomosis.
3 Closure of the rectal stump and creation of an end ileostomy.

The end or loop ileostomy is delivered through the premarked site, which according to the patient's body habitus may be used for one of the ports. When an ileo-anal reservoir is created, a pelvic drain is usually placed and brought out through the left iliac fossa port.

Figures 16.9 and 16.10 show the immediate and late postoperative appearance of a patient who underwent a laparoscopically assisted total proctocolectomy with

Figure 16.8
Exteriorization of the abdominal colon through a Pfannenstiel incision in laparoscopic total abdominal colectomy.

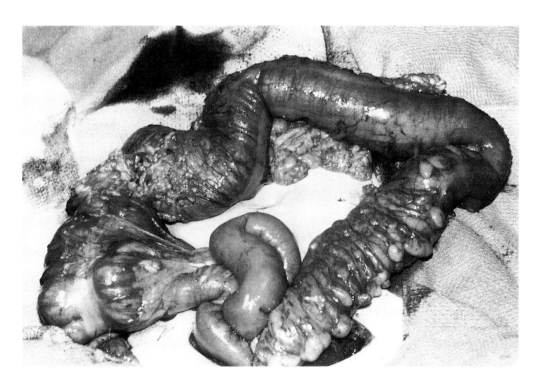

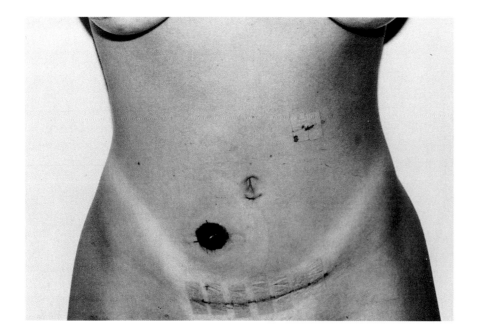

Figure 16.9
Immediate postoperative appearance of a patient who underwent a laparoscopically assisted total proctocolectomy and creation of an ileo-anal reservoir with a loop ileostomy.

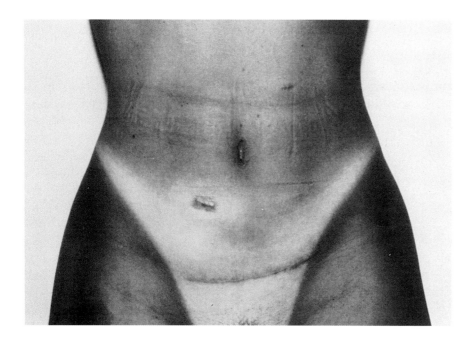

Figure 16.10
The same patient as in Fig. 16.9, 3 months later. The loop ileostomy was closed 6 weeks after surgery.

creation of an ileo-anal reservoir and a temporary loop ileostomy. Although the markedly improved cosmetic results are appreciated by both patients and surgeons, no other advantages relative to the length of ileus, hospitalization and return to normal activity have been shown to date [26]. Moreover, laparoscopically assisted total abdominal colectomy has been shown to be associated with a significantly higher morbidity when compared with segmental colonic resections [28,29].

Abdominoperineal resection

Benign disorders which may require an abdominoperineal resection include intractable perianal or rectal Crohn's disease and cases of severe irradiation proctitis. In general, abdominoperineal resection is a well-suited procedure for the laparoscopic technique. The procedure consists of a complete laparoscopic mobilization of the rectosigmoid which may be carried out to the levator muscles. If the colon is still intact, the sigmoid descending junction should be divided prior to the rectal dissection. The rectal dissection should be undertaken in the presacral loose areolar tissue plane after ligation of the inferior mesenteric or superior haemorrhoidal artery. Although high ligation of the inferior mesenteric artery is not necessary, dissection closer to the rectal wall may be tedious as multiple mesenteric vessels are anticipated. In male patients, the identification and preservation of the presacral sympathetic nerves is of utmost importance to avoid impotence. The nerves are quite well visualized through the laparoscope. The deep pelvic dissection may be facilitated by retraction of the small bowel out of the pelvis while the patient is placed in a steep Trendelenburg position. Alternative manoeuvres include anterior retraction of the urinary bladder and manual manipulation of the posterior vaginal wall by the assistant's finger. As the laparoscope may be placed deep in the pelvis, excellent exposure and visualization is usually achieved. The lateral stalks are usually divided by electrocautery.

After the mobilization of the rectum is completed, the perineal phase of the procedure is started. Since the procedure is performed for benign disease, the perineal dissection is undertaken in an intersphincteric plane with preservation of the external anal sphincter. The rectosigmoid is removed through the perineal incision, and careful laparoscopic inspection of the pelvis is undertaken. Temporary occlusion of the perineal incision to prevent leakage of the pneumoperitoneum may be achieved by using a moist laparotomy pad. Placement of a pelvic drain through the left lower port site may be performed without losing the pneumoperitoneum, using a technique described elsewhere [30]. Creation of an end colostomy at the premarked stoma site is the next step. Maturation of the colostomy and closure of the perineal incision and the port sites conclude the procedure.

Laparoscopic surgery for rectal prolapse

Although it is uncommon, complete rectal prolapse is a severely debilitating condition which may be treated only by surgical repair. The various surgical procedures may be divided into two main categories: (i) abdominal approach; and (ii) perineal approach. Laparoscopy may have a role in both approaches [31–35].

Laparoscopic abdominal rectopexy with or without resection

One of the more frequently performed abdominal procedures for complete rectal prolapse is rectopexy as initially described by Ripstein [36] or as later modified by Wells [37]. The rectum is completely mobilized after which a prosthetic rectopexy is undertaken using a Marlex mesh (C.R. Bard, Massachusetts, USA) for fixation of the rectum to the presacral fascia. When performed laparoscopically, the rectum is completely mobilized to the pelvic floor; after completion of the mobilization, a folded Marlex mesh rectangle is introduced through one of the 10–12 mm ports. The mesh is then unfolded and sutured or clipped to the posterior rectal wall and presacral fascia on both sides of the rectum. Alternatively, a Marlex sling may be placed anterior to the rectal wall and fixed to the presacral fascia. However, this technique is associated with a higher incidence of constipation and sling-related complications [37].

Another abdominal approach, which both avoids the use of foreign material and is associated with a reduced incidence of postoperative constipation, is the Frykman–Goldberg procedure [38,39]. This procedure consists of complete mobilization of the rectum down to the levators, combined with sigmoid resection with colorectal anastomosis at the level of the promontory, and a sutured rectopexy of the rectum to the presacral fascia. The Frykman–Goldberg procedure is well suited for the laparoscopic technique. The sigmoid and rectum are completely mobilized, the sigmoid is resected and an end-to-end double stapled colorectal anastomosis is performed. The lateral stalks on each side of the rectum are sutured to the presacral fascia with non-absorbable suture material. Alternatively, the sutured rectopexy phase of the procedure may be done through a small suprapubic incision. If this approach is chosen, transection of the rectosigmoid may be carried out using a standard linear stapler device, introduced through the suprapubic incision. The sigmoid may then be delivered through the same incision and transected, and the anvil of a circular stapler device may be introduced into the proximal colon. The double stapled end-to-end anastomosis may be fashioned under direct vision.

Laparoscopic assistance in perineal procedures for rectal prolapse

If a perineal approach is preferred for the surgical treatment of a complete rectal prolapse, laparoscopic assistance may be used for the perineal rectosigmoidectomy. This manoeuvre may be used in a combined fashion using transabdominal laparoscopic mobilization of the rectum to facilitate a more extensive perineal resection of the rectosigmoid [34]. Alternatively, while performing a perineal rectosigmoidectomy, the laparoscope may be inserted transperineally anterior to the prolapsed rectum for visualization and assessment of residual redundancy of the sigmoid colon or to confirm that the maximal length of the rectosigmoid is resected [35].

Ileocolic and small bowel resection

These procedures are usually performed as laparoscopically assisted ones with a small transumbilical or paramedian incision used for specimen delivery and creation of an extracorporeal anastomosis [40–42]. The laparoscopic principles of an ileocolic resection are similar to those of a right hemicolectomy. However, since this procedure is most commonly performed in patients with Crohn's disease, thorough inspection of the small bowel is mandatory. This may be performed using a two-handed technique with two atraumatic Babcock clamps for systematic inspection of the small bowel starting at the terminal ileum and moving proximally to the ligament of Treitz. An inflamed bulky mesentery of the terminal ileum may be anticipated in patients with Crohn's disease. The size of the phlegmon may require extension of the planned incision or, alternatively, converting the procedure to an open standard laparotomy. In addition, common complications of Crohn's disease such as phlegmon, fistulae, and abscesses, alter the procedure or the size of the incision. In general, however, a 2–3 cm transumbilical incision will permit vascular ligation, specimen delivery and anastomosis (Fig. 16.11).

Ileostomy/colostomy

Procedures to create an end or loop ileostomy or colostomy for temporary or permanent faecal diversion are well-suited to the laparoscopic technique. Indications include faecal incontinence, acute sphincter injury, rectovaginal fistulae, colovesical or rectovesical fistulae, perineal sepsis due to Crohn's disease or necrotizing fasciitis, and irradition proctitis [4,43–47].

Two or three ports are usually required for the creation of a loop ileostomy (Fig. 16.12). Initially, all ports are 10–12 mm in size, the first one placed in a supra-umbilical midline position, and a second one placed in the premarked stoma site which is usually in a right lower position. A steep Trendelenburg position with a tilt to the left side of the patient is used to facilitate exposure of the terminal ileum. In the presence of adhesions or unclear anatomy, a third port in the left lower position is mandatory to facilitate adhesiolysis and mobilization of the terminal ileum. The most distal segment of ileum that can easily reach the anterior abdominal wall without tension is chosen for creation of the stoma. The proximal and distal directions are marked using hernia staples. The proximal loop is marked by two staples placed at the mesentery, close to the bowel wall, and the distal loop is marked by one staple. This manoeuvre will ensure proper orientation of the terminal ileal loop after its exteriorization. Before the ileal loop is exteriorized, the existing cannula at the stoma site is replaced with an 18 mm cannula (Ethicon Endosurgery Inc.) using the Seldinger techique. This wider port will enable the withdrawl of the ileal loop, under laparoscopic guidance, without loss of pneumoperitoneum. If the loop is too bulky to fit into the

Figure 16.11
This 72-year-old patient with Crohn's disease underwent an ileocolic resection. The specimen was removed through a 3 cm midline incision.

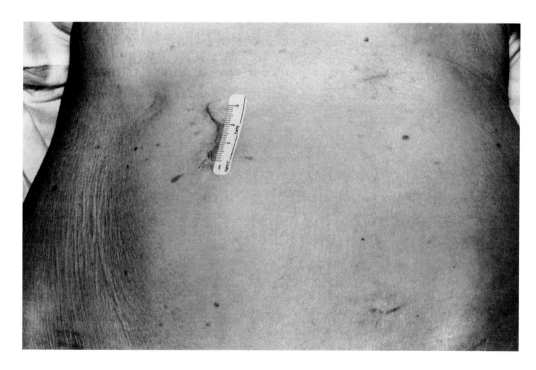

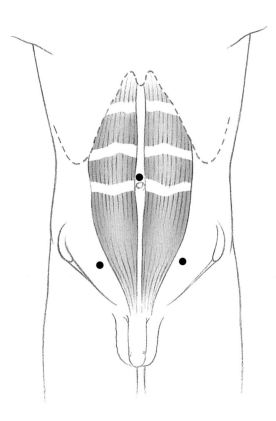

Figure 16.12
*Port site placement for
laparoscopic loop ileostomy.
The right lower port is placed
in the premarked stoma site.*

18 mm cannula, the adjacent fascia and skin are incised and the cannula with the loop of bowel held by the Babcock clamp is withdrawn as a unit. Once the loop is exteriorized and proper alignment is ensured according to the hernia staples which were previously placed, the ileostomy is matured over a plastic rod in the standard fashion. Even if the loop of ileum fits the 18 mm cannula, after its exteriorization, the skin and fascia must be incised to prevent stoma outlet obstruction. This incision may be performed with electrocautery, cutting against the insulated shaft of the Babcock clamp which holds the loop of ileum. After the ileostomy is matured, the abdominal cavity is re-insufflated and inspected for haemostasis and orientation of the loop of ileum is verified. Similarly to 'open' loop ileostomy, laparoscopic loop ileostomy has been shown to be a safe and attractive alternative for temporary faecal diversion [44–47].

The principles of laparoscopic creation of a colostomy are similar to those of a laparoscopic ileostomy. After sufficient mobilization of the colonic loop it is delivered through the port at the previously marked colostomy site. Again, care should be taken to incise the skin and fascia sufficiently to enable safe delivery of the colon and prevent later colostomy outlet obstruction. After maturation of the colostomy, the abdomen is now re-insufflated for final inspection to confirm proper alignment.

Appendicectomy

Laparoscopic appendicectomy is one of the most frequently performed laparoscopic surgical procedures. It is usually performed as an emergency procedure for acute appendicitis or right lower quadrant peritonitis [48–50].

However, it may also be performed as an elective procedure for interval appendicectomy in patients who have recovered from a peri-appendicular abscess or in patients who suffer from familial Mediterranean fever with recurrent episodes of peritonitis [51,52]. One of the major advantages of laparoscopic appendicectomy versus open appendicectomy through the traditional McBurney incision is the opportunity to perform an exploratory laparoscopy with thorough inspection of the pelvis and the entire abdominal cavity to rule out other concomitant or primary pathology. Various techniques for laparoscopic appendicectomy have been described to date with similar good results. The detailed technique of laparoscopic appendicectomy is described elsewhere in this book and therefore will not be discussed in this chapter.

Adhesiolysis

Until recently, previous abdominal surgery and suspected intestinal adhesions were considered a contraindication for laparoscopic procedures. However, as more experience has been gained and improved surgical instrumentation, optics and video montoring equipment have been made available, this contraindication has been generally abandoned.   Today, laparoscopic procedures are universally performed in patients who have had previous abdominal surgery and have intestinal adhesions. The concept of laparoscopic adhesiolysis for intestinal obstruction evolved after surgeons became experienced in laparoscopic adhesiolysis performed as the initial step in other laparoscopic surgical procedures. Since adhesions due to previous abdominal surgery are the most frequent cause of intestinal obstruction [53–55], laparoscopic adhesiolysis as a treatment for recurrent intestinal obstruction may have a wide application in selected patients. Ideally, laparoscopic adhesiolysis should be performed as an elective procedure in patients with documented recurrent intestinal obstruction after previous abdominal surgery [56–60]. The preparation for surgery in such cases is similar to that for other laparoscopic colorectal procedures including a standard bowel preparation. However, recent reports have shown that laparoscopy with adhesiolysis alone or followed by another laparoscopic surgical procedure may be successfully performed in acute intestinal obstruction as well [60,61]. In such cases, bowel resection, or repair of an incarcerated internal abdominal wall or an inguinal hernia which caused the obstruction may be performed. However, severe abdominal distension with massively dilated bowel loops, diffuse peritonitis and the presence of extremely dense adhesions with fused loops of bowel, which may compromise the safety of the laparoscopic adhesiolysis, should all be considered contraindications and warrant open laparotomy.

The preparation, patient's positioning, operating room setup and technical principles of laparoscopic adhesiolysis are similar to the previously discussed laparoscopic colorectal procedures. Intraoperative insertion of ureteric stents (standard or illuminated) is extremely helpful for fast and safe laparoscopic identification of the ureters. The initial step of pneumoperitoneum creation should be carefully planned and executed. An open Hasson technique, using a blunt tip trocar or a 10 mm cannula without the trocar, should be performed to avoid inadvertent injury to the bowel, mesentery or omentum. Alternatively, a Veress needle may be inserted in a 'virgin' area, remote from previous surgical and laparoscopic scars. In such cases, sweeping the needle in different directions while insufflating may disclose the presence of closure adhesions which should be avoided when inserting the first cannula. When the tip of the needle touches the adhesions, a sudden increase in pressure and interruption of CO_2 flow will occur. Hence, when placing the first trocar, it should be directed away from the suspected area of adhesions.

After establishment of pneumoperitoneum by either the open or the Veress needle technique, careful inspection of the abdominal cavity is attempted. Most often, visibility is limited due to adhesions and at least one more port should be inserted under vision before exploration may be carried out. This second port is used for initial lysis of adhesions in the vicinity of the first port, and enables additional port placement as more exposure is gained. A pair of 10 mm laparoscopic scissors (Ethicon Endosurgery Inc.) connected to electrocautery is used for sharp, blunt and electrocautery dissection and lysis of the adhesions. Dense vascular adhesions may also be lysed by using haemostatic clips or endoloops. Frequent repositioning of the camera and instruments are usually required while performing this procedure.

After the abdominal wall is cleared from intestinal or omental adhesions, careful inspection of the bowel may be carried out. This inspection may be facilitated by positioning the operating table in different steep angles, according to the inspected area. Two atraumatic Babcock clamps are used to run the bowel in a retrograde fashion starting from the terminal ileum and moving proximally towards the ligament of Treitz using a two-handed technique. Although it may be difficult to assess which of the adhesions are responsible for the clinical symptoms, especially in elective cases, sound surgical judgement should be used and all suspected symptomatic adhesions should be lysed. According to the intraoperative findings, resection of a small bowel loop may be required in addition to the adhesiolysis.

Although laparoscopic adhesiolysis for intestinal obstruction has been performed for only a short period of time, early reports are promising. Nevertheless, the laparoscopic option must not alter the indications for surgical intervention in intestinal obstruction nor sound surgical judgement while performing the procedure. Laparoscopic adhesiolysis is technically challenging and, therefore, should be performed only by a highly skilled and experienced laparoscopic surgical team. Larger series with longer follow-up are mandatory before final conclusions concerning the role of laparoscopy in the treatment of intestinal obstruction can be reached.

The Cleveland Clinic Florida experience with laparoscopic colorectal procedures for benign colorectal disease

Between August 1991 and late 1994, 137 laparoscopic or laparoscopically assisted colorectal procedures were performed in the Department of Colorectal Surgery at the Cleveland Clinic Florida. The vast majority of these procedures were performed by one of two surgeons, Dr Steven D. Wexner or the late Dr David G. Jagelman. One hundred and eighteen of these procedures were performed for benign colorectal disease. There were 65 male and 53 female patients, of a mean age of 48 years (range: 12–88 years). All patient information, including demographics, diagnosis, type and length of procedure, conversion to open laparotomy, complications and length of hospitalization were entered in a laparoscopic registry database for analysis. Indications for surgery included inflammatory bowel disease in 47 patients, including mucosal ulcerative colitis in 25 and Crohn's disease in 22, benign colonic polyps in 15, diverticular disease in 16, faecal incontinence in 11, familial adenomatous polyposis in six, colonic inertia in seven, sigmoidocele in three, irradiation proctitis in four, rectal prolapse in two, rectovaginal fistulae in three, and volvulus, ischaemic colitis, severe anal stenosis and endometriosis in one patient each. Procedures included total abdominal colectomy in 38 patients, including ileo-anal reservoir in 28, ileorectal anastomosis in eight and creation of an end ileostomy in two. Segmental colonic resection was performed in 39 patients, abdominoperineal resection in one, small bowel resection in 13, diverting stoma in 15, reversal of the Hartmann procedure in 10 and rectopexy in two patients. Eleven cases (9%) were converted to open laparotomy due to bleeding in five, severe adhesions in four, and technical difficulties in two patients. Twenty-six patients (22%) sustained 32 complications including bleeding in nine, prolonged ileus in five, enterotomies in four, pelvic abscess in four, wound infection in four, small bowel obstruction in two, and four miscellaneous complications. There was no mortality. When divided by the type of procedure, the overall complication rate in total abdominal colectomy cases was significantly higher (42%) when compared with that of all other procedures (segmental resection 19%, other miscellaneous procedures 12%) ($P<0.02$). The mean length of surgery was 4 h (range: 2.5–6.5 h) for total abdominal colectomies, 2.6 h (range: 1.5–5.5 h) for segmental resection and 1.7 h (range: 0.7–4 h) for all other procedures. The mean length of hospitalization was 6.4 days (range: 2–40 days) (8.4, 6.7 and 6.6 days for total abdominal colectomy, segmental resections and other procedures, respectively). In our series, the right-sided colonic or small bowel segmental resections were performed in a laparoscopically assisted fashion while the left-sided procedures were performed in a complete laparoscopic fashion with creation of an intracorporeal end-to-end double stapled anastomosis. Due to these results, we no longer perform laparoscopically assisted total abdominal colectomies.

Conclusion

The feasibility of laparoscopic colorectal surgery has been well established as more complex and larger surgical procedures have been safely and successfully performed. In contrast to laparoscopic colorectal procedures for malignancy, the management of benign colorectal disorders is free of concerns such as distant and local recurrences, long-term survival and port site recurrences. However, the final role of laparoscopic colorectal surgery in general has yet to be determined as the results of more controlled prospectively randomized studies become available.

References

1   Wexner SD, Johansen OB. Laparoscopic bowel resection: advantages and limitations. *Ann Med* 1992; **24**: 105–10.
2   Monson JRT, Darzi A, Carey PD, Guillou PJ. Prospective evaluation of laparoscopic assisted colectomy in an unselected group of patients. *Lancet* 1992; **340**: 831–3.
3   Phillips EH, Franklin M, Caroll BJ *et al.* Laparoscopic colectomy. *Ann Surg* 1992; **216**: 703–7.

4   Wexner SD, Cohen SM, Johansen OB *et al.* Laparoscopic colorectal surgery: a prospective assessment and current perspective. *Br J Surg* 1993; **80**: 1602–5.

5   Wexner SD, Reissman P. Laparoscopic colorectal surgery: a provocative critique. *Int J Surg* 1994; **70**: 235–9.

6   Falk PM, Beart RW, Wexner SD *et al.* Laparoscopic colectomy: a critical appraisal. *Dis Colon Rectum* 1993; **36**: 28–34.

7   Franklin ME, Ramos R, Rosenthal D, Schuessler W. Laparoscopic colonic procedures. *World J Surg* 1993; **17**: 51–6.

8   Larach SW, Salomon MC, Williamson PR *et al.* Laparoscopic assisted colectomy: experience during the learning curve. *Coloproctology* 1993; **1**: 38–41.

9   Cohen SM, Reissman P, Wexner SD. Laparoscopic colorectal surgery: are we being honest with our patients. *Dis Colon Rectum* (in press).

10 Shallman RW, Shaw TJ, Roach JM. Colonoscopically assisted intracorporeal–laparoscopic wedge resection of a benign right colon lesion. *Surg Laparosc Endosc* 1993; **3**: 482–4.

11 Reissman P, Piccirillo M, Teoh TA, Nogueras JJ, Wexner SD. Colonoscopic assisted laparoscopic colectomy. *Surg Endosc* 1994; **8**: 1352–3.

12 Hasson HM. Modified instrument and method for laparoscopy. *Am J Obstet Gynecol* 1971; **110**: 886–7.

13 Teoh TA, Reissman P, Weiss EG, Verzaro R, Wexner SD. Enhancing cosmesis in laparoscopic colorectal surgery. *Dis Colon Rectum* 1995; **38**: 213–14.

14 Hass BE, Schrager RE. Small bowel obstruction due to Richter's hernia after laparoscopic procedures. *J Laparoendosc Surg* 1993; **3**: 421–3.

15 Reissman P, Shiloni E, Gofrit O *et al.* Incarcerated hernia in lateral trocar site: an unusual early postoperative complication of laparoscopic surgery. *Eur J Surg* 1994; **160**: 191–2.

16 Binderow SR, Cohen SM, Wexner SD *et al.* Must early postoperative oral intake be limited to laparoscopy. *Dis Colon Rectum* 1994: **37**: 584–9.

17 Reissman P, Wexner SD, Teoh TA *et al.* Is early oral feeding safe after elective colorectal surgery. *Ann Surg* (in press).

18 Sharpe DR, Redwine DB. Laparoscopic segmental resection of the sigmoid and rectosigmoid colon for endometriosis. *Surg Laparosc Endosc* 1992; **2**: 120–4.

19 Scoggin SD, Frazee RC. Laparoscopically assisted resection of colonic lipoma. *J Laparoendosc Surg* 1992; **2**: 185–9.

20 Reissman P, Wexner SD. Laparoscopic Hartmann's and Hartmann's reversal procedures. In: Phillips EH, Rosenthal R (eds) *Operative Strategies in Laparoscopic Surgery*. Springer Verlag, New York (in press).

21 Larach SW, Hellinger MD. The evolving role of laparoscopic technique in the performance of Hartmann's procedure. *Surg Oncol Clin North Am* 1994; **3**: 717–30.

22 Roe AM, Prabhue S, Ali A *et al.* Reversal of Hartmann's procedure: timing and operative technique. *Br J Surg* 1991; **78**: 1167–70.

23 Sosa JL, Sleeman D, Puente I, McKenney MG, Hartmann R. Laparoscopic assisted colostomy closure after Hartmann's procedure. *Dis Colon Rectum* 1994; **37**: 149–52.

24 Lointier PH, Lautard M, Massoni C *et al.* Laparoscopically assisted subtotal colectomy. *J Laparoendosc Surg* 1993; **3**: 439–53.

25 Peters WR. Laparoscopic total proctocolectomy with creation of ileostomy for ulcerative colitis: report of two cases. *J Laparoendosc Surg* 1992; **2**: 175–8.

26 Wexner SD, Johansen OB, Nogueras JJ, Jagelman DG. Laparoscopic total abdominal colectomy: a prospective trial. *Dis Colon Rectum* 1992; **35**: 651–5.

27 Cohen SM, Wexner SD. Laparoscopic restorative proctocolectomy. In: Lezoche E, Paganini AM, Cuschieri A (eds) *Minimally Invasive Colorectal Surgery*. Documento Editoriale Srl, Milan, 1994: 62–5.

28 Reissman P, Wexner SD, Cohen SM *et al.* Complications of laparoscopic colorectal surgery (abstract). *Surg Endosc* 1994; **8**: 562.

29 Reissman P, Cohen SM, Weiss EG, Nogueras JJ, Wexner SD. Laparoscopic colorectal surgery: ascending the learning curve. *World J Surg* (in press).

30 Reissman P, Cohen SM, Weiss EG, Wexner SD. Simple technique for pelvic drain placement in laparoscopic abdominoperineal resection. *Dis Colon Rectum* 1994; **37**: 381–2.

31 Munro W, Avramovic J, Roney W. Laparoscopic rectopexy. *J Laparoendosc Surg* 1993; **3**: 55–8.

32 Cuschieri A. Laparoscopic rectopexy for complete prolapse. In: Lezoche E, Paganini AM, Cuschieri A (eds) *Minimally Invasive Colorectal Surgery*. Documento Editoriale Srl, Milan, 1994: 69–71.

33 Berman IR. Sutureless laparoscopic rectopexy for procidentia. Technique and implications. *Dis Colon Rectum* 1992; **35**: 689–93.

34 Lointier P, Lechner C, Larpent JL, Chipponi J. Laparoscopic assisted perineal rectosigmoidectomy with pull through. *J Laparoendosc Surg* 1993; **3**: 547–56.

35 Reissman P, Weiss EG, Teoh TA, Wexner SD. Laparoscopic assisted perineal rectosigmoidectomy for rectal prolapse. *Surg Laparosc Endosc* 1995; **5**: 217–18.

36 Ripstein CB. Treatment of massive rectal prolapse. *Am J Surg* 1952; **83**: 68–71.

37 Wells C. New operation for rectal prolapse. *Proc R Soc Med* 1959; **52**: 602–3.
38 Frykman HM, Goldberg SM. The surgical treatment of procidentia. *Surg Gynecol Obstet* 1969; **129**: 1225–30.
39 Sayfan J, Pinho M, Alexandre-Williams J, Keighley MRB. Sutured abdominal rectopexy with sigmoidectomy compared to Marlex rectopexy. *Br J Surg* 1990; **77**: 143–5.
40 Schlinkert RT. Laparoscopic assisted ileocolectomy. *Dis Colon Rectum* 1991; **34**: 1030–1.
41 Milsom JW, Lavery IC, Bohm B, Fazio VW. Laparoscopically assisted ileocolectomy in Crohn's disease. *Surg Laparosc Endosc* 1993; **3**: 77–80.
42 Bauer JJ, Harris MT, Gorfine SR *et al*. Laparoscopic assisted intestinal resection for Crohn's disease: initial experience (abstract). *Surg Endosc* 1994; **8**: 231.
43 Romero CA, James KM, Cooperstone LM *et al*. Laparoscopic sigmoid colostomy for perianal Crohn's disease. *Surg Laparosc Endosc* 1992; **2**: 148–51.
44 Furhman G, Ota DM. Laparoscopic intestinal stomas. *Dis Colon Rectum* 1994; **37**: 444–9.
45 Lange V, Meyer G, Shardey M, Schildberg FW. Laparoscopic creation of a loop ileostomy. *J Laparoendosc Surg* 1991; **1**: 307–12.
46 Khoor E, Montrey J, Cohen MM. Laparoscopic loop ileostomy for temporary fecal diversion. *Dis Colon Rectum* 1993; **36**: 966–8.
47 Teoh TA, Reissman P, Cohen SM, Weiss EG, Wexner SD. Laparoscopic loop ileostomy (letter). *Dis Colon Rectum* 1994; **37**: 514.
48 Pier A, Gotz F, Bacher C. Laparoscopic appendectomy in 625 cases: from innovation to routine. *Surg Laparosc Endosc* 1991; **1**: 8–13.
49 Welch NT, Hinder RA, Fitzgibbons RJ. Laparoscopic incidental appendectomy. *Surg Laparosc Endosc* 1991; **1**: 116–18.
50 Saye WB, Rives DA, Cochrane B. Laparoscopic appendectomy: three years experience. *Surg Laparosc Endosc* 1991; **1**: 109–15.
51 Reissman P, Gofrit O, Rivkind A. Exploratory laparoscopy: a crucial advantage of laparoscopic versus open appendectomy (letter). *South Med J* 1994; **87**: 576.
52 Reissman P, Durst AL, Rivkind A *et al*. Elective laparoscopic appendectomy in patients with familial Mediterranean fever. *World J Surg* 1994; **18**: 139–42.
53 Manyies D, Ellis H. Intestinal obstruction from adhesions: how big is the problem? *Ann R Coll Surg Engl* 1990; **72**: 60–3.
54 Fabri PJ, Rosemurgy A. Reoperation for small bowel obstruction. *Surg Clin North Am* 1991; **71**: 131–46.
55 Ellis H. The cause and prevention of intestinal adhesions. *Br J Surg* 1982; **69**: 241–3.
56 Reissman P, Ligumsky M, Bloom A, Durst AL. Laparoscopic adhesiolysis: a treatment for recurrent intestinal obstruction due to adhesions. *Min Inv Ther* 1994; **3**: 103–4.
57 Reissman P, Wexner SD. Laparoscopic surgery for intestinal obstruction. In: Wexner SD, Jager R (eds) *Laparoscopic Colorectal Surgery*. Churchill Livingstone, New York (in press).
58 Daniell JF. Laparoscopic enterolysis for chronic abdominal pain. *J Gynecol Surg* 1989; **5**: 61–6.
59 Silva PD, Coghill TH. Laparoscopic treatment of recurrent small bowel obstruction. *Wis Med J* 1991; **90**: 169–70.
60 Francois Y, Mouret P, Tomaoglu K, Vignal J. Postoperative adhesive peritoneal disease. *Surg Endosc* 1994; **8**: 781–3.
61 Franklin ME Jr, Dorman JP, Pharand D. Laparoscopic surgery in acute small bowel obstruction. *Surg Laparosc Endosc* 1994; **4**: 289–96.

Chapter 17

Retroperitoneoscopy and retroperitoneal colonic mobilization in the era of laparoscopic colonic surgery

R. Stacey and A. Darzi

Introduction

Laparoscopic colonic surgery has not developed at the same pace as other laparoscopic procedures because of the requirement for advanced skills in laparoscopic surgery and concerns regarding the technique. In particular these include increased operating time, risk of damage to vital retroperitoneal structures and concerns that laparoscopic resections may not be adequate for neoplasia.

Although the colon is a retroperitoneal structure, in most descriptions of colonic mobilization, either laparoscopic or open, colectomy is performed via a transperitoneal route. This chapter describes a combined technique involving both laparoscopic and retroperitoneoscopic approaches to colonic mobilization using specially designed balloons and operating in the retroperitoneal space.

Surgical technique

Full video endoscopic facilities are required, including the provision of a camera, television monitor and insufflation system for both laparoscopy and retroperitoneoscopy (Fig. 17.1).

Laparoscopy

Standard preoperative preparations are employed including antithrombotic measures, routine bowel preparation and antibiotic prophylaxis. A nasogastric tube and urinary catheter are passed after anaesthesia and the patient is positioned in a modified Lloyd-Davies position with minimal hip flexion. A pneumoperitoneum is established using a standard method for insufflation, with a Veress needle, and is maintained at 12–16 mmHg by an automatic carbon dioxide (CO_2) insufflator. A 10 mm 0° laparoscope is inserted through a subumbilical port and initial laparoscopy is performed. At this stage the feasibility of resection is assessed.

Figure 17.1
Theatre setup for both laparoscopy and retroperitoneoscopy.

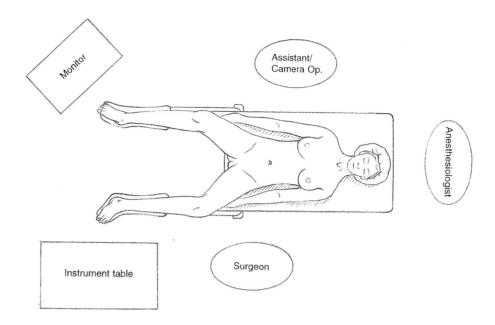

Retroperitoneoscopy

A 2 cm incision is made just above the anterior superior iliac spine, and the subcutaneous and fascial layers are dissected down to the iliacus and quadratus lumborum muscles. Continuous laparoscopic monitoring ensures that the peritoneum is not violated. A modified preperitoneal latex balloon is then inserted into the retroperitoneal space behind either the ascending or descending colon, depending on the operation site (Fig. 17.2).

Figure 17.2
Retroperitoneal balloon distension resulting in colonic mobilization.

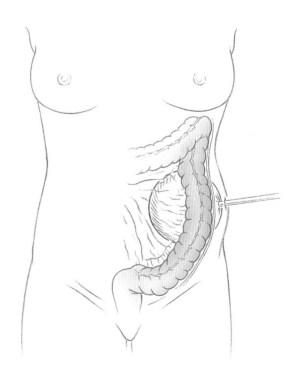

At this stage, the laparoscope is passed through the retroperitoneal 'balloon' port (Fig. 17.3) and gentle dissection is commenced by distending the balloon with a handheld bulb insufflator. The transparent balloon surrounds the retroperitoneal laparoscope allowing direct visualization of vital retroperitoneal structures including the ureter, gonadal vessels and, on the right side, the duodenum. The retroperitoneal distension process is simultaneously monitored by a second laparoscope inserted through the umbilicus. Careful balloon distension is used initially to create a small lateral space into which CO_2 may be introduced for further dissection. This avoids the possibility of trapping the ureter and gonadal vessels against the posterior abdominal wall. After initial mobilization the balloon port is replaced by a 10 mm occlusion port and the cavity thus formed is distended with CO_2. The retroperitoneal endoscope is passed through the retroperitoneal port and, under direct vision, two further 5 mm ports are inserted. This allows the introduction of grasping forceps which are used to carefully peel off any structures which are adherent to the undersurface of the peritoneum (Fig. 17.4). In this way vital structures are identified and gently placed against the posterior abdominal wall, well away from the now mobilized peritoneum.

As dissection proceeds the colonic mesentery is elevated and particularly good views are obtained of the aortic origins of the vascular pedicle (Fig. 17.5). This allows flush ligation, under direct vision, using the Endo-GIA (Autosuture, Ascot, UK) stapling device. When this has been achieved, complete and accurate excision of the lymphatic drainage field is now possible. Once mobilization is complete, two further intraperitoneal ports are inserted under direct vision in the contralateral hypochondrium and iliac fossa for the use of laparoscopic hooked scissors and graspers.

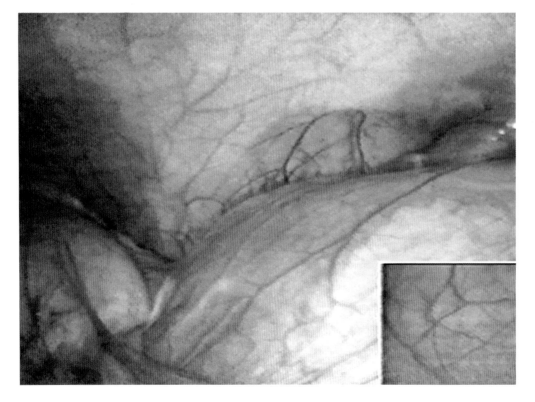

Figure 17.3
Laparoscopic view of retroperitoneal balloon distension. The insert is the view from the retroperitoneal camera.

Figure 17.4
The view via the retroperitoneal camera once distension is complete, showing the psoas muscle, ureter and gonadal vessels.

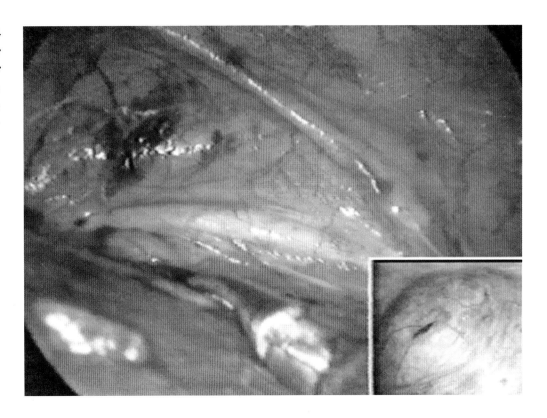

Figure 17.5
The inferior mesenteric vessels mobilized to their origin.

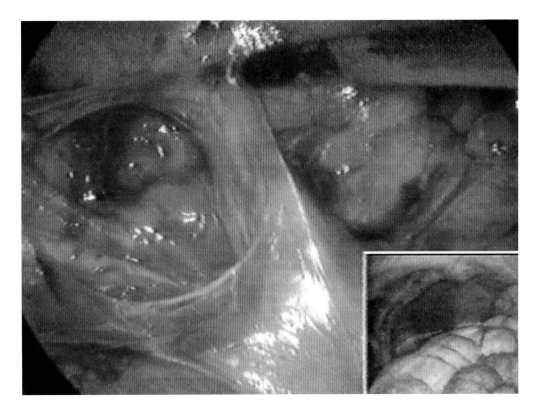

Standard laparoscopically assisted colectomy involves bowel retraction, mobilization, division of mesenteric vessels and delivery of the bowel to the skin surface for resection and subsequent anastomosis [1,2]. Using the retroperitoneal approach, colonic mobilization is almost complete except for division of the peritoneal reflection (Fig. 17.6). With the retroperitoneal space distended with CO_2, the colonic peritoneal reflection is divided accurately with scissors, operating from the laparoscopic ports, without risk to retroperitoneal structures (Fig. 17.7). High mesenteric vascular ligation has already been performed and the relevant bowel section, thus mobilized, is delivered through a small skin incision for resection and anastomosis. Thus far this method of colonic mobilization has been performed successfully via an open laparotomy wound and as a fully laparoscopic procedure in patients who have given fully informed consent [3].

Discussion

Laparoscopic colonic surgery has the same potential benefits of decreased postoperative pain and shorter postoperative stay as those associated with laparoscopic cholecystectomy [4]. The technique has, however, been criticized for doubts over oncological safety, increased operating time and problems with accurate identification and preservation of vital retroperitoneal structures [5,6]. With the use of retroperitoneoscopy and balloon-assisted blunt colonic mobilization, the potential for sharp or diathermy-related injuries and the overall operating time are reduced. This technique also provides particularly clear views of the mesenteric vessels allowing division at their origin and thus complete excision of the lymphatic drainage field. Colonic mobilization, whether open or laparoscopic, is traditionally performed by sharp division of the peritoneal reflection. This is followed by blunt mobilization of the colon and its mesentery

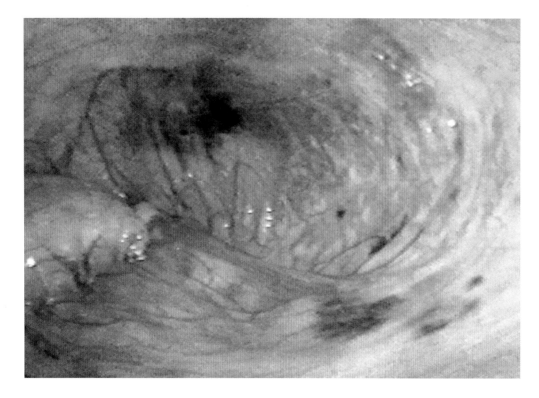

Figure 17.6
A laparoscopic view of the mobilized colon with the peritoneal reflection intact.

Figure 17.7
Division of the peritoneal reflection via the laparoscopic ports.

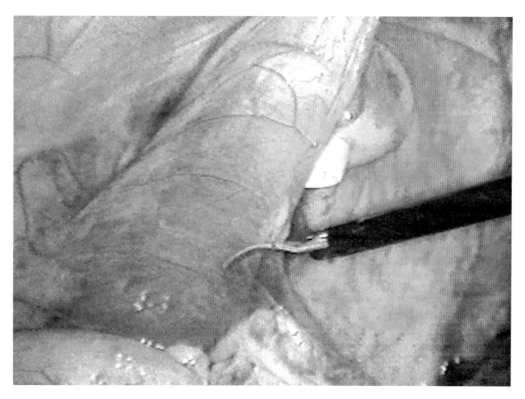

off the retroperitoneal structures [7]. In laparoscopic colonic mobilization, retraction of the colon at two fixed points is essential to achieve adequate tension on the peritoneal reflection. This has the disadvantage of adding extra ports and also requiring the use of Babcock-type grasping forceps which might traumatize the bowel. In our experience the time required to achieve adequate colonic mobilization is shorter when employing balloon dissectors. Similar balloon dissectors are now being employed in extraperitoneal hernia repair and most reports suggest that this technique facilitates the procedure and shortens the operating time.

Retroperitoneoscopy is an exciting new approach in endoscopic surgery. Recent reports of the extraperitoneal technique in hernia repair, nephrectomy, lumbar sympathectomy and even adrenalectomy [8] have revolutionized this approach to retroperitoneal structures. The colon and rectum, with the exception of the transverse colon, are retroperitoneal structures and the authors feel that retroperitoneoscopy and balloon dilatation have unique advantages especially in identifying vital retroperitoneal structures early in the procedure. It is obvious that caution should be employed when dealing with colonic neoplasias. If the initial laparoscopy suggests that the tumour is fixed, then we feel that an open approach is best adopted.

References

1   Darzi A, Hill ADK, Henry MM, Guillou PJ, Monson JRT. Laparoscopic surgery of the colon — operative technique. *Endosc Surg Allied Technol* 1993; **1**: 13–15.
2   Fowler DL, White SA. Laparoscopic assisted sigmoid resection. *Surg Laparosc Endosc* 1991; **1**(3): 283–8.
3   Stacey RJ, Hunt N, Darzi AW. Retroperitoneoscopy and retroperitoneal colonic mobilisation: a new approach in laparoscopic colonic surgery. *Br J Surg* (in press).

4   Southern Surgeons Club. A prospective analysis of 1518 laparoscopic cholecystectomies. *N Engl J Med* 1991; **324**: 1073–8.

5   Guillou PJ, Darzi A, Monson JRT. Experience with laparoscopic colorectal surgery for malignant disease. *Surg Oncol* 1993; **2** (Suppl.): 43–9.

6   Warshaw AL. Reflections on laparoscopic surgery (editorial). *Surgery* 1993; **114**: 629–30.

7   Monson JRT, Darzi A, Carey PD, Guillou PJ. Prospective evaluation of laparoscopic assisted colectomy in an unselected group of patients. *Lancet* 1992; **340**: 831–3.

8   Brunt LM, Molmenti EP, Kerbl K, Stone MS, Clayman RV. Retroperitoneal endoscopic adrenalectomy: an experimental study. *Surg Laparosc Endosc* 1993; **3**: 300–6.

H.J. Espiner

Introduction

The revolution in abdominal surgery which has followed the introduction of video endoscopy has been due entirely to the replacement of painful incisions in the abdominal wall by simple punctures. Even now, 7 years after the first laparoscopic cholecystectomy, the difference in the postoperative course between the open and the laparoscopic case is striking. While a number of laparoscopically assisted techniques have appeared which result in smaller incisions and proportionately less disturbance for the patient, there can be no doubt that an operation which avoids any division of muscle and fascia requiring suture will always be the most acceptable to the patient.

Possible sites for retrieval

The majority of operations on the colon result in resection of tissue and this poses the new problem of retrieval. In contrast with simple cholecystectomy, it is not possible to stretch a 10–15 mm puncture site to allow extraction of a piece of bowel: the risk of contamination and rupture with traction is too great. In cases of cancer the possibility of implantation in the wound cannot be allowed. For these reasons most reports of laparoscopic colonic surgery [1,2] include details of small incisions through which the specimen is removed and the procedures are better described as laparoscopically assisted. We are thus in a position where the real advantages of a fully laparoscopic procedure are not being exploited [3]. In a small number of cases extraction is possible without incision: laparoscopic abdominoperineal resection [4,5] is well established; a small carcinoma of the rectosigmoid or a large villous adenoma can be prolapsed through the anus and resection and anastomosis completed externally without risk of splitting the rectum or causing anal incontinence [6]; similarly, a small mid-rectal lesion may also be excised and removed through the rectal stump [7]. Extraction through the vagina after a posterior colpotomy has been described [8]. If, however, a tumour involves much of the rectal wall the risk of splitting the rectal stump is considerable and the possibility of tumour implantation on the cut edge must be taken into account [9]. Buess *et al.* [10] have proposed using a large rectoscope with a sleeve of impermeable material to avoid this latter risk, but tumour size will always be a limiting factor. Figures 18.1 to 18.5 illustrate these methods.

It is thus possible to envisage two approaches evolving in this early phase of laparoscopic colonic surgery. The first has the aim of preserving all the advantages of minimal access, but this requires a proper solution to the problem

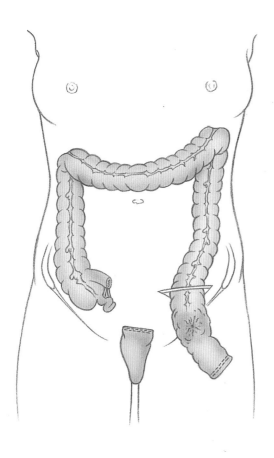

Figure 18.1
In laparoscopically assisted colonic surgery, a small incision is placed appropriately for easy resection, extraction and reconstruction. In this case, a muscle-splitting incision in the left iliac fossa is used for a sigmoid resection.

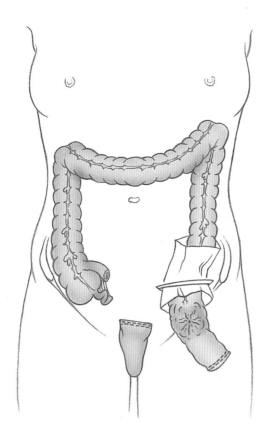

Figure 18.2
A wound-protecting sleeve should reduce the risk of contamination during extraction. When used in conjunction with a pneumatic cuff, the surgeon can insert his or her hand early in the procedure to assist dissection.

Figure 18.3

It is possible to remove a resected segment of sigmoid colon through an incision in the posterior vaginal fornix. If this procedure is carried out for carcinoma of the colon, enclosure within a retrieval sac is advisable.

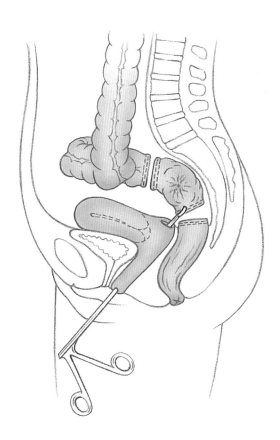

Figure 18.4

A mobile small lesion of the sigmoid colon may be removed externally by intussusception of the colon through the rectum to the exterior. The anastomosis can then be completed without the need for any abdominal wall incision.

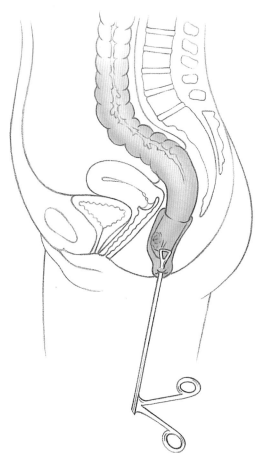

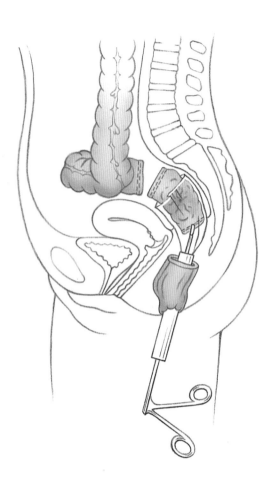

Figure 18.5
A resected lesion of the rectum may be removed through the rectum itself provided it is not too bulky. This illustration shows how a large rectoscope may be used with an incorporated sleeve to protect the walls of the rectum and the cut margin from contamination during removal.

of retrieval without incision. The second is the acceptance of a modest incision and using it for the division of the mesentery, excision of the bowel and anastomosis; this has the advantage of reduced costs in terms of operating time and resources. If the incision is made at the beginning of the operation conventional instruments can be used; Meijer *et al.* [11] have extended this assisted approach to incorporate the incision as a port using a pneumatic sleeve to retain the pneumoperitoneum and to allow the surgeon to use his or her hand internally. It would be the author's view that in the longer term as techniques are standardized and instruments refined the total laparoscopic approach will be preferred.

The need for a secure retrieval system

For the present, however, the problem of retrieval for right and left hemicolectomy for cancer remains and with it the genuine concerns regarding the risks of tumour dissemination. The desire to minimize the parietal incision to preserve the advantage of minimal access is in direct conflict with the risk of tumour metastasis, both directly into the wound site by contact and remotely in the abdominal cavity by shedding of surface cells with the friction of removal [12,13]. Protection of the wound margins with plastic film might reduce the risk of direct contact, but will not eliminate the shedding of cells as the bowel is stripped through a restricting aperture.

As yet, no clear account has been offered for the disturbing incidence of port site recurrence encountered by some surgeons [14]. Direct handling of the tumour surface causing exposure of cancer cells to the pneumoperitoneum must be an important possibility. Shedding of single cells or clumps of cells could also account for deposits found on sites of surgical trauma within the abdomen, and with the outward flow of gas and fluid via the ports the sites of puncture could easily become points of implantation. The high level of carbon dioxide throughout the operation might favour the survival of clumps of tumour cells with predominately anaerobic respiration. The problem of wound recurrence is not new to colorectal surgery, but it is uncommon, occurring in 1% of cases [15]. There is evidence that tumour cells are more proliferative in healing tissues such as wounds and anastomoses [16] and this could account for the appearance of metastases at these sites before more generalized secondary growths are detected. The prudent surgeon will ensure that extraction is easy and will avoid the use of any force. For a readily palpable tumour, an incision of at least 5 cm in length would usually be required.

There is clearly a need for a secure retrieval system applicable to all forms of colorectal surgery and ultimately it should be possible to eliminate the need for any incision.

Retrieval sacs

Various pouches and sacs have been developed for renal surgery [17] and cholecystectomy [18] and one system offers a range of sacs for small procedures, such as lymph node biopsy and appendicectomy and larger procedures including splenectomy, ovariectomy and colonic resection [19].

The problems of gallbladder retrieval in laparoscopic cholecystectomy are particularly relevant to colonic surgery. Already there are reports of port site metastasis of unexpected carcinoma of the gallbladder [20], usually in the umbilicus, the site selected for extraction. There is a strong likelihood that direct contact of the cancer cells with the exposed tissue during extraction leads to implantation. It is clear that placing the gallbladder in an impermeable sac would prevent this rare complication. In addition, when dealing with very large friable gallbladders containing multiple stones and mucopus, extraction is safe and simple when a retrieval sac is used and the risk of dissemination of stones and infected material in the peritoneal cavity is completely avoided. By using a sac specially designed for these difficult cases, it is possible to disrupt and fragment the gallbladder and its contents from the outside so that there is no need for an incision in the abdominal wall.

The simplest system would be a plastic bag, but sheet films have no resistance to tear; an accidental puncture would destroy any protection the moment even modest force were applied during extraction. The material must, therefore, be strong and able to resist tearing yet be light enough in weight to allow construction of a sac large enough to hold the considerable bulk of a tumour including the adjacent bowel and mesentery. The bulk of the sac itself should be small enough to pass through a 12 or 15 mm cannula. Currently the most suitable material for a colon retrieval sac is ripstop nylon, which is extremely strong and light and has a very high resistance to tearing. It can be covered with polyurethane to render it impermeable and it can be worked to create any shape without reliance on heat sealing. An early prototype sac made from this material was used for the extraction of the whole of the right colon, including a tumour of the caecum and 15 cm of terminal ileum, and was deployed through a 10 mm cannula. The whole operation was completed intraperitoneally and a 2.5 cm incision was made at the umbilicus to extract the specimen which was securely retained in this device [18]. The simple sac, however, has proved awkward to use in spite of its more than ample capacity and a very wide mouth for easy encapture; manipulation of a mass of tissue into the sac in the confined space of the right abdomen and anterior surface of the liver has proved difficult. There is the additional tendency of the specimen to become rolled up within the pouch making extraction through a small aperture rather tedious.

Retrieval sleeves: a concept for the future

A better design has been a sleeve rather than a sac, made in the same material and with the same ample capacity, but much easier to use. The wide mouth is still retained, but the truncated fundus continues as a tube and the system can then be deployed from one puncture site and retrieved through another (Figs 18.6 and 18.7). Typically the right upper quadrant is chosen for deployment and the umbilicus for extraction. This design offers the distinct advantage of allowing placement of the specimen in the sleeve by traction, and because the sleeve is always longer than the specimen the tendency to 'roll up' is eliminated. A considerable traction force can be applied to the bowel as it lies securely within its sleeve, but in most cases a modest incision is necessary to complete extraction unless the tumour is small and confined to the mucosa.

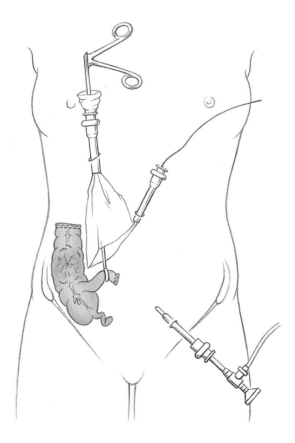

Figure 18.6
For a right hemicolectomy for carcinoma and for bulky specimens, a retrieval sleeve offers a possible solution for extraction. Here the sleeve has been deployed through the right upper quadrant port and held by a tail incorporated in its construction which is withdrawn through the umbilical cannula. A snare is used to hold the terminal ileum at the end of the resected specimen and to draw it into the open mouth of the sleeve.

Figure 18.7
The sleeve is sufficiently long to draw the extended specimen fully inside. If the specimen is small, a modest extension of the umbilical puncture would allow removal of the specimen from within the impermeable sac, so preventing any contact whatsover with the abdominal wall tissues.

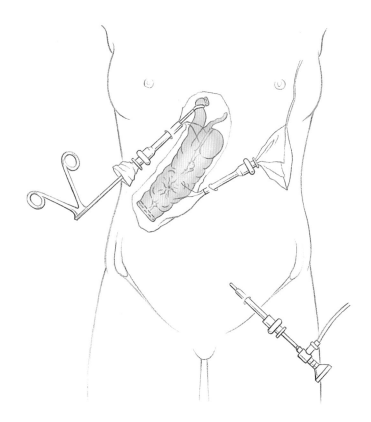

This sleeve design offers the further possible advantage that the bowel could be dissected within the sleeve when it is in its fully drawn out position and still within the abdomen. Studies are being undertaken to determine if adequate pathology data can be secured in this way before morsellation homogenization or fine shredding progressively reduces the whole mass to become sufficiently amorphous for removal without any parietal incision whatsoever. Considerable experience with this approach has already been gained from gallbladder extraction. A grossly thickened gallbladder can be cut to pieces within the sac under direct endoscopic control: it is possible to use heavy duty scissors passed from the outside to cut the wall into strips while the procedure is closely observed on screen with the video endoscope. The sac material is semitranslucent when wet and the cutting surfaces and points of the scissors can be easily seen and kept clear of the wall of the sac. Distension with fluid can assist the process. Another tactic which is often quicker is to cut open the gallbladder and release the stones as it lies within the sac still inside the abdomen. The telescope is advanced into the sac and grasping forceps and endoscopic scissors used to cut the gallbladder wall into pieces small enough to remove with ease. The contents can then be quickly removed with forceps and suction irrigation after the sac has been drawn further up to the abdominal wall. There is no reason why similar procedures should not be carried out on the colon within the sleeve as it lies inside the abdomen. Direct inspection by an endoscope in the abdominal cavity would monitor the progress of dissection, which could also be conducted directly in the view of a second endoscope placed within the sac as outlined in Fig. 18.8.

The techniques described here have already been applied in the clinical setting except for the disintegration of the specimen before extraction. It should be

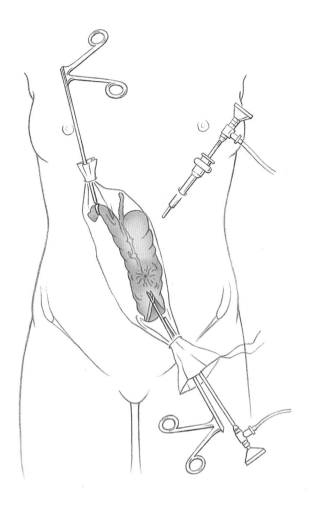

Figure 18.8
This illustration shows one of the ways in which tissue retrieval may be developed. With the cancerous specimen drawn out within the abdominal cavity, but completely enclosed in an impermeable sac, a video endoscope can be placed inside the sac to observe progressive sampling of the tissue and reduction of the bulk of the specimen. The whole process can be monitored on a second video endoscope within the abdominal cavity making certain that the operative procedure does not compromise the integrity of the sac.

possible to mark the apical lymph nodes without compromise of the no-touch technique before the specimen is placed in the impermeable sleeve. With both ends of the sleeve exteriorized and the wounds well protected, dissection within the sleeve could be completed: the mesentery could be excised and removed intact and longitudinal strips of bowel could be cut through the tumour to give histological details of depth of mural penetration. When all the necessary sampling had been completed the remainder of the specimen could be disintegrated and withdrawn. The narrow tubular end of the sleeve could then be sealed and washed in cytocidal fluid and capped. For absolute security of removal, the end would be drawn into a long cannula and this cannula passed to the exterior through the main cannula; the sleeve would then be taken clear of the whole operation field.

References

1   Wexner SD, Cohen SM, Johansen OB, Nogueras JJ, Jagelman DG. Laparoscopic colorectal surgery: a prospective assessment and current perspective. *Br J Surg* 1993; **80**: 1602–5.
2   Monson JR, Darzi A, Carey PD, Guillou PN. Prospective evaluation of laparoscopic-assisted colectomy in an unselected group of patients. *Lancet* 1992; **340**: 831–3.
3   Soper NJ, Brunt LM, Kerbl K. Laparoscopic general surgery. *N Engl J Med* 1994; **330**: 409–19.
4   Sackier JM, Berci G, Hiatt JR, Hartunian S. Laparoscopic abdominoperineal resection of the rectum. *Br J Surg* 1992; **79**: 1207–8.

5 Köckerling, Gastinger I, Schneider B, Krause W, Gall FP. Laparoscopic abdominoperineal excision of the rectum with high ligation of the inferior mesenteric artery in the management of rectal carcinoma. *Endosc Surg* 1993; **1**: 16–19.

6 Lointier P, Lechner C, Larpent JL, Chipponi JD. Laparoscopic-assisted perineal rectosigmoidectomy with pullthrough. *J Laparoendosc Surg* 1993; **3**: 547–56.

7 Darzi A, Super P, Guillou PJ, Monson JR. Laparoscopic sigmoid colectomy: total laparoscopic approach. *Dis Colon Rectum* 1994; **37**: 268–71.

8 Peiper M, Emmermann A, Zornig C. Removal of the specimen in laparoscopic spleen and colon surgery via colpotomy. *Surg Endosc* 1994; **8**: 967.

9 Cohen SM, Wexner SD. Laparoscopic colorectal resection for cancer, the Cleveland Clinic Florida experience. *Surg Oncol* 1993; **2** (Suppl. 1): 35–42.

10 Buess G, Manncke K, Merhan J, Lirici M. State of the art of laparoscopic colorectal surgery. *Endosc Surg* 1993; **1**: 3–12.

11 Meijer D, Bannenberg J, Leahy P, Klopper P. Helping hand for laparoscopic sigmoid-resection (abstract). *Min Invasive Ther* 1994; **3** (Suppl. 1): 43.

12 O'Rourke NA, Heald RJ. Laparoscopy for colorectal cancer. *Br J Surg* 1993; **80**: 1229–30.

13 Guillou PJ, Darzi A, Monson JRT. Experience with laparoscopic colorectal surgery for malignant disease. *Surg Oncol* 1993; **2** (Suppl. 1): 43–9.

14 Alexander RJT, Jaques BC, Mitchell KG. Laparoscopic assisted colectomy and wound recurrence. *Lancet* 1993; **341**: 249–50.

15 Hughes ES, McDermott FT, Polglase AI, Johnson WR. Tumour recurrence in the abdominal wall scar tissue after large bowel cancer surgery. *Dis Colon Rectum* 1983; **26**: 571–2.

16 Skipper D, Jeffrey MJ, Cooper AJ, Alexander P, Taylor I. Enhanced growth of tumour cell in healing colonic anastomoses and laparotomy wounds. *Int J Colorect Dis* 1989; **4**: 172–7.

17 McDougall EM, Clayman RV. Laparoscopic organ entrapment sac. *Min Invasive Ther* 1993; **2**: 97–101.

18 Espiner HJ. Laparoscopic cholecystectomy. In: Keen G, Farndon JR (eds) *Operative Surgery and Management*. Butterworth-Heinemann, Oxford, 1994; 304–7.

19 Roe AM, Harper R, Eltringham WK, Espiner HJ. Intracorporeal laparoscopic resections for colorectal cancer: report of cases of abdominoperineal rectal excision and right hemicolectomy with 2 year follow-up. *J R Soc Med* 1994; **87**: 519–21.

20 Pezet D, Fondrinier E, Rotman N *et al*. Parietal seeding of carcinoma of the gall bladder after laparoscopic cholecystectomy. *Br J Surg* 1992; **79**: 230.

Chapter 19

Design and assessment of clinical trials in laparoscopic colorectal surgery

P.J. Guillou

Introduction

The adoption of laparoscopic cholecystectomy as the 'gold standard' of management for patients with gallstones occurred rapidly following its development in 1987 [1]. So precipitously was this procedure embraced by the surgical community that the window of opportunity was lost to assess the procedure by the time-honoured method of the clinical randomized trial. In the face of valiant efforts in a few quarters, the claim was eventually made that such a randomized trial would be unethical because of the very 'obvious' benefits of the procedure [2], despite the fact that at the time the incidence of complications such as bile duct injury were reportedly higher than with the conventional open procedure [3]. Surgeons have since sought to justify this posture by claims that many individuals were 'on their learning curve' during the early period of reporting the results of this operation, that the current incidence of bile duct injury has fallen to levels equivalent to those of the prior 'gold standard' which pertained when peroperative cholangiography was performed routinely during open cholecystectomy, and that subsequent data have borne out the initial optimism which led laparoscopic surgery to be offered routinely to patients despite the absence of prospective comparative trials.

The purpose of this rather circuitous preamble is to suggest that never again should surgeons allow themselves to jeopardize their own reputations as objective observers (to say nothing of jeopardizing the development of a promising technique) by assuming that randomized trials would inevitably confirm their personal prejudices about the procedure, and that these trials would therefore become obsolete before they reached maturity. After all, our colleagues in internal medicine would rarely adopt a particular regimen of medical therapy without having it confirmed prospectively within the context of a randomized clinical trial. It should be a matter of some satisfaction that prospective trials have confirmed the value of laparoscopic appendicectomy and they are already being conducted in order to compare the laparoscopic and open procedures for inguinal hernia repair. This review attempts to outline some of the aspects of prospective evaluation which need now to be applied to laparoscopic colorectal surgery before it, too, has proceeded so far into routine clinical application as to make prospective studies impossible to procure. It is, however, interesting to observe that surgical caution applies, understandably, rather more to the adoption of the more time consuming procedures such as colorectal resection than it does to cholecystectomy or hernia repair. There currently exists a healthy scepticism among some surgeons [4–7] for the enthusiastic claims for laparoscopic colorectal surgery which have been expressed by others [8–10].

In both the United States and the United Kingdom, registers of laparoscopic colorectal surgical procedures have been established and will undoubtedly contribute to our understanding of the place of laparoscopic surgery in colorectal disease. However, it is interesting to speculate that if the concept of the 'average quality of life-adjusted survival' had been applied to the first 3 years of a register of laparoscopic cholecystectomy cases, the procedure would have been regarded as hazardous and might have been abandoned. Registers of procedures have their limitations since by their very nature the data they accrue must be interpreted cautiously as they are non-comparative.

Here, therefore, I begin to make the argument for the randomized clinical trial of laparoscopic surgery for colorectal disease, particularly for cancer, which, rightly, is the area of laparoscopic colorectal surgery which concerns most surgeons. Nevertheless, even in the surgery of some benign conditions some series have suggested that the complication rate might be higher than with conventional open surgery [11], again underscoring the importance of randomized clinical comparisons. If, for the moment, it is accepted that prospective comparative evaluations of laparoscopic colorectal surgery are required then a number of questions present themselves and these will be addressed below. However, the rate at which these questions can be answered has a significant impact on the design of such trials. Conventional trials can be used to answer questions about the value of, for example, laparoscopic rectopexy for rectal prolapse over a number of years dependent on the rate of patient accrual, whereas others, such as those surrounding the value of laparoscopic surgery for colorectal cancer, oblige us to provide the most accurate answers in the quickest time possible. The latter therefore need modified designs and will be described below.

The design of clinical trials of laparoscopic colorectal surgery for cancer

Which surgeons should participate in the trials?

This is an intriguing question and may be so for some years. It would seem obvious to suggest that trials of laparoscopic colorectal surgery should be confined to pre-approved, designated surgeons. The question is, which surgeons should be so designated? The laparoscopic revolution has been led (after the gynaecologists) by general surgeons who developed laparoscopic cholecystectomy and have that particular expertise and possess the corresponding track record in laparoscopic surgery. However, there is an increasing trend towards the development of specialized coloproctologists who would rightly claim particular expertise in rectal dissection, particularly the all-important total mesorectal excision for rectal cancer popularized by Heald et al. [12,13]. It has been repeatedly demonstrated that, in general, the outcome from colorectal surgery for cancer is consistently better in the hands of specialized colorectal surgeons [14] and so it might be argued that trials of a particular surgical technique are best conducted by such specialists. The dilemma is that, with notable exceptions, such specialized surgeons have not acquired laparoscopic skills because, in a purely coloproctology practice, neither the time nor the opportunity has been generally available. The situation may be analogous to that of laparoscopic cholecystectomy where there was an initially high complication rate, which fell as the technique became more practised and expertise became disseminated by surgeons who had already obtained the necessary skills over a large number of patients.

Accordingly, one is left with the compromise that designated surgeons are defined as those who have completed a predetermined number of laparoscopic colorectal operations to enable them to have become proficient. The current best estimate is that this should be a minimum of 20 procedures [15]. However, the implication of this is that the evaluation will take place in the hands of surgeons who are not all necessarily pure coloproctologists. This pragmatic solution is perhaps not so far removed from the real world because in the United Kingdom only 10–15% of colorectal resections for cancer are performed by surgeons who are pure coloproctologists.

Which patients should participate in the trials?

It is perhaps easier to define the criteria for those patients who should not be included in a trial of laparoscopic colorectal surgery, rather than to define those for whom positive criteria exist. Age alone does not appear to be a bar. The oldest patient included in our own series was 92 years old and had a successful outcome [16]. Indeed, there is some suggestion that the minimally invasive approach may be the least physiologically perturbing and might be a preferential approach in the elderly; clearly this requires verification by trial. The inclusion of patients with pre-existing cardiovascular or respiratory disease requires careful consideration because of the influence of the carbon dioxide pneumoperitoneum on those with cardiorespiratory compromise. Some consideration of bodily habitus (for example weight in excess of 90 kg) may be pertinent to patient selection as has been suggested by others [17] and this requires prospective evaluation. A number of authors have excluded patients who have undergone multiple operations, whereas others have not [18].

In patients with colorectal cancer, the inclusion of patients with large tumours may require that the tumour size be determined by such preoperative imaging techniques as computed tomography (CT), magnetic resonance imaging (MRI) or intraluminal ultrasound in order to determine the suitability or otherwise of the tumour, particularly of the rectum, for laparoscopic dissection. Finally, it has been the policy of some surgeons to reserve laparoscopic colorectal surgery for cancer for those patients in whom the resection will inevitably be palliative, i.e. those with identified liver metastases. Such a policy has been questioned and emphasizes the importance of the surgeon's assessment of whether such a resection is considered to be curative or palliative as defined by pre-arranged criteria. Most authors concur that tumours which involve other organs are unsuitable for laparoscopically assisted resection and clearly this would be an intrinsic bias in any comparative clinical trial.

Which tumours should be included in the trials?

All will agree that in any trial of a new surgical technique there must be no compromise of current surgical standards, and nowhere is this more important than in colorectal resection for cancer where complete surgical excision is the only opportunity for cure. At the same time sphincter-preserving resections for rectal cancer are being performed for lower and lower tumours and with shorter distal and proximal resection margins than were previously considered acceptable. Accordingly, many would argue that patients with middle or lower third rectal tumours should be excluded from prospective trials of laparoscopic surgery for fear of compromising the lateral and mesorectal dissection. Similarly, it is argued that such is the difficulty of laparoscopic dissection of the gastrocolic omentum that tumours involving an extensive transverse colon dissection, and of course tumours of the transverse colon, should be excluded from such trials.

Again it is difficult to adopt anything other than a pragmatic approach to this issue. In so far as tumours of the rectum are concerned, experience with laparoscopic abdominoperineal resection of the rectum has led some, including the author, to the conclusion that such is the view obtained within the pelvis during laparoscopic rectal dissection that the dissection of the mesorectum and lateral pelvic tissues is arguably better than with conventional open surgery [8,19]. I would therefore suggest that no analysis of the value of the laparoscopic approach would be complete without the inclusion of rectal cancer. After all, the anastomotic procedure for a low anastomosis is identical whichever procedure is used to perform the dissection, and if the tumour is so low as to require an abdominoperineal resection then it might be hypothesized that the true combination of laparoscopic intra-abdominal and perineal resection might be oncologically more complete. As for tumours within the transverse colon, here again personal experience will be called into play as to the advisability of including such patients in a trial. There is no doubt that with practice both the splenic and hepatic flexures can be readily dissected. To extend these dissections to the lesser sac requires a commitment of time, effort and technology which may be beyond many. Accordingly, the exclusion of such tumours from a randomized trial is understandable.

How can the surgical techniques be evaluated?

It is difficult to divorce the assessment of surgical technique from the assessment of the feasibility of a particular procedure, which in turn will be a reflection of the individual surgeon's threshold for abandoning the laparoscopic procedure and converting to open surgery. Having established the criteria for acceptance into the 'designated surgeon' category, however, one must simply accept that an individual's judgement is commensurate with a will to subscribe to the aims of the trial as loyally as is compatible with patient safety. Scrutiny of randomly selected video films of complete procedures represents one way in which to assess this, but this requires that a panel of 'judges' is selected who are acceptable to all participants. This would still leave an element of surgical preference which may be influenced by the necessity to complete the operating theatre list, personal preference or fatigue, or simply equipment availability. Although the procedures for left colectomy, right colectomy, sigmoid colectomy and rectal dissection have been described in sufficient detail to be prescriptive [16,18], this still leaves the trial designer with a number of questions concerning the degree of flexibility which should be written into the guidelines laid down for a particular procedure.

1 Should there be a measure of personal preference for the number and position of port sites used for each operation? These have largely evolved from personal experience rather than dogma but on the whole adhere to well-developed laparoscopic principles such as the angle between instruments required for the optimal entry of long-instrument working port sites, avoidance wherever possible of opportunities for 'fencing' between instruments, and the optimum site of camera insertion to enable visualization of the structures being dissected.

2 It would be important to standardize whether mesenteric or intestinal division should be performed intracorporeally or extracorporeally. For both the left and the right colon it is a simple matter to prolapse the dissected colon through a small appropriately placed incision to accomplish these components of the procedure. However, for sigmoid and rectal dissections, high division of the inferior mesenteric vessels can, and perhaps should, be accomplished laparoscopically. For all tumours the terms 'curative' and 'palliative' resection need to be defined prior to induction of the trial so that all concerned are working to the same definition. This definition may occasionally mandate conversion from a laparoscopic to a conventional open operation.

3 Should the anastomoses be performed intracorporeally or extracorporeally? Within a clinical trial one can only suggest that, with the exception of those rectal anastomoses which may be stapled, most anastomoses will be performed extracorporeally following the creation of an incision to prolapse and remove the surgical specimen. Although techniques have been described for intracorporeal stapled anastomoses using linear staplers after, for example, right hemicolectomy, their routine performance is too time consuming to be acceptable to most surgeons even within a clinical trial.

4 The adequacy of tumour staging during laparoscopic colorectal surgery for cancer is another factor which required consideration during the evolution of these procedures. Many surgeons now use peroperative ultrasound to examine the liver for the presence of metastases during conventional open surgery for colorectal cancer. This should be done with laparoscopic ultrasound probes during laparoscopic surgery; such probes are available but the resolution still requires further refinement. The loss of tactile sensation also partially deprives the laparoscopic surgeon of the ability to determine the fixity or otherwise of the primary tumour at the time of operation. The author is currently exploring the value of laparoscopic ultrasound in combination with Doppler colour imaging to determine the relationship of the tumour to vascular structures and its degree of fixity. An additional factor in colon cancer is the size of the primary tumour, which determines the size of the ultimate incision required for the removal of the surgical specimen, and we are interested to know whether ultrasound is of assistance in this regard. Current data suggest that this modality may not be appropriate but it requires further research to determine the validity of this conclusion and this should be written into any prospective trial. Equally, because of the loss of tactile sensation, peroperative evaluation of the whole colon is compromised by laparoscopic surgery and so the use of pre- or peroperative colonoscopic localization of lesions which do not extend to the serosal surface also requires incorporation into clinical trials. Indeed, the whole issue of the indications for conversion to a conventional open operation demands analysis which goes beyond the discretion of the individual surgeon to be acting in the safe interests of the patient.

5 The reported incidence of conversion from a laparoscopic to an open operation for a mixed series varies between 8 [20] and 48% [17]. It is of interest to note that higher conversion rates are reported in the more recent and mature reports which contain larger numbers of laparoscopically assisted procedures. However, this may be because these larger studies are of longer duration and were initiated when reasons for abandoning the laparoscopic approach were very stringent. For example, if the duodenum and/or the ipsilateral ureter were not adequately visualized then in some series [17] the protocol determined that this was an absolute indication for abandoning the laparoscopic procedure in favour of an open operation. Other briefer series failed to define their criteria for conversion [9,20]. However, it is self evident that the design of any comparative trial of open and laparoscopic colorectal surgery requires these factors to be categorized in the protocol. Many of these factors are readily identified (for example adhesions, haemorrhage or obesity) but, regrettably, they are rather badly quantified. Most series identify that the time required to perform laparoscopic colorectal procedures is far greater than that required to perform the equivalent open procedure. Those involved in trial design need to acknowledge these factors and in particular should predetermine whether or not a time limit should be imposed on a particular procedure so that if the operation has not been completed within the predetermined time limit then this should be an acceptable reason for completing the procedure by conventional open surgery. This has practical implications for the health-care economics of laparoscopic colorectal surgery within the context of operating theatre utilization.

How can the role of anaesthetic technique be evaluated?

This issue is raised simply because the role of anaesthesia and appropriate analgesia is frequently underplayed in reports of the success of laparoscopic procedures. It is important because the method of surgery — conventional or laparoscopic — may have a major impact on immediate postoperative recuperation. In particular the use of epidural analgesia may ameliorate the metabolic response to surgical injury [21] and play an important role in determining some of the traditional parameters of outcome, such as the overall analgesic and opiate requirement, the day of discharge and the resumption of oral intake. In reality such comparisons are only of importance if their use applies to one group and not another. Within a clinical trial this aspect of patient management requires that both treatment groups are treated identically, which is probably not possible where patients are actively selected for laparoscopic or conventional open surgical treatment. Again this underscores the importance of data accumulated from prospective trials as opposed to registry data.

Outcome measures

The measurement of outcome in patients undergoing laparoscopic surgery for colorectal cancer requires rather more than the conventional outcome parameters (e.g. 30-day mortality, complication rates, recurrence rates, and overall and disease-free survival) that are generally regarded as critical parameters for the success of cancer surgery. Additional factors, which migrate into non-traditional surgical domains, such as quality of life and overall recuperation times, also need to be considered. Some of these assessment parameters are self evident but others require the use of instruments not usually associated with the analysis of surgical outcomes.

The timing of the assessments requires careful consideration but falls broadly into three chronologically defined categories.

Immediate parameters of outcome

This encompasses the traditional measures of clinical outcome from surgical procedures, as follows.

1 Time to resumption of oral intake as an indicator of the duration of postoperative ileus. In general, this is also accompanied by recording the postoperative day upon which flatus is first passed, thus providing a dual check on the day upon which the patient recovers from postoperative ileus. The proportion of cases whose period of primary ileus exceeds 10 days (secondary ileus) is an important parameter of the effectiveness of the surgical procedure. The incidence of secondary ileus (defined as ileus occurring after peristalsis has recovered, which occurs more than 10 days after surgery and which requires intervention by restoration of the nasogastric tube or re-operation) is an important mirror of technical complications.

2 The cumulative intravenous fluid requirement is a composite measurement which reflects not only the recovery from postoperative ileus but also the patient's desire to resume oral refreshment, and thus recovery from ileus which might otherwise render the patient nauseated.

3 Measurement of pain. Quantification of pain following laparoscopic procedures is an important parameter to measure in comparisons with conventional open surgery because it reflects important aspects of the physiological response to surgical injury which are otherwise difficult to quantify without laborious laboratory measurements of metabolites of the neuroendocrine response to surgical injury. A number of studies of this aspect of laparoscopic surgery have been reported, largely suggesting that the response is attenuated [22,23]. However, these need to be included in prospective studies of the place of advanced surgical procedures in surgical management, and they usually take the form of linear analogue scales. It is emphasized that the trial design needs to ensure that as far as possible the anaesthetic techniques are equivalent between the two groups.

4 It has become conventional to record the day of discharge as a measure of the immediate clinical outcome. This is rational because, again, it reflects a

composite of factors such as physiological perturbation induced by the surgery itself and any associated complications.

5 It is unimaginable to conduct a trial of a novel surgical technique without recording the comparative incidence of technical complications of the procedures. The complications of conventional surgery for colorectal cancer are well documented, but in this context the frequency of ureteric and duodenal injury needs to be observed. In addition, laparoscopic surgery carries its own procedural complications, such as diathermy injury to the bowel outside the field of view, which have been reviewed elsewhere [24]. These need to be recorded because they may ultimately have an impact on such measures as quality of life years.

6 Blood transfusion requirements. In patient with benign colorectal disease this may serve as an indicator of the complexity of the procedure, particularly if conversion to an open operation was required. More importantly, in patients undergoing surgery for malignant disease, this is an important consideration because there is increasing evidence that blood transfusion exerts a significant impact on long-term survival from surgery for colorectal cancer [25]. It is frequently claimed that laparoscopic surgery has to be bloodless in order that videoscopic vision is maintained [9]. Hence the individual blood transfusion requirements for laparoscopic surgery may less than those for conventional open surgery. This potentially beneficial effect of laparoscopic surgery for colorectal cancer surgery requires prospective verification.

Intermediate parameters of outcome

A number of conventional measures of surgical outcome are included under this heading. It is clearly important to determine the mortality and morbidity from thromboembolic disease and pulmonary and wound infection, in addition to conventional indicators of surgical technical efficacy such as anastomotic leak rates and 30-day mortality and morbidity. Although the duration of hospitalization has been included under the heading of immediate outcome measures above, it is important to record the total duration of hospitalization which should include re-admission for complications.

Other conventional measures of outcome (such as the total time from the operation to return to useful work or normal household activity) are essential because they have an important impact on the economic evaluation of these procedures. The quantification of overall recovery time, as determined by the time of return to work and the resumption of normal activity, are incorporated into analyses which described the overall usefulness of a procedure (see below).

Long-term parameters of outcome

Again, these relate to conventional measures of outcome following cancer therapies, such as recurrence rates, disease-free survival and overall survival rates. However, in the case of laparoscopic surgery some modification of these may be required because of the conflicting evidence that the site of recurrence, i.e. at port sites, might be different in those patients undergoing a laparoscopic approach [6,26]. Here pathological analysis is critical to the interpretation of data on local, especially port site, recurrences.

Pathological analysis

The final arbiters of the value or otherwise of laparoscopic surgery for colorectal cancer are local recurrence and disease-free survival rates. However, it is possible to obtain information on likely local recurrence rates by detailed review of the pathological specimens; this requires more detailed study than has been reported so far. Obviously it is important to obtain cancer clearance in terms of the length of normal bowel above and below the tumour as well as mesenteric and lymphatic clearance. Most series have claimed that the longitudinal distal and proximal resection margins and the numbers of lymph nodes excised within the mesentery are equivalent to those which are excised by conventional open surgery [16,27,28]. However, justification of laparoscopic approaches on these grounds is unacceptable. The well-documented studies of Quirke *et al.* [29] have reliably demonstrated that for rectal cancer at least, it is the circumferential resection margins which are an important determinant of local recurrence. If the lateral resection margins are positive then there is an 87% chance of local recurrence at 2 years. Surprisingly, the same information is not available for colonic cancer. However, it seems reasonable to assume that the same principle applies.

Thus by using the pathological technique described by Quirke and Dixon [30], with 0.5 cm slicing of the surgical specimen and assessment of the maximum extent of tumour spread from the outer limit of the muscularis propria, it should be possible to evolve a 'best estimate' of the likelihood of local recurrence rates following laparoscopic surgery in something less than the 8–10 years which would be required by a conventional multicentre trial. This is important because we need to determine the value of laparoscopic colorectal cancer surgery before the window of assessment opportunity is lost.

Economic outcomes, cost analysis and quality of life assessments

Purchasers of health care are increasingly requesting clinicians to justify their selection of one particular therapeutic option or another on the basis of economic evaluations of clinical options. Within the design of clinical trials this now requires considerable effort to determine not just clinical effectiveness but also the cost-effectiveness of a particular procedure in order to obtain the most value for the expenditure. Many surgeons will be familiar with the expression 'cost-effectiveness' but may be unable to distinguish this from the term 'cost–benefit'. These are distinct but interrelated evaluations of economic activity. Cost–benefit analyses are comparable to the determination of a financial return on an investment whose financial return cannot be quantified by non-monetary parameters such as social and physical factors [31]. In the determination of cost-effectiveness, the aim is to choose the procedure which achieves a given outcome for the lowest cost [32]. The determination of cost-effectiveness in oncology requires the precise definition of economic terminology [32]. Models exist which can be utilized for the determination of the costs and benefits of a given clinical scenario [33]. It is insufficient simply to quantify the expenditure of a particular procedure as has recently been done with laparoscopic cholecystectomy [34] because cost–benefit and cost-efficiency determinations require models which incorporate modifications of survival rates as well as treatment and care costs for recurrent admissions. Furthermore, the impact of shifting care costs from a hospital-based to a community-based environment (which is hopefully one of the more desirable aspects of laparoscopic surgery) also requires modelling. There are very few data on this subject.

The development of these assessments of outcome of surgical procedures will be unfamiliar to most surgeons. Indeed, their quantification has been an issue of some dispute between health care economists. At its simplest level, summation of the operating theatre costs should be a relatively straightforward issue and indeed it is. In general, overall costs for laparoscopic colorectal surgery have been described as either equivalent to [18] or slightly less than [35] those of conventional open surgery. However, the overall cost-benefit evaluation must take into account not just these costs but also the theoretical benefit of a shorter postoperative hospital stay. Those data from the United States which indicate that the overall costs of the laparoscopic procedure are less than those incurred during conventional open surgery appear to do so because although theatre costs are higher, because of the use of disposable instruments and longer operating times, overall costs are lower because of the shorter hospital stay [35]. However, in the published literature, such as it is, these differences are relatively small and have not been encompassed by a true global assessment of the cost–benefit. These costs not only include the fixed costs such as those for durable equipment, but may require the estimation of indirect costs such as wages lost as a result of time off work. (It might be argued that some of these latter costs should be disregarded because most of these patients will be retired from the workforce and this, together with the costs of pain and suffering, will be taken into account in the assessment of quality-adjusted survival (see below).) However, these costs will inevitably fall to the community services and will require quantification. For example, although elderly patients may be discharged earlier to the community as a result of clinical wellbeing following laparoscopic surgery, there is an as yet unquantified burden on community services which has been shifted from the hospital ward.

The position remains fluid because of the development of re-useable instruments, which are now required by law to possess some form of flushing channel or to be readily dismantled for appropriate cleaning. In the author's own unit we now do not routinely employ any disposable ports or instruments whatsoever for laparoscopic surgery and clearly this factor reduces the overall theatre costs. However, such re-useable instruments have an outlay cost and this needs to be incorporated into the capital costs for the performance of laparoscopic surgery. The changing picture of laparoscopic instrumentation is yet another argument for the conduct of a prospective clinical trial rather than placing reliance on registry data. An additional question is related to the cost implications of embarking on a laparoscopically assisted colorectal procedure which requires conversion to an open operation for its completion.

Any economic analysis must presume the null hypothesis that the open and the laparoscopic procedures provide equivalent clinical benefit which may, of course, not be true. Thus, the financial aspects need to quantify the marginal costs of the more expensive procedure over the cheaper operation rather than a simple comparison of the costs of the two procedures. Inevitably, therefore, the analysis must focus on the costs incurred during the perioperative period where there is likely to be the most difference between the two groups. This invites the risk of ignoring the long-term life costs if either procedure proves to have disadvantageous characteristics in terms of the adequacy of surgical clearance as determined, for example, by the pathological findings and ultimately by the local recurrence and survival rates. Despite these difficulties there is considerable merit in comparing the costs of performing laparoscopic and conventional open surgery during the perioperative period because in reality this is the time at which the requirement for resources is the greatest in both procedures. Furthermore, if there are no differences between these procedures in terms of recurrence and disease-free survival rates, then clearly these economic issues may have a significant impact on the adoption of one or other procedure. Conversely, if the disease-free survival rate is found to be superior in one procedure, then these cost evaluations will probably be irrelevant unless they happen to be in favour of the more successful procedure.

Current estimates suggest that a minimum of 1000 patients would require entry into a trial of the two procedures. Because of the potential loss of patients from the laparoscopic arm of the trial who have to be converted to an open operation (currently averaging around 15% from published data [9,27,35,36]), the randomization procedure could be weighted in favour of the laparoscopic arm in the ratio of, say, 3:2. However, it would be difficult and probably unnecessary to recruit data from all of these patients for the cost-analysis of the trial and these studies could be performed on subgroups of the two cohorts of patients being compared.

However, one further difficulty in analysing the benefit of one procedure against another lies in the determination of the impact of adjuvant therapy on clinical outcomes. The use of adjuvant therapy with 5-fluorouracil and levamisole for Dukes' stage C colonic cancer is reported to provide a 30% survival advantage at 5 years. Similarly the use of radiotherapy as an adjunct to surgery for rectal cancer is considered to provide a significant advantage in relation to local recurrence and possibly survival. The use of these adjuncts, particularly in the context of other clinical trials such as the AXIS and QUASAR trials, may be confounding factors in a trial of surgical technique which uses survival and disease-free interval as end points. It is a simple enough matter to exclude the costs of adjuvant therapy from the analysis but it is difficult to disentangle the clinical impact of these adjuvants on the survival data unless the trial forbids the use of adjuvant therapy. Such a stricture would be unethical and unacceptable to those surgeons who have accepted the data on adjuvant therapy and use it routinely. It must be said that in the United Kingdom opinion on this is much more heterogeneous than it is in the United States where consensus views have almost completely eliminated clinical choice in this area. Nevertheless, stratification of patients within a trial of surgical technique which permits adjuvant therapy to be administered according to a surgeon's personal preference places serious restrictions on such a trial because it greatly increases the number of patients required to stratify sufficient patients into the various subgroups which are required to answer the questions concerning the surgical approach. The use of pathological end points such as the lateral resection margins which have a quantified relationship with local recurrence and survival rates may partially act as a useful surrogate for these clinical parameters.

Instruments utilized in economic and quality of life assessments

Integral to these cost–benefit analyses is the need to compare the quality of life advantages (or disadvantages!) of the two trial procedures. Within randomized clinical trials, subgroups of the two trial arms could be selected for this rather than the whole cohort because of the detail required for many of the socioeconomic instruments utilized in such studies. These require questionnaire-based data which assess patient self-referred symptoms as well as quantification of the recovery of functional abilities. This could therefore include two important instruments, the McCorkle symptom distress scale and a quality of life index (QLI). These are both evaluated from self-completed postal questionnaires and they both accrue data on symptoms, functional abilities and patient-perceived complications. The timing of these assessments is important. A reasonable schedule to be adopted might be that the symptom distress score should be quantified at 48 h, 14 days and 2 months after the procedure and the QLI performed on day 14 and then repeated at 2 and 18 months after the procedure.

The QLI instrument is extremely difficult to predetermine for a randomized clinical trial of laparoscopic colorectal surgery. Fortunately in Europe there has emerged a quality of life questionnaire (Euroqol) which seems to be applicable to most patients who might be eligible for recruitment into a randomized clinical trial of laparoscopic versus conventional open surgery. This is replacing the Nottingham health profile which in the past has been a useful tool for evaluating quality of life within clinical trials but has some limitations for surgical and oncological trials.

There also exists a tool for re-calculating survival in a way which incorporates parameters of quality of life measurements into the survival time so as to provide an overall view of the benefits of the two procedures. This is known as quality-adjusted time without symptoms of disease and toxicity of treatment (Q-TWiST) [37]. Q-TWiST requires the identification of periods of health states for the specific disease under study and the treatments being evaluated. For the present purposes, for example, four health states could be designated as: (1) the perioperative period (i.e. 30 days after the operation); (2) the time without symptoms or side effects ('toxicity') of the surgery (TWiST); (3) late complications; and (4) recurrent disease. TWiST would be defined as the period from the end of the first 30 postoperative days to disease relapse or study closure. Late complications are those which require hospitalization and may be arbitrarily assigned a period of 1 month; the recurrent disease period extends from the time of diagnosis of the recurrence to death or termination of the study. The next procedure is to partition the overall survival of each of the patients in the study into each of these health states and then to weight the time spent by each patient in these health states by a predetermined coefficient (U) which is obtained from the QLI reported by the patients in each arm of the trial for each health state. Thus, by summating the weighted survival times, the average quality-adjusted survival in each trial arm can be determined by multiplying the time spent by trial patients in each health state by the mean patient-reported utility (U) for that state according to the formula:

$$\text{Q-TWiST} = [U_{\text{periop}} \times 30 \text{ days}] + [U_{\text{TWiST}} \times \text{duration}_{\text{TWiST}}] +$$

$$[U_{\text{complications}} \times \text{duration}_{\text{complications}}] + [U_{\text{recurrence}} \times \text{duration}_{\text{complications}}]$$

The calculation of U for each health state is determined by the average QLI for each health state for each arm of the trial. Thus for the perioperative period the average score of the 0–100 quality of life score at 14 days for each arm is transformed to a 0–1 scale and utilized as U_{periop} in the formula described above; and similarly for each value of U for each health state.

A perceived additional advantage of the use of the Q-TWiST value for each procedure is that it permits a single figure evaluation of the relative cost-effectiveness of the two procedures by dividing the marginal cost of the procedure by the marginal benefit measured in quality-adjusted survival. This figure is thus a cost (in pounds sterling) per quality-adjusted year of life. The difficulty at this stage is deciding what constitutes a threshold of cost-effectiveness, i.e. should a cost of UK £10 000 per quality-adjusted year of life be regarded as cost-effective, but a figure of UK £20 000 per quality-adjusted year of life be regarded as cost-ineffective?

Conclusion

It seems unlikely that in the current economic climate surgeons will ever again have the opportunity to introduce a surgical procedure without submitting it to the most intense evaluations of cost-effectiveness and cost–benefit. Purchasers of health care will require proof that the operative procedures for which they are paying possess both these attributes and it is interesting that the national research and development initiative is now using its resources to commission research into procedures whose value has been unquestioned for years. Some may see this economic approach as an intrusion into their personal clinical freedom. However, all surgeons would agree that it is their responsibility to ensure that the treatments they advise are clinically effective and thus by the same token it must also, in this cost-conscious environment, be at least partly our responsibility to determine the economic value of new procedures. Surely, knowing the clinical imperatives, we are in a much stronger position to dictate these values than economists with no medical insights. Unless we contribute to these debates in an informed manner undesirable restrictions will be imposed upon us from without and this certainly will result in an erosion of our clinical freedom which will stifle technological development and be deleterious to patient care.

References

1   Dubois F. Laparoscopic cholecystectomy: historical perspective and personal experience. *Surg Laparosc Endosc* 1991; **1**: 52–7.
2   Neugebauer E, Troidl H, Spangenberger W, Dietrich A, Lefering R, the Cholecystectomy Study Group. Conventional versus laparoscopic cholecystectomy and the randomised controlled trial. *Br J Surg* 1991; **78**: 150–4.
3   The Southern Surgeons Club. A prospective analysis of 1518 laparoscopic cholecystectomies. *N Engl J Med* 1991; **324**: 1073–8.
4   Guillou PJ. Laparoscopic surgery for diseases of the colon and rectum — quo vadis? *Surg Endosc* 1994; **8**: 669–71.
5   Wexner SD, Johansen OB. Laparoscopic bowel resections: advantages and limitations. *Ann Med* 1992; **24**: 105–10.
6   Cirocco WC, Schwartzman A, Golub RW. Abdominal wall recurrence after laparoscopic colectomy for colon cancer. *Surgery* 1994; **116**: 842–6.
7   O'Rourke NA, Heald RJ. Laparoscopic surgery for colorectal cancer. *Br J Surg* 1993; **80**: 1229–30.
8   Monson JRT, Darzi A, Carey PD, Guillou PJ. Prospective evaluation of laparoscopic-assisted colectomy in an unselected group of patients. *Lancet* 1992; **340**: 831–3.

9   Phillips EH, Franklin M, Carroll BJ, Fallas MJ, Ramos R, Rosenthal D. Laparoscopic colectomy. *Ann Surg* 1992; **216**: 703–7.

10 Franklin ME, Ramos R, Rosenthal D, Scheussler W. Laparoscopic colonic procedures. *World J Surg* 1993; **17**: 51–6.

11 Wexner SD, Cohen SM, Johansen OB, Nogueras JJ, Jagelman DG. Laparoscopic colorectal surgery: a prospective assessment and current perspective. *Br J Surg* 1993; **80**: 1602–5.

12 Heald RJ. The 'holy plane' of rectal surgery. *J R Soc Med* 1988; **81**: 503–8.

13 MacFarlane JK, Ryall RD, Heald RJ. Mesorectal excision for rectal cancer. *Lancet* 1993; **341**: 457–60.

14 McArdle CS, Hole D, Hansell D, Blumgart LH, Wood CB. Prospective study of colorectal cancer in the west of Scotland: 10-year follow-up. *Br J Surg* 1990; **77**: 280–2.

15 Larach SW, Saloman MC, Williamson PR, Goldstein E. Laparoscopic assisted colectomy: experience during the learning curve. *Coloproctology* 1993; **1**: 38–41.

16 Guillou PJ, Darzi A, Monson JRT. Experience with laparoscopic colorectal surgery for malignant disease. *Surg Oncol* 1993; **2**(Suppl. 1): 43–50.

17 Dean PA, Beart RW, Nelson H, Eltmann TD, Schlinkert RT. Laparoscopic-assisted segmental colectomy: early Mayo Clinic experience. *Mayo Clin Proc* 1994; **69**: 834–40.

18 Elftmann TD, Nelson H, Ota DM, Pemberton JH, Beart RW. Laparoscopic-assisted colectomy: surgical techniques. *Mayo Clin Proc* 1994; **69**: 825–33.

19 Sackier JM, Berci G, Hiatt JR, Hartunian S. Laparoscopic abdominoperineal resection of the rectum. *Br J Surg* 1992; **79**: 1207–8.

20 Tate JJ, Kwok S, Dawson JW, Lau JY, Li AKC. Prospective comparison of laparoscopic and conventional anterior resection. *Br J Surg* 1993; **80**: 1396–8.

21 Kehlet H. Surgical stress response — effects of pain and analgesia. *Br J Anaesth* 1989; **63**: 189–95.

22 McMahon AJ, Russell IT, Ramsay G *et al.* Laparoscopic and minilaparotomy cholecystectomy: a randomized trial comparing postoperative pain and pulmonary function. *Surgery* 1994; **115**: 533–9.

23 Carey PD, Thayeb A, Wakefield CH, Darzi A, Monson JRT, Guillou PJ. The effects of minimally invasive surgery on neutrophil hypochlorous acid production. *Br J Surg* 1994; **81**: 557–60.

24 Guillou PJ. The scope of diagnostic and interventional laparoscopy for malignant disease. In: Taylor I, Guillou PJ, Cooke TC (eds) *General Surgical Oncology*. Churchill Livingstone, London, 1995 (in press).

25 Heiss MM, Mempel W, Delanoff C *et al.* Blood transfusion-modulated tumour recurrences: first results of a randomized study of autologous versus allogenic blood transfusion in colorectal cancer surgery. *J Clin Oncol* 1994; **12**: 1859–67.

26 Ramos JM, Gupta S, Anthone GJ, Ortega AE, Simons AJ, Beart RW. Laparoscopy and colon cancer; is the port site at risk? *Arch Surg* 1994; **129**: 897–9.

27 Van Ye T, Cattey RP, Henry LG. Laparoscopically assisted colon resections compare favourably with open technique. *Surg Laparosc Endosc* 1994; **1**: 25–31.

28 Cohen SM, Wexner SD. Laparoscopic colorectal resection for cancer: the Cleveland Clinic Florida experience. *Surg Oncol* 1993; **2**(Suppl. 1): 35–42.

29 Quirke P, Durdey P, Dixon MF, Williams NS. Local recurrence of rectal adenocarcinoma due to inadequate surgical resection. *Lancet* 1986; **2**: 996–9.

30 Quirke P, Dixon MF. The prediction of local recurrence in rectal adenocarcinoma by histopathological examination. *Int J Colorect Dis* 1988; **3**: 127–31.

31 Pearce CW, Nash CA. *The Social Appraisal of Projects*. John Wiley, New York, 1981.

32 Smith TJ, Hillner BE, Desch CE. Efficacy and cost-effectiveness of cancer treatment: rational allocation of resources based on decision analysis. *J Natl Cancer Inst* 1993; **85**: 1460–74.

33 Eddy DM. A computer-based model for designing cancer control strategies. In: Greenwald P, Sondik EJ (eds) *Cancer Control Objectives for the Nation 1985–2000*. NCI publication No. 86–2880. 2. NCI, Bethesda, Maryland, 1986.

34 Fullarton GM, Darling K, Williams J, MacMillan R, Bell G. Evaluation of the cost of laparoscopic and open cholecystectomy. *Br J Surg* 1994; **81**: 124–6.

35 Musser DJ, Boorse RC, Madera F, Reed JF. Laparoscopic colectomy: at what cost? *Surg Laparosc Endosc* 1994; **4**: 1–5.

36 Peters WR, Bartels TL. Minimally invasive colectomy: are the potential benefits realized? *Dis Colon Rectum* 1993; **36**: 751–6.

37 Gelber RD, Gelman RS, Goldhirsch A. A quality-of-life-oriented endpoint for comparing therapies. *Biometrics* 1989; **45**: 781–95.

Index

(Page numbers in *italic* and **bold** indicate, respectively, an illustration or table appearing away from its relevant text. LCRS = laparoscopic colorectal surgery.)